T0249451

Food Allergy

Editor

AMAL H. ASSA'AD

IMMUNOLOGY AND ALLERGY CLINICS OF NORTH AMERICA

www.immunology.theclinics.com

May 2021 • Volume 41 • Number 2

ELSEVIER

1600 John F. Kennedy Boulevard • Suite 1800 • Philadelphia, Pennsylvania, 19103-2899

http://www.theclinics.com

IMMUNOLOGY AND ALLERGY CLINICS OF NORTH AMERICA Volume 41, Number 2

May 2021 ISSN 0889-8561, ISBN-13: 978-0-323-81319-8

Editor: Katerina Heidhausen

Developmental Editor: Jessica Cañaberal

Immunology and Allergy Clinics of North America (ISSN 0889–8561) is published quarterly by Elsevier Inc., 360 Park Avenue South, New York, NY 10010-1710. Months of issue are February, May, August, and November. Periodicals postage paid at New York, NY and additional mailing offices. Subscription prices are $347.00 per year for US individuals, $827.00 per year for US institutions, $100.00 per year for US students and residents, $423.00 per year for Canadian individuals, $100.00 per year for Canadian students, $864.00 per year for Canadian institutions, $447.00 per year for international individuals, $864.00 per year for international institutions, $220.00 per year for international students. To receive student/resident rate, orders must be accompanied by name of affiliated institution, date of term, and the *signature* of program/residency coordinator on institution letterhead. Orders will be billed at individual rate until proof of status is received. Foreign air speed delivery is included in all *Clinics* subscription prices. All prices are subject to change without notice. **POSTMASTER:** Send address changes to *Immunology and Allergy Clinics of North America,* Elsevier Health Sciences Division, Subscription Customer Service, 3251 Riverport Lane, Maryland Heights, MO 63043. **Customer Service: 1-800-654-2452 (U.S. and Canada); 314-447-8871 (outside U.S. and Canada). Fax: 314-447-8029. E-mail: journalscustomerservice-usa@elsevier.com (for print support); journalsonlinesupport-usa@elsevier.com (for online support).**

Reprints. For copies of 100 or more, of articles in this publication, please contact the Commercial Reprints Department, Elsevier Inc., 360 Park Avenue South, New York, New York 10010-1710. Tel. 212-633-3874, Fax: 212-633-3820, E-mail: reprints@elsevier.com.

Immunology and Allergy Clinics of North America is covered in MEDLINE/PubMed (Index Medicus), Current Contents/Life Sciences, Science Citation Index, ISI/BIOMED, Chemical Abstracts, and EMBASE/Excerpta Medica.

Contributors

EDITOR

AMAL H. ASSA'AD, MD
Professor of Pediatrics, Division of Allergy and Immunology, Cincinnati Children's Hospital Medical Center, University of Cincinnati, Cincinnati, Ohio, USA

AUTHORS

AMAL H. ASSA'AD, MD
Professor of Pediatrics, Division of Allergy and Immunology, Cincinnati Children's Hospital Medical Center, University of Cincinnati, Cincinnati, Ohio, USA

SULTAN ALBUHAIRI, MD
Consultant, Allergy and Immunology, Department of Pediatrics, Allergy and Immunology Section, King Faisal Specialist Hospital and Research Centre, Riyadh, Saudi Arabia

STEFANIA ARASI, MD, PhD
Translational Research in Pediatric Specialities Area, Division of Allergy, Bambino Gesù Children's Hospital, IRCCS, Rome, Italy

SAMI L. BAHNA, MD, DrPH
Professor of Pediatrics and Medicine, Chief of Allergy and Immunology Section, Reddy Professor of Allergy and Immunology, Louisiana State University Health Sciences Center in Shreveport, Shreveport, Louisiana, USA

BERBER VLIEG–BOERSTRA, PhD, RD
Department of Pediatrics, OLVG Hospital, Amsterdam, the Netherlands

AUDREY G. BREWER, MD, MPH
Center for Food Allergy and Asthma Research, Department of Pediatrics, Northwestern University Feinberg School of Medicine, Department of Medicine, Ann and Robert H. Lurie Children's Hospital, Chicago, Illinois, USA

BRYAN J. BUNNING, MS(c)
Department of Biostatistics, Mailman School of Public Health, Columbia University, New York, New York, USA

SHERRY COLEMAN COLLINS, MS, RDN, LD
Southern Fried Nutrition Services LLC, Marietta, Georgia, USA

ASHLEY LYNN DEVONSHIRE, MD, MPH
Assistant Professor, Department of Pediatrics, Division of Allergy and Immunology, Cincinnati Children's Hospital Medical Center, Cincinnati, Ohio, USA

RAQUEL DURBAN, MS, RDN, LDN
Carolina Asthma & Allergy Center, Charlotte, North Carolina, USA

AMY A. EAPEN, MD, MS
Senior Staff Allergist, Division of Allergy and Clinical Immunology, Henry Ford Health System, Detroit, Michigan, USA

WENDY ELVERSON, RD, LDN
Division of Gastroenterology, Hepatology and Nutrition, Center for Nutrition, Senior Clinical Nutritionist, Boston Children's Hospital, Boston, Massachusetts, USA

MELISSA L. ENGEL, MA
Department of Psychology, Emory University, Atlanta, Georgia, USA

MICHELLE M. ERNST, PhD
Professor, Department of Pediatrics, University of Cincinnati College of Medicine, Division of Behavioral Medicine and Clinical Psychology, Cincinnati Children's Hospital Medical Center, Cincinnati, Ohio, USA

ALESSANDRO GIOVANNI FIOCCHI, MD
Translational Research in Pediatric Specialities Area, Division of Allergy, Bambino Gesù Children's Hospital, IRCCS, Rome, Italy

ALYSSA FRIEBERT, MS, RD
Section of Allergy, Department of Pediatrics, Children's Hospital Colorado, University of Colorado School of Medicine, Allergy and Immunology Clinic, Aurora, Colorado, USA

LEAH GREENFIELD, BS
Department of Internal Medicine, Allergy and Immunology Division, Rush University Medical Center, Rush Medical College, Chicago, Illinois, USA

BENJAMIN GROBMAN
Center for Food Allergy and Asthma Research, Northwestern University Feinberg School of Medicine, Chicago, Illinois, USA

MARION GROETCH, MS, RDN
Division of Allergy and Immunology, Icahn School of Medicine at Mount Sinai, New York, New York, USA

RUCHI S. GUPTA, MD, MPH
Center for Food Allergy and Asthma Research, Department of Pediatrics, Northwestern University Feinberg School of Medicine, Department of Medicine, Ann and Robert H. Lurie Children's Hospital, Chicago, Illinois, USA

XIAORUI HAN, PhD
Sean N. Parker Center for Allergy and Asthma Research, Stanford University, Stanford, California, USA

ZIYUAN HE, PhD
Sean N. Parker Center for Allergy and Asthma Research, Stanford University, Stanford, California, USA

JIALING JIANG, BA
Center for Food Allergy and Asthma Research, Northwestern University Feinberg School of Medicine, Chicago, Illinois, USA

ELISABET JOHANSSON, PhD
Division of Asthma Research, Department of Pediatrics, Cincinnati Children's Hospital Medical Center, University of Cincinnati, Cincinnati, Ohio, USA

KASSIDY M. JUNGLES, BS
Department of Pharmacology, University of Michigan, Ann Arbor, Michigan, USA

KYLIE N. JUNGLES, MD
Department of Pediatrics, University of Michigan C.S. Mott Children's Hospital, Ann Arbor, Michigan, USA; Department of Internal Medicine, Allergy and Immunology Division, Rush University Medical Center, Chicago, Illinois, USA

JAMIE KABOUREK, MS, RD
University of Nebraska-Lincoln, Food Innovation Center, Lincoln, Nebraska, USA

HAEJIN KIM, MD
Senior Staff Allergist, Division of Allergy and Clinical Immunology, Henry Ford Health System, Detroit, Michigan, USA

JAMES WALTER KREMPSKI, PhD
Sean N. Parker Center for Allergy and Asthma Research, Stanford University, Stanford, California, USA

STÉPHANIE LEJEUNE, MD
Sean N. Parker Center for Allergy and Asthma Research, Stanford University, Stanford, California, USA

ADORA A. LIN, MD, PhD
Assistant Professor, Department of Pediatrics, Division of Allergy and Immunology, Children's National Hospital, Washington, DC, USA

MAHBOOBEH MAHDAVINIA, MD, PhD
Department of Internal Medicine, Allergy and Immunology Division, Rush University Medical Center, Chicago, Illinois, USA

STEPHANIE M. MARCHAND, PhD, RD, CNSC, CLC, LDN
Clinical Assistant Professor, Department of Pediatrics, The Warren Alpert School of Medicine at Brown University, Senior Clinical Pediatric Dietitian, Food and Nutrition Services, Hasbro Children's Hospital, Providence, Rhode Island, USA

VICKI McWILLIAM, PhD, AdvAPD
Dietitian, Department of Allergy and Immunology, Royal Children's Hospital, Researcher, Murdoch Children's Research Institute, Melbourne, Australia

MAURIZIO MENNINI, MD, PhD
Translational Research in Pediatric Specialities Area, Division of Allergy, Bambino Gesù Children's Hospital, IRCCS, Rome, Italy

TESFAYE B. MERSHA, PhD
Division of Asthma Research, Department of Pediatrics, Cincinnati Children's Hospital Medical Center, University of Cincinnati, Cincinnati, Ohio, USA

ROSAN MEYER, PhD, RD
Paediatric Research Dietitian, Honorary Senior Lecturer, Department of Pediatrics, Imperial College, London, United Kingdom

KARI NADEAU, MD, PhD
Sean N. Parker Center for Allergy and Asthma Research, Stanford University, Stanford, California, USA

MERRYN NETTING, PhD, AdvAPD
Women and Kids Theme, South Australian Health and Medical Research Institute, Department of Pediatrics, University of Adelaide, Adelaide, South Australia, Australia; Nurition Department, Women's and Children's Health Network, North Adelaide, South Australia, Australia

RIMA RACHID, MD
Associate Professor of Pediatrics, Division of Immunology, Boston Children's Hospital, Department of Pediatrics, Harvard Medical School, Boston, Massachusetts, USA

CHRISTINE J. RUBEIZ, MD
Resident Physician, Department of Pediatrics, Cincinnati Children's Hospital Medical Center, Cincinnati, Ohio, USA

ISABEL SKYPALA, PhD, RD
Imperial College, Department of Allergy and Clinical Immunology, Royal Brompton & Harefield NHS Foundation Trust, Royal Brompton Hospital, London, United Kingdom

TARYN VAN BRENNAN, RD
Department of Allergy and Immunology, Aurora, Colorado, USA

EMILLIA VASSILOPOULOU, PhD, RD
Department of Nutritional Sciences and Dietetics, International Hellenic University, Thessaloniki, Greece

CARINA VENTER, PhD, RD
Section of Allergy, Department of Pediatrics, Children's Hospital Colorado, University of Colorado School of Medicine, Associate Professor of Pediatrics, Section of Allergy & Immunology, University of Colorado Denver School of Medicine, Children's Hospital Colorado, University of Colorado, Aurora, Colorado, USA

CHRISTOPHER WARREN, PhD
Sean N. Parker Center for Allergy and Asthma Research, Stanford University, Stanford, California, USA

CHRISTOPHER M. WARREN, PhD
Center for Food Allergy and Asthma Research, Northwestern University Feinberg School of Medicine, Chicago, Illinois, USA

WENMING ZHANG, PhD
Sean N. Parker Center for Allergy and Asthma Research, Stanford University, Stanford, California, USA

Contents

Preface: Focus on the Patient with Food Allergy   xiii

Amal H. Assa'ad

Food Allergies: An Example of Translational Research   143

James Walter Krempski, Christopher Warren, Xiaorui Han, Wenming Zhang,
Ziyuan He, Stéphanie Lejeune, and Kari Nadeau

Food allergies have been rising in prevalence since the 1990s, imposing substantial physical, psychosocial, and economic burdens on affected patients and their families. Until recently, the only therapy for food allergy was strict avoidance of the allergenic food. Recent advances in translational studies, however, have led to insights into allergic sensitization and tolerance. This article provides an overview of cutting-edge research into food allergy and immune tolerance mechanisms utilizing mouse models, human studies, and systems biology approaches. This research is being translated and implemented in the clinical setting to improve diagnosis and reduce food allergy's public health burden.

The Phenotype of the Food-Allergic Patient   165

Amy A. Eapen and Haejin Kim

Food allergy's increasing prevalence across the globe has initiated research into risk factors associated with the disease and coexistence with other allergic diseases. Longitudinal birth cohorts have identified food allergy phenotypes of patients based on genetic background, racial diversity, and environmental factors. Identifying food sensitization patterns and coexistence of other allergic diseases allows physicians to provide appropriate care for food allergy and personalized anticipatory guidance for the appearance of other allergic diseases. The authors seek to detail key findings of 4 longitudinal allergy birth cohorts that investigate food allergy and other allergic diseases to further characterize food allergy phenotypes.

Psychosocial Aspects of Food Allergy: Resiliency, Challenges and Opportunities   177

Christine J. Rubeiz and Michelle M. Ernst

Food allergy is a public health concern and has been found to be increasing in prevalence; however, psychosocial factors differentiate challenges related to management throughout the lifespan. Resilience has been found to improve quality of life in other chronic diseases, but little has been published regarding increasing resilience in food allergy. The psychosocial impacts of food allergy vary by age group and developmental stage. This article reviews developmental milestones within the context of food allergy in infancy, school-age children, adolescents, and adults. Recommendations for promoting resilience in patients with food allergy are provided.

Racial/Ethnic Differences in Food Allergy

189

Christopher M. Warren, Audrey G. Brewer, Benjamin Grobman, Jialing Jiang, and Ruchi S. Gupta

Immunoglobulin E–mediated food allergy is an increasingly prevalent public health concern globally. In North America, particularly in the United States, racial and ethnic differences in food allergy prevalence and rates of sensitization have become apparent. Black and Hispanic children in the United States have been estimated to have the highest rates of food allergy. Beyond rates of prevalence, food allergy outcomes, such as health care utilization, psychosocial outcomes, and economic burden, also vary considerably by race and ethnicity. It is important to consider socioeconomic status in conjunction with race and ethnicity in studying differences in food allergy outcomes.

Tackling Food Allergy in Infancy

205

Ashley Lynn Devonshire and Adora A. Lin

Atopic dermatitis and food allergy are the most common allergic conditions affecting the infant population. Both immunoglobulin E (IgE)-mediated and non-IgE-mediated food allergy are seen in infancy. Early life feeding guidelines have changed dramatically over the past 30 years, more recently because of an improved understanding of IgE-mediated food allergy. This article focuses on identification, diagnosis, management, and prevention of food allergy in the infant population.

Developing National and International Guidelines

221

Maurizio Mennini, Stefania Arasi, Alessandro Giovanni Fiocchi, and Amal Assa'ad

Food allergy (FA) is considered an emerging public health problem. The development of evidence-based guidelines aims to help health care professionals in an accurate diagnosis and management of such diseases. It is proven that there are differences in the factors that determine FA in the different regions of the world. It is necessary to encourage standardization processes of guidelines development. Nevertheless, in the future it will be necessary to take into consideration not only a methodologically correct analysis of the evidence but also the socio-economic realities where the guidelines will be applied.

Dietary Management of Food Allergy

233

Raquel Durban, Marion Groetch, Rosan Meyer, Sherry Coleman Collins, Wendy Elverson, Alyssa Friebert, Jamie Kabourek, Stephanie M. Marchand, Vicki McWilliam, Merryn Netting, Isabel Skypala, Taryn Van Brennan, Emillia Vassilopoulou, Berber Vlieg–Boerstra, and Carina Venter

Food allergy prevalence is increasing worldwide, especially in children. Food allergy management strategies include appropriate avoidance strategies and identifying suitable alternatives for a nutritionally sound diet. Individualized dietary intervention begins with teaching label reading. Food allergens and labelling laws differ among countries. Dietary intervention should include a nutritionally sound plan with alternatives to support optimal growth and development. Inadequate dietary advice may increase the risk of adverse reactions, growth faltering, and nutrient deficiencies. Evidence indicates input from a registered dietitian improves nutritional outcomes.

Biologics and Novel Therapies for Food Allergy

271

Sultan Albuhairi and Rima Rachid

Food allergy is a significant public health burden affecting around 10% of adults and 8% of children. Although the first peanut oral immunotherapy product received Food and Drug Administration approval in 2020, there is still an unmet need for more effective therapeutic options that minimize the risk of anaphylaxis, nutritional deficiencies, and patient's quality of life. Biologics are promising modalities, as they may improve compliance, target multiple food allergies, and treat other concomitant atopic diseases. Although omalizumab has been evaluated extensively, most biologics are more novel and have broader immunologic impact. Careful evaluation of their safety profile should therefore be conducted.

The Infant Microbiome and Its Impact on Development of Food Allergy

285

Kylie N. Jungles, Kassidy M. Jungles, Leah Greenfield, and Mahboobeh Mahdavinia

The prevalence of food allergy (FA) has been increasing over the past few decades; recent statistics suggest that FA has an impact on up to 10% of the population and 8% of children. Although the pathogenesis of FA is unclear, studies suggest gut microbiome plays a role in the development of FA. The gut microbiome is influenced by infant feeding method, infant diet, and maternal diet during lactation. Breastfeeding, Mediterranean diet, and probiotics are associated with commensal gut microbiota that protect against FA. This area of research is essential to discovering potential preventive methods or therapeutic targets against FA.

Genetics of Food Allergy

301

Elisabet Johansson and Tesfaye B. Mersha

The risk factors for food allergy (FA) include both genetic variants and environmental factors. Advances using both candidate-gene association studies and genome-wide approaches have led to the identification of FA-associated genes involved in immune responses and skin barrier functions. Epigenetic changes have also been associated with the risk of FA. In this chapter, we outline current understanding of the genetics, epigenetics and the interplay with environmental risk factors associated with FA. Future studies of gene-environment interactions, gene-gene interactions, and multi-omics integration may help shed light on the mechanisms of FA, and lead to improved diagnostic and treatment strategies.

The Unmet Needs of Patients with Food Allergies

321

Melissa L. Engel and Bryan J. Bunning

This article reviews the unmet needs of patients with food allergies. Anxiety is common among patients with food allergies and their caregivers, which naturally stems from the avoidance, exposure, and uncertainty involved in care. Anxiety associated with allergen avoidance can have both adaptive and detrimental effects on overall health. Anxiety has implications for transitioning the responsibility of health and well-being from caregivers to the patients. As more children with food allergies become adults with food allergies, this will be an urgent topic. Moreover, as more exposure-based therapies become available, understanding patients' psychological expectations and experiences of exposure is vital.

Food Allergy: Catering for the Needs of the Clinician　　　　331

Sami L. Bahna and Amal H. Assa'ad

The practice of food allergy (FA) for clinicians has boomed, with a dramatic rise in the number of patients and families seeking care and with many advances on several fronts. The practice itself sometimes is evidence-based science and sometimes an art of pattern and phenotype recognition. This article examines the tools for diagnosis and management and therapy options available to physicians providing care for patients with FA. The article touches on pressing needs of clinicians and highlights the rapid and important movements in national and international support and advances that will have a positive impact on the field of FA.

IMMUNOLOGY AND ALLERGY CLINICS OF NORTH AMERICA

FORTHCOMING ISSUES

August 2021
Skin Allergy
Susan T. Nedorost, *Editor*

RECENT ISSUES

February 2021
Climate Change and Allergy
Jae-Won Oh, *Editor*

SERIES OF RELATED INTEREST

Medical Clinics
https://www.medical.theclinics.com/

THE CLINICS ARE AVAILABLE ONLINE!
Access your subscription at:
www.theclinics.com

Preface

Focus on the Patient with Food Allergy

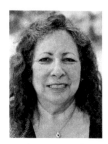

Amal H. Assa'ad, MD
Editor

Much has been written about food allergy in scientific journals and in the lay press. This issue takes a novel and different view in that the focus is on the patient with food allergy. The issue opens with a most comprehensive review by Krempski and colleagues from Dr. Nadeau's group of the bidirectional flow between clinical knowledge and basic research, how mouse studies complement human studies, how both generate novel diagnostics and therapeutics and utilize novel systems biology, making food allergy an excellent example of translation research. Eapen and Kim introduce the physical phenotype of the patient with food allergy as deducted from 4 large and racially diverse cohorts of food allergy, which elucidate the interaction of race, genetics, and environment to produce sensitization and clinical allergy in a way that challenges the traditional atopic march concept. Rubeiz and Ernst follow with an examination of the psychological milestones and challenges of patients with food allergy during different stages of their lives and highlight how allergists can strengthen resilience in their patients to enhance quality of life. Warren and colleagues from Dr. Gupta's group expose the large burden of food allergy that falls disproportionately on patients from racial and ethnic minority populations and propose that, to advance equity in food allergy outcomes and management, a rigorous and standardized characterization of socioeconomic status be incorporated in future studies. Devonshire and Lin delve into the unique presentations of food allergy in infants and toddlers, specifically disorders that bridge immunoglobulin E (IgE) and non-IgE mechanisms. Mennini and colleagues from Dr. Fiocchi's group review the recent guidelines for food allergy generated by multiple international organization and call for the guidelines to not only abide by the evidence but also consider the socioeconomic realities of the countries and the patients where the guidelines will be applied. Durban and colleagues from Dr. Venter's group assembled the largest group of expert dietitians from around the world to demonstrate how dietary intervention is not limited to avoidance advice, but should

Immunol Allergy Clin N Am 41 (2021) xiii–xiv
https://doi.org/10.1016/j.iac.2021.02.003
0889-8561/21/© 2021 Published by Elsevier Inc.

immunology.theclinics.com

expand to a nutritionally sound plan that includes suitable alternatives to support optimal growth and development and to improve quality of life. Albuhairi and Rachid shine a ray of hope for patients with food allergy by reviewing the only Food and Drug Administration–approved therapy for peanut allergy and a promising pipeline of biologics that are considered for food allergy. Jungles and colleagues from Dr. Mahdavinia's group enlighten us by the notion of a close interaction between the human microbiome and the susceptibility to food allergy and how the microbiome can be changed to a more favorable profile. Johannson and Mersha delve into the genetics of food allergy and the interaction of the genetic background in patients with food allergy with the environment and other atopic conditions. Engel and Bunning write from the science and from the heart about the daily difficulties faced by patients with food allergy and their caregivers and the unmet needs for this population. Finally, Dr Bahna and I, 2 academic allergists and immunologists with more than three-quarters of a century of practice experience between us, wrap up the issue with a discussion of the past, present, and future as seen from the point of view of clinicians serving patients with food allergy and how to cater to their needs so they can provide the best care.

This issue is written not only by leaders in the field in the United States and internationally but also by young faculty and residents who have answered the call to study food allergy and serve patients by carving a niche for their research. They are the future of food allergy research and clinical care.

It has been my honor to be invited to be the editor of this issue of *Immunology and Allergy Clinics of North America* on food allergy. I recall that, as an allergy and immunology fellow, I waited impatiently for each new issue of this journal and as soon as I would get it, I would not put it down until I read it cover to cover. Later, as a professor and educator, I have used many amazing issues to teach residents and fellows about allergy and immunology. I sincerely thank all the contributors to this issue and hope that it will be used to teach generations of learners about food allergy and that the patients with food allergy find and see themselves on its pages.

Amal H. Assa'ad, MD
Professor of Pediatrics
Division of Allergy and Immunology
Cincinnati Children's Hospital
Medical Center
3333 Burnet Avenue
Cincinnati, OH 45229, USA

E-mail address:
amal.assaad@cchmc.org

Food Allergies
An Example of Translational Research

James Walter Krempski, PhD*, Christopher Warren, PhD,
Xiaorui Han, PhD, Wenming Zhang, PhD, Ziyuan He, PhD,
Stéphanie Lejeune, MD, Kari Nadeau, MD, PhD

KEYWORDS

- Food allergy • Translational • Mouse models • Allergy diagnosis • System biology

KEY POINTS

- Translational studies of food allergy include mouse studies, human studies, and computation methods and understanding how they complement each other.
- Two areas in which mouse studies complement human studies are in determining the immunologic processes sensitization and tolerance.
- Novel diagnosis approaches include component-resolved diagnostics, basophil activation test, histamine-release assays, mast cell activation test, and novel algorithms to predict the severity of reaction during oral food challenge.
- System biology approaches, including genomics, epigenomics, transcriptomics, proteomics, metabolomics, and microbiomics, are being used in food allergy research.

INTRODUCTION
The Recent Rise of Food Allergies

Over the past few decades, IgE-mediated food allergy has become a chronic condition of increasing concern for clinicians, allergists/immunologists, and affected patients and their families. Food allergy constitutes a key step along the allergic march—the natural history of allergic disease manifestations that often progresses from allergic sensitization early in infancy to atopic dermatitis, food allergy, asthma, and allergic rhinitis. Although fatalities are rare relative to the number of people affected,[1] recent epidemiologic data suggest that the population-level burden of food allergy is substantial. A recent survey of a nationally representative sample of more than 50,000 US households estimated that approximately 8% of US children[2] and 10% of adults[3] have a current food allergy—with 40% of affected children and 45% of adults allergic to multiple foods. When placed in the context of previous prevalence estimates, these data suggest that the prevalence of food allergies still may be

Sean N. Parker Center for Allergy and Asthma Research, Stanford University, Stanford, CA, USA
* Corresponding author.
E-mail address: jwkremp@stanford.edu

Immunol Allergy Clin N Am 41 (2021) 143–163
https://doi.org/10.1016/j.iac.2021.01.003   immunology.theclinics.com
0889-8561/21/© 2021 Elsevier Inc. All rights reserved.

on the rise in North America. A meta-regression of food allergy surveillance data collected by the US Centers for Disease Control and Prevention from 1988 to 2011 concluded that reported prevalence of pediatric food allergy had increased by 1.2 percentage points per decade (95% CI, 0.7–1.6).[4] Given that a majority of patients with food allergy are not expected to naturally develop tolerance, particularly to the most common allergens (ie, peanut, tree nut, and seafood), it is likely that the prevalence of food allergies across the US general population is likely to continue rising until their etiology is better understood and effective prevention and/or treatment interventions are widely implemented.

The Recent Rise of Food Allergies—National Healthcare Utilization Data

The aforementioned cross-sectional survey data indicating rising food allergy prevalence in the United States are corroborated via examination of temporal trends in food allergy–related health care utilization. This includes a recent longitudinal analysis of national health insurance claims data,[5] which demonstrated the incidence of peanut allergy increased steadily from 2001 to 2016. Another analysis of national claims data found that, from 2007 to 2016, the percent of claim lines with diagnoses of anaphylactic food reactions rose 377%.[6] The most common eliciting allergic foods were peanut and tree nut, which are consistent with other US studies showing these as among the most frequent causative foods of severe allergic reactions and emergency department (ED) visits.[7] Other studies of large private and publicly available[8] administrative claims databases[7] have found that rates of pediatric ED visits and hospitalizations for food-induced anaphylaxis have risen substantially over the past 2 decades. One study of the Healthcare Cost and Utilization Project Kids' Inpatient Database—the only all-payer pediatric inpatient care database in the United States—estimated a doubling of food-induced anaphylaxis hospitalization rates from 2000 to 2009.[8] Another analysis of a private administrative care database concluded that rates of ED visits for food-induced anaphylaxis more than doubled from 2005 to 2014 among all segments of the US pediatric population—particularly among adolescents, where they rose more than 4-fold.[7] Overall, the specific allergen responsible for the greatest increase in ED visitation was for reactions to tree nuts/seeds, rates of which increased more than 3.5-fold over the 9-year study period.

The Recent Rise of Food Allergies—Psychosocial Burden

In light of the relatively low fatality rates associated with food allergy and general lack of symptoms experienced by patients in the absence of acute allergenic food exposure—food allergies arguably impose their greatest burden in the psychosocial domain. Previous research describes how the stress of daily food allergy management compounded by a dearth of effective, accessible treatment options can have an adverse impact on family relationships and limit social activities, ultimately contributing to impaired food allergy–related quality of life.[9] Previous studies have indicated that patients with a greater number of food allergies reported lower quality of life compared with their counterparts with fewer food allergies—likely a function of the greater degree of vigilance required for allergen avoidance.[10–12] Among patients with specific allergies, those with milk and egg allergy report lower quality of life compared with children with more easily avoidable allergens, such as peanut and tree nut.[13,14] Food allergy–related quality of life also is worse among children and caregivers for those with a history of severe food-allergic reactions, more symptoms during a previously reported food allergic reaction, and a prior history of epinephrine use.[10,12,15] Similarly, individuals who believe themselves more likely to experience potentially life-threatening anaphylaxis report worse quality of life than their counterparts who are less concerned about potentially fatal anaphylaxis. Due to the ubiquity of food, management of food allergies remains a daily challenge for many patients, as they seek to strike an appropriate balance between vigilance, preparedness, and stress management.

The Recent Rise of Food Allergies—Economic Impact

Beyond its effects on physical and psychological health, food allergy patients also incur substantial economic burden in their efforts to diagnose, treat, and manage this chronic condition on a daily basis. Although little is known about the economic burden of food allergies on adult patients, in 2013, the annual economic cost of pediatric food allergy was estimated to be $24.8 billion, approximately $4184 per child.[16] Estimated annual direct medical costs totaled $4.3 billion; annual out-of-pocket costs related to food allergy were $5.5 billion; and annual opportunity costs, such as a caregiver leaving/changing jobs and missing work to care for their food-allergic child, were estimated to be $14.2 billion. A 2019 systematic review of 11 studies addressing the economic burden of food allergy supported this conclusion that household-level lost opportunity costs appear to be a major driver of food allergy–related economic burden.[17]

Challenges Posed by the Rise of Food Allergies—Lack of Treatment Options

The rise of food allergies poses numerous challenges for patients and their families, chief among them is the current dearth of Food and Drug Administration (FDA)-approved treatment options. Although evidence for the safety and efficacy of numerous food allergen immunotherapeutic modalities continues to accumulate, as of Fall 2020, the only FDA-approved immunotherapy is an oral peanut allergy treatment—Palforzia—indicated for use in pediatric patients 4 years to 17 years of age. The epidemiologic data summarized previously, however, suggest that fewer than 1 in 10 US food allergy patients are peanut-allergic children (most are adults and/or allergic to allergens besides peanut). Furthermore, more than half of peanut allergy patients have multiple food allergies.

Challenges Posed by the Rise of Food Allergies—Lack of Understanding About Mechanisms

Although much has been learned about the etiology of food allergies in recent years,[18] major knowledge gaps remain. For example, although recent data indicate that many adults develop new-onset allergies to foods in adulthood, which formerly were tolerated, it still is not fully understood how or why this occurs.[3] Conversely, much remains unknown about the exact mechanisms through which some patients gain tolerance to foods that previously induced allergic reactions, whereas others remain allergic, and still others experience a progressive worsening of allergy symptoms. Improving scientific understanding of how to promote and sustain immune tolerance at molecular and cellular levels is fundamental to the success of emerging food allergen immunotherapies, including oral, sublingual, and epicutaneous approaches.

Challenges Posed by the Rise of Food Allergies—How to Prevent Them?

Over the past decade, findings from numerous studies investigating the safety and efficacy of earlier introduction of allergenic solids have been translated into revised guidelines for the prevention of peanut allergy.[19–22] Much remains unknown, however, about the optimal timing, format, frequency, quantity, order, and/or dietary context (eg, probiotic, vitamin D, and/or fiber supplementation) in which "early" introduction of allergenic solids should occur to maximize preventive effects—particularly for allergens besides peanut. Although encouraging parents to incorporate allergenic solids earlier and more often into their diet perhaps is the most widely studied food allergy prevention modality—others currently are being explored. These include (1) vitamin D supplementation among patients with vitamin D insufficiency; (2) aggressive, early emollient treatment of infant eczema (a key determinant of subsequent food allergy development)[23,24] and other efforts to optimize early life skin barrier function; and (3) promoting exposure to a diverse array of environmental microbiota to help ensure colonization of the gastrointestinal tract by commensal microbes[25] believed to play a role in inducing a balanced, tolerogenic immune response.

Broad Areas of Study

Ongoing research into the molecular and cellular mechanisms of food allergy and immune tolerance is poised to provide key insights into why food allergies have apparently risen so dramatically in prevalence over recent decades. Improving understanding of how environmental influences interact with genetic risk to predispose individuals to developing food allergies has the potential to inform further advances in food allergy prevention and treatments. Moreover, learning more about predictors of both natural and treatment-induced tolerance to food allergens can help inform clinical management, including identification of patients who are most likely to potentially benefit from emerging immunotherapies.

Translating Food Allergy Research from Bench to Bedside

The National Center for Advancing Translational Sciences defines translation as "the process of turning observations in the laboratory, clinic and community into interventions that improve the health of individuals and the public—from diagnostics and therapeutics to medical procedures and behavioral changes." The translational science spectrum (**Fig. 1**)[26] shows the process of scientific research from knowledge about the biological basis of health and disease to delivery of interventions that improve the health of individuals and the public. The field of food allergy research currently is at an inflection point, where advances in cellular and molecular immunology are being translated into FDA-approved targeted food allergen immunotherapies and prevention interventions.[22] This article aims to provide an overview of how cutting-edge research into the mechanisms of food allergy and immune tolerance currently is being translated and implemented in the clinical setting in order to reduce the public health burden of IgE-mediated food allergy.

OBSERVATIONS AND MECHANISMS

Mouse models are instrumental in deepening an understanding of immune mechanisms that human samples alone cannot accomplish. This section aims to demonstrate how mouse models can illuminate sensitization and tolerance mechanisms of food allergy.

Pros and Cons of Using Mouse Models

Awareness of the strengths and weaknesses of mouse studies facilitates a balanced interpretation of their results (**Table 1**).
Advantages of mouse modeling for food allergy studies:

1. Mouse models allow for tissue-specific analysis, such as lungs, gastrointestinal (GI) tract, and lymph nodes.
2. Mouse models provide mechanistic insight into food allergy sensitization, prevention, and persistence by identifying connections between essential cells, molecules, and conditions.

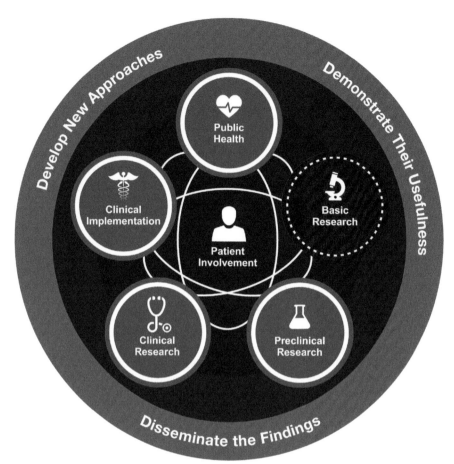

Fig. 1. The translational science spectrum illustrates the nonlinear, multidirectional process of scientific research from knowledge about the biological basis of health and disease to delivery of interventions that improve the health of individuals and the public. (*From* the NIH National Center for Advancing Translational Sciences (NCATS); with permission.)

3. Genetic models allow for specific studies on the roles of specific cell types and cytokines by inducing mutations, such as gain of function, loss of function, and conditional. Transfer of specific cells or microbes also is useful.
4. Mice live in carefully controlled conditions, reducing confounding factors inherent in human studies.

   Some disadvantages include

1. Mouse models may not represent human disease accurately.
2. Several colliding factors likely are responsible for food allergy, such as environment, genetics, diet, and microbiome changes.[27,28] Oversimplification and overestimation of individual factors are likely to minimize other factors' roles.
   a. Allergic disease processes may be different in mice than in humans due to biological differences.

Table 1
Strengths and weaknesses of using mouse models for food allergy

Strength	Weakness
Allows for tissue-specific analysis, such as lungs, gastrointestinal tract, and lymph nodes.	The model may not accurately represent human disease.
Provides mechanistic insight into food allergy sensitization, prevention, and persistence by identifying connections between essential cells, molecules, and conditions	Several colliding factors are responsible for food allergy, such as environment, genetic, diet, and microbiome changes.[27,28] Oversimplification and overestimation of individual factors are likely to minimize other factors' roles.
Genetic models allow for specific studies on the roles of specific cell types and cytokines by inducing mutations, such as gain of function, loss of function, and conditional. Transfer of specific cells or microbes also are useful.	
Mice live in carefully controlled conditions, reducing confounding factors inherent in human studies.	

b. Human behavior at the individual, family, and societal levels is critical to understanding food allergy etiology such that mouse studies cannot provide the insights necessary to address the food allergy epidemic fully.

Translation—modeling human disease
Key areas that mouse studies contribute to understanding mechanisms of tolerance and sensitization to food allergens are studies investigating the microbiome and route of allergen exposure.

Microbiome
The microbiome is a vital piece of the food allergy puzzle. A healthy microbiome helps prevent food allergy.[18,27,28] *Clostridia* species have several benefits to human gut health[29] and mouse studies flesh out potential mechanisms. For example, a mouse study showed that *Clostridia* species promote gut integrity by inducing interleukin (IL)-22 secretion from innate lymphoid cells and helper T cells (T_H), thereby regulating intestinal epithelial permeability.[30] *Clostridia*-enriched microbiota transferred into germ-free mice induce higher levels of Foxp3 expressing regulatory T cells (Tregs) in the colon, which helps promote tolerance.[18] Certain *Clostridia* species promote a transforming growth factor (TGF)-β and IL-10–rich cytokine milieu in mouse colons, essential for a tolerogenic gut environment.[31]

Clostridia also have therapeutic benefits for at least 2 food allergy models. For example, introduction of *Clostridia* species into gnotobiotic mice reduced levels of peanut-specific and total IgE relative to germ-free controls.[29] Another study examined whether commensal bacteria play a causal role in the cow's milk allergy (CMA) allergic response. Investigators colonized germ-free mice with feces from infants with CMA or healthy infants and sensitized them to β-lactoglobulin. Sensitization occurred in the CMA colonized mice but not the healthy control mice. The investigators identified the *Clostridia* species *Anaerostipes caccae* as a protective species that may be therapeutically relevant for infants with CMA.[32]

Certain bacteria also play a role in sensitization to food allergy. Mice with gain of function mutations in the IL-4α subunit have elevated STAT-6 signaling of IL-4 and IL-13, leading to increased food allergy susceptibility. Food allergy sensitized mice show altered abundance of the bacterial species *Lactobacillaceae, Rikenellaceae,* and *Porphyromonadaceae.*[33] Transfer of the microbiota from these mice into germ-free mice transferred increased susceptibility of food-mediated anaphylaxis.

The surface has barely been scratched on the microbiome's contribution to food allergy. Further research using mouse models will allow researchers to identify other beneficial and harmful microbes, their mechanisms, and how they translate to human disease.

Environmental exposure in sensitization

Current hypotheses suggest that the route of initial bodily exposure to food allergens is a significant contributor to sensitization or tolerance. Initial allergen exposure via nonoral routes, such as through the airway or skin, is likely to lead to sensitization. In contrast, initial exposure via oral consumption is likely to be tolerogenic.[19,34] Models are needed that take these observations into account.

Mouse models are most effective when they model the human condition as closely as possible. An excellent example of this are models investigating peanut allergy.

Multiple mouse studies have examined peanut skin sensitization by epicutaneous exposure on the ear pinna of mice with crude peanut extract or the peanut protein components Ara h1 and Ara h2 or by utilizing abdominal tape stripping and peanut flour exposure to the tape stripped area.[35,36] Sensitization also occurs through airway peanut exposure.[37] In each study, sensitized mice exhibit elevated peanut-IgE levels and induction of anaphylaxis upon peanut protein challenge, thus modeling the human condition. None of these models uses adjuvants and likely is closer to how environmental exposure occurs in infants.

Type 2 helper T cells and follicular helper T cells cells drive peanut-specific antibody responses and anaphylaxis

Both the airway and tape-stripping with peanut flour models demonstrate that sensitization to peanut depends on follicular T_H (T_{FH}), whereas the ear pinna sensitization model indicates T_H2 cells are required for sensitization. As the tape stripping skin and airway models show, T_{FH} cells are essential for peanut-IgE and anaphylaxis. This likely is because T_{FH} cells are specialized to interact with germinal center B cells in the lymph nodes, thus generating somatic hypermutation and affinity maturation.[38] Additionally, IL-13 derived from type 2 innate lymphoid cells is indispensable for T_{FH} cells generation and plasma peanut-IgE.[39]

The method and route of sensitization and allergen itself may induce differing immune pathways because the use of specific proteins leaves out other components of peanut, such as fats and carbohydrates. Although the peanut proteins Ara h1, Ara h2, Ara h3, and Ara h6 are the main targets of peanut-specific antibody responses, peanut is a complex molecule, and the other components may have unique roles in initiating the direction of the immune response.

Tolerance

Models of mouse tolerance can help define mechanisms of tolerance generated and loss. Foods typically are well tolerated; however, a breakdown of tolerance to the same food sensitizes, thus acting as either an agent of sensitization or tolerance. The phenomenon of oral tolerance has long been an area of scientific interest. In 1907, guinea pigs' sensitization to vegetable proteins resulted in violent anaphylaxis and death.[40] In 1911, Wells[41] demonstrated that guinea pigs raised on a daily diet of corn before sensitization protected them from anaphylaxis and death. Since then, several studies have assessed how tolerance develops. Many of these studies used the protein ovalbumin (OVA) with an adjuvant.[42–45] Whether these observations from OVA hold for real-world food allergens is unknown. OVA is not a natural allergen; sensitization can only occur when OVA is coupled to an adjuvant, or by use of transgenic mice with genetically modified T-cell receptors (TCRs) specifically engineered to react against OVA peptides. Real-world allergens are more biologically complex, and tolerance induction may differ depending on the allergen's nature.

A mouse model can examine how oral tolerance protects from sensitization, both immunologic and clinically. For example, using a model of milk casein allergy, Kim and colleagues[46] showed that IL-10–producing B-regulatory cells from the mesenteric lymph nodes, but not from the spleen of peritoneal lymph nodes, protected mice from casein-induced allergic responses through Tregs. Another study showed that feeding mice peanut butter before skin or airway exposure mice protected them from sensitization, mirroring the Learning Early About Peanut (LEAP) study results.[47] Examining T cells in the lung draining lymph nodes revealed that tolerance was dependent on the inhibitory molecule CTLA-4 (**Fig. 2**).

Conclusions and future directions of mouse modeling

Mouse studies have helped generate novel ideas and insights that translate well to human food allergy. Areas in which mouse studies have helped significantly are the microbiome's role and how environmental exposure has an impact on immunologic mechanisms of sensitization and tolerance.

Skin or airway T-cell–mediated sensitization to peanut

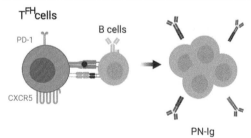

Oral-induced T-cell–mediated tolerance to peanut

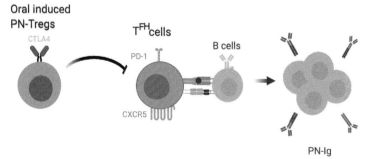

Fig. 2. T-cell–mediated sensitization and tolerance.

Clostridia species appear to promote immune tolerance, whereas sensitized mice demonstrate alterations in *Lactobacillaceae*, *Rikenellaceae*, and *Porphyromonadaceae* species. Further work to clarify beneficial and harmful species is needed.

Mouse work also helps confirm the hypothesis that allergen exposure's initial route plays a significant role in sensitization and tolerance. Mice exposed to peanut via the nonoral skin or airway routes are sensitized. At the same time, tolerance occurs when mice are exposed to peanut butter orally before skin or airway exposure. Mouse modeling also demonstrated immunologic mechanisms of sensitization and tolerance. Key roles for T_{FH} cells, CTLA4-expressing Tregs, and IL-10–producing B-regulatory cells are described.

Mouse models can continue to assist in other areas of food allergy. The initiating events of how allergens engage with innate immunity are unknown. Appropriate mouse models can help clarify these early events in a way that human samples cannot. Insights from these studies may help provide ideas for therapeutics to stave off food allergy in at-risk children.

It is unknown how food allergies persist. For example, the contributions of memory T cells, memory B cells, plasma cells, and microbes are unknown in maintaining food allergy. These studies are well suited for mouse modeling because many studies may involve tissue-specific analysis and bone marrow extraction. Insight from these studies likely would generate novel directions in therapeutic ideas to reverse sensitization.

Lastly, the effectiveness of mouse modeling in food allergy is related directly to how well it models the human condition.

Mechanisms learned from human studies

IgE-mediated food allergy accounts for the vast majority of food-induced allergic reactions.

The knowledge of mechanisms behind the induced desensitization in allergen immunotherapy has been advancing largely through investigating peripheral blood of human patients undergoing oral immunotherapy (OIT) trials, with changes occurred at local tissues including gastrointestinal tract and skin barrier as peripheral subjects of interest.

This section focuses on findings emerged in recent human studies of food allergy, including OIT trials.

Timing of allergen introduction

For decades, allergen avoidance remained the standard clinical practice of preventing food allergies. Since the American Academy of Pediatrics issued a revised infant feeding policy in 2008,[48] early introduction of highly allergenic foods has been increasingly recommended for all infants. Results from the LEAP trial demonstrated early introduction of peanut allergen in high-risk infants can reduce the risk of developing peanut allergy.[19] A meta-analysis of 5 trials showed that early egg introduction at 4 months to 6 months was associated with reduced egg allergy.[49] New clinical guidelines are under implementation, with physicians facing challenges in offering evidence-based recommendations.[50]

Immunoglobulins and basophils

The key factor that inhibits effector cell activation mediated by IgE comes from an increase in allergen-specific IgG4 level, which is a common feature of and a response to allergen immunotherapy.[51] Although allergen-specific IgE (sIgE) level is not a predictive biomarker to clinical reactivity,[51] IgE antibodies to Ara h2 have been reported to efficiently differentiate clinical peanut allergy from asymptomatic peanut sensitization.[52] Lower peanut-induced basophil activation and higher peanut allergen–specific IgG4/sIgE before treatment is associated with OIT-induced sustained effects in patients undergoing a double-blind, randomized, placebo-controlled, phase 2 peanut OIT trial.[53,54]

T cells
Activation and polarization of T-cell subsets are the main effectors in allergic inflammation and tolerance. Desensitization to allergens often is associated with a shift away from a T_H2-skewed phenotype toward a T_H1-skewed response, together with restored suppressor function of allergen-specific Tregs, as reported in multiple reports of OIT clinical trials.[55,56] Expression of skin and gut homing receptors on the surface of allergen-specific T cells has been found to increase in patients with milk allergy and other atopic conditions.[57,58]

Microbiome and epithelial barrier
There has been an increase of interest in studying the interplay between commensal bacteria and the gastrointestinal tract mucosal surface, which serves as the first physical layer of protection against foreign antigens. Intestinal bacteria are now known to play a role in regulation allergic responses to dietary antigens. Intestinal bacteria of healthy infants have demonstrated a protective effect against anaphylactic responses to a cow's milk allergen in colonized mice.[59] As a recent report showed in peanut-allergic adult patients, an increase of gut microbiota diversity was observed during active oral immunotherapy.[60]

DIAGNOSIS: CHALLENGES AND FUTURE PROSPECTS

A safe and accurate diagnosis of food allergy is extremely important to guide safe and yet not overly restrictive dietary management. Currently, the cornerstone of the diagnosis of IgE-mediated allergy is the clinical history followed by in vitro or in vivo tests, including the skin prick test (SPT), sIgE test, cellular test, and oral food challenges (OFCs).[61] These methods of diagnostic testing for allergy often are inconclusive and, in cases of food challenges, sometimes stressful and scary. **Table 2** shows the advantages and disadvantages of diagnostic approaches. Researchers are trying to identify more safe and precise diagnostic methods, including developing new approaches, improving current tests, and combining diagnostic tools together to improve the accuracy of the predictive performance of diagnosis.

Double-blind placebo-controlled food challenge (DBPCFC) still is the only gold standard for definitive diagnosis and sometimes cannot be avoided,[62] except when a patient has suffered an anaphylactic shock. OFC, however, is time-consuming, costly, and burdened by the risk of life-threatening anaphylactic reactions.[62,63] Therefore, reliable prognostic markers for predicting severity of allergic reactions during OFC are needed.[64,65] Chinthrajah and colleagues[66] proposed an integrated approach combining laboratory values (ratio of peanut-stimulated basophils to anti–IgE-stimulated basophils), along with clinical variables (exercise-induced asthma and forced expiratory volume in the first second of expiration/forced vital capacity ratio at time of DBPCFC) to be incorporated into a novel algorithm for assigning challenge severity score to predict the severity of reaction during peanut OFC. This decision rule is under a clinical trial (NCT02103270) for further testing before it can be considered outside research settings.

For many patients, conventional allergy tests like SPT and sIgE to allergen extracts that indicate they might react to a food are misinterpreted to mean that they do react to that food. This can lead to unnecessary avoidance of foods, which increases costs,

Table 2
Advantages and disadvantages of diagnostic approaches for food allergy

Diagnosis Approaches		Advantages	Disadvantages
Conventional approaches	SPT	Fast; cheap; no risk of allergen exposure	High false-positive rate
	Serum IgE test: Total IgE, specific-IgE	Fast; no risk of allergen exposure	High false-positive rate
	OFC	The only gold standard for definitive diagnosis	Time-consuming; costly; risk of life-threatening anaphylactic reactions
Novel approaches	CRD: Single or multiplex molecular allergens assays	More accurate diagnosis, capable of discriminating cosensitization vs cross-sensitization phenomena	CRD offered increased specificity but decreased sensitivity, when compared with traditional S FT and serum-specific IgE testing
	Cellular test: BAT	Shows advantage compared with HRA and MAT	BAT requires fresh blood samples for testing; not applicable for subjects with low basophil number
	MAT	Adds significant diagnostic value to conventional methods and reduces the need for OFC testing; no risk of allergen exposure	Lower sensitivity than BAT
	HRAs	Using serum instead of fresh blood; applicable to subjects whose basophils do not respond to the BAT / Diagnoses subjects with low basophil number in contrast to HRA	Lower sensitivity than BAT
	Novel algorithm: Novel algorithm to predict the severity of reaction during peanut OFC	Reduces the risk of life-threatening anaphylactic reactions caused by OFC	Might need further testing and optimization

adds to anxiety, and limits food choices and nutrition options. To improve current diagnostic tests, researchers are trying to use pure allergens instead of food allergen extracts for the SPT and sIgE tests. With pure allergens, it is possible to overcome the problem of low concentration and low stability of the allergens that may be lost when making a food allergen extract. The advanced antigen-based tests like component-resolved diagnostics (CRD) characterize the molecular components of each allergen involved in a sIgE-mediated response. In the clinical practice, CRD can lead to more accurate diagnosis and selection of therapeutic intervention[67,68] and increasingly is incorporated into clinical workflows.[69] A recent systemic review suggested that sIgE to Ara h2 can enhance the certainty of diagnosis and reduce the number of OFCs necessary to rule out clinical peanut allergy in unclear cases.[70] A Europe-wide hazelnut allergy study suggested that combinations of CRD-based approaches with clinical history and extract data are superior to CRD alone.[71] Another advanced technology for allergy diagnosis based on CRD is multiplex molecular allergens assays, such as Madx ALEX[72] and Euroimmun Multiplex immunoblot assay,[73] which enable clinicians to simultaneously detect multiple sIgE test in a single test that requires only a small amount of blood. This will be useful particularly for younger children from whom only small amounts of blood may be taken for testing. The multiplex CRD also will enable clinicians to discriminate cosensitization versus cross-sensitization phenomena and can be useful to stratify the clinical risk associated with a specific sensitization pattern, in addition to the OFC.

Another recent area of research is to improve the allergy diagnosis by using cellular allergy tests, such as the basophil activation test (BAT),[74,75] histamine-release assays (HRAs),[76] and, more recently, the mast cell activation test (MAT),[77,78] which use cell activity as a measure of allergic responsiveness. Those tests have been reported to add significant diagnostic value to SPT and IgE-based test methods and reduce the need for OFC testing. BAT was compared with histamine release (HR) and passive HR and did not show a significant advantage but could diagnose subjects with low basophil number in contrast to HR.[76] The reports on the usage of passive sensitization strategies using the mast cell lines[12] or mast cell precursors[13] showed promising potential on distinguishing peanut allergy from peanut sensitization but lower sensitivity than BAT. MAT has the advantage, however, of using serum instead of fresh blood, overcoming the limitation that BATs require fresh blood. In addition, the MAT provides results for patients whose basophils do not respond to the BAT.

Although an increasing number of advanced diagnostic methods are under development, no currently available tests can predict the severity of a patient's next food allergy reaction. Identifying new diagnostic tests that are easy, safe, accurate, and stress-free still is an unmet need. Novel diagnostic methods integrating data from different sources and technologies together with a better understanding of mechanisms of allergic inflammation may contribute to developing sophisticated precision medicine tools for better diagnosis.

FOOD ALLERGEN AND SYSTEM BIOLOGY

Another example of translational research in food allergy is the application of omics technologies and systems biology approaches. Systems biology studies biological process through comprehensive interrogations of the biomolecules at different levels to gain insights into complex biological systems[79] (**Fig. 3**). In food allergy, multiple players at different scales, including food proteins, gut microbiome, host gastrointestinal tract, host immune system, and more, interact with each other dynamically and contribute to the process. The high individual heterogeneity and complex nature of

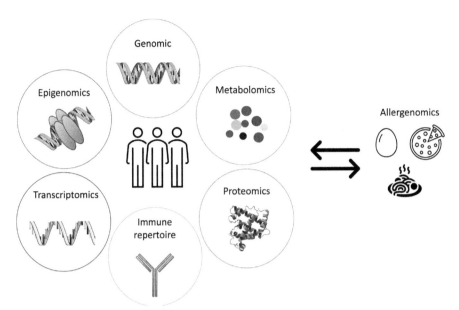

Fig. 3. Genomic, epigenomic, transcriptomics, metabolomics, proteomics, and immune studies are part of a comprehensive interrogations of the biomolecules at different levels to gain insight of the complex biological system to study food allergies.

food allergy make it an especially suitable target for systemic biological approaches. With the rapid advance of omics technologies, massive data now can be generated at relatively low cost. Systemic approaches have been used to not only better understand the mechanisms behind food allergy but also show potential for identifying biomarkers to better diagnose, prevent, and treat food allergy.[80] Omics technologies, including genomics, epigenomics, transcriptomics, proteomics, metabolomics, and microbiomics, have been or are being used in food allergy research (**Table 3**).[81]

Although the contribution of heritable factors to food allergy remains to be determined, a body of evidence has identified certain genetic predispositions to food allergy. In genomic-wide association studies, genetic variants, typically single-nucleotide polymorphisms (SNPs), are examined across the whole genome. Several loci have been linked to the risk of food allergy.[82] SNPs mapping to the HLA regions have been shown to be associated with peanut allergy[83] and wheat allergy.[84] Genetic background also was found to be associated with total IgE level as well as sIgE levels.[83] Immune repertoire, referring to the genetic diversity of B-cell receptors (ie, immunoglobulins) and TCRs, also is under intense investigation in food allergy. Studies of IgE-producing B-cell receptors have revealed the mechanism of IgE class switching during allergen-specific immune responses.[85,86] Another study found certain TCR clones in CD4$^+$ T cells that recognized peanut epitopes were shared among peanut allergic individuals.[87]

Epigenetic modifications, including DNA methylation, histone modification, and nucleosome positioning, induced by environmental factors, can affect the expressional profiles of the genomes.[88] The increasing risk of food allergy in the recent generations could be linked with environmental changes through epigenetic modifications. One study of Dutch children found that DNA methylation generally was increased with CMA.[89] Peanut allergic individuals who were desensitized through immunotherapy had hypomethylation of FOXP3 gene in Tregs compared with those who were nontolerant.[90]

Table 3
Genomics, epigenomics, transcriptomics, proteomics, metabolomics, and microbiomics applied to food allergy

Platforms	Targets	Application Examples in Food Allergy
Genomics	SNPs across genome	SNPs at HLA regions associated with food allergy
Immune Rrepertoire	TCR and B-cell receptor diversities	Identified origin of IgE–producing B cells; identified common TCR recognizing peanut
Epigenomics	DNA methylation, histone modification, and nucleosome positioning	DNA methylation associated with CMA
Transcriptomics	Gene expression profiles	Immune gene clusters were associated with allergic response in peanut allergy
Proteomics	Protein expression at cellular level	Identify immune cells population and functions associated with allergy response
Metabolomics	Metabolites and metabolic pathway in host and microbes	Food allergy associated with decreased sphingolipid levels in serum
Allergenomics	Protein/peptides in the food	Identify allergens and epitopes

Transcriptomics examine the RNA molecules and provide the information of the current gene expression profile of the sample. Immune cells, usually from peripheral blood samples, from allergic individuals were isolated with or without the stimulation of relevant food allergens and analyzed for gene expressions. Gene clusters related to acute and inflammatory pathway were identified in peanut allergic children following OFCs.[91] Single-cell RNA sequencing also was applied to examine circulating immune cells before and during OIT for peanut allergy and observed a transient increase of TGF-β–producing cells and changes in T_H2 cells.[92]

Proteomics aim to measure all the protein components in the samples. Mass cytometry detects heavy metal ions instead of fluorescent dyes in the traditional flow cytometry and allows for measuring more than 40 protein markers simultaneously within a single cell.[93] This permits more detailed and efficient investigation of immune cells than allowed by previous approaches. In peanut allergy, investigators have found increased frequency of activated B cells and peanut-specific memory CD4 T cells using mass cytometry.[94] Another application of proteomics in food allergy is to identify and characterize allergens in the offending food using mass spectrometry, also called allergenomics, which is important in food safety.[95]

Metabolomics measure the collection of metabolites (generally small molecules) including sugar, lipids, amino acids, fatty acids, and so forth. This is an emerging field and studies applying metabolomic approaches to food allergy are relatively scarce. In an asthma/food allergy pediatric cohort, Crestani and colleagues[96] found food allergy was uniquely associated with decreased sphingolipid levels in serum. Metabolomics also is particularly interesting to consider in combination with microbiomics approaches because microbiota may affect host immune system through metabolites they secrete. (The microbiome in food allergy are discussed extensively previously.)

Despite the decreasing cost of omics technologies, the implications of omics technologies still are mainly in the research setting because these technologies generally require highly trained expertise to both acquire and analyze data.[80] Automated sample processing and artificial intelligence–aided data analysis may make these tools more available in the future within routine clinical settings. The application of systemic biology in food allergy can lead to identifications of novel biomarkers and hints to inspire new prevention strategy or treatments.

CLINICS CARE POINTS

- Food allergies are among allergic disorders, including atopic dermatitis, asthma, and allergic rhinitis. Many individuals with a single allergic disorder eventually develop other atopic comorbidities, suggesting common underlying mechanisms. Classically, the earliest manifestation of allergic diseases starts with atopic dermatitis in infancy and preschool years, and these individuals then may develop food allergy, allergic rhinitis, and/or asthma in subsequent years.[97,98] This natural progression of allergic disorders is termed the allergic or atopic march.

- Food allergies are adverse antigen-specific immune-mediated responses upon exposure to a given food, affecting 8% of children and 5% of adults in the United States.[99] Common allergenic foods include milk, eggs, peanuts, tree nuts (such as almonds, cashews, and walnuts), fish, shellfish, soy, and wheat. Prevalence of peanut allergy is estimated to be 2% to 3%.[100–102] IgE-mediated food allergies are characterized by the rapid onset of symptoms (typically observed within minutes to approximately 2 hours) after ingestion of the suspected allergen, generally proteins in foods.[103] Food allergy reactions can lead to anaphylaxis, a rapid and systemic allergic reaction, involving the upper and lower airways, skin, conjunctiva, gastrointestinal tract, and cardiovascular systems. Untreated, anaphylaxis can be fatal, most often due to upper or lower airways obstruction or to cardiovascular collapse.[103,104] Cofactors, such as concomitant infection, medication, alcohol intake, and exercise, may influence the occurrence of anaphylaxis.

- Other subtypes of food allergy include oral allergy syndrome, a hypersensitivity reaction to plant-based foods, usually mild, due to cross-reactivity between food proteins and inhalant allergens, with usually mild symptoms (eg, PR-10 syndrome); alpha-gal allergy, a reaction to an oligosaccharide present in red meats and tick saliva[105]; eosinophilic esophagitis, a chronic, local, immune-mediated esophageal disease,[103] whose pathophysiology is unclear but involves food allergy[106]; and non–IgE-mediated food allergies, such as food protein–induced allergic proctitis, food protein–induced enteropathy, food protein–induced enterocolitis.

- Until recently, the only effective therapy for food allergy was strict avoidance of the allergenic food. New approaches with disease-modifying properties, including allergen immunotherapy and the use of biologics, most of which are humanized monoclonal antibodies targeting the T_H2 inflammatory pathway, have been developed in the past 20 years, leading to a revolution in the field.[107] Preventive strategies to limit risk factors and their impact on the mechanism of food allergy also are encouraged by a growing body of research. The most effective preventive strategy might be early introduction of solid foods at 4 months to 6 months of age, and guidelines no longer recommend allergen avoidance.[108] Consistent with the dual-allergen hypothesis and atopic march, prevention of allergen exposure through maintaining skin barrier integrity also could serve as an effective preventive strategy in the future. Finally, findings on the role of the microbiota in allergic disorders and immune tolerance have led to the idea of probiotic supplementation as a preventive intervention, although current evidence does not indicate that probiotic supplementation reduces the risk of developing food allergy in children, as opposed to a possible benefit in the primary prevention of atopic dermatitis.[109]

- From bench to bedside, fully understanding the mechanisms leading to food allergy and tolerance will provide deeper comprehension of the relevant clinical outcomes in food allergy patients. Studying the modifications induced by novel therapeutics may improve overall comprehension of their mechanisms and allow introducing them in the standard of care.

DISCLOSURE

Dr K. Nadeau reports grants from National Institute of Allergy and Infectious Diseases (NIAID), National Heart, Lung, and Blood Institute (NHLBI), National Institute of Environmental Health Sciences (NIEHS), and Food Allergy Research & Education (FARE); is director of World Allergy Organization (WAO) Center of Excellence at Stanford; advisor at Cour Pharma; cofounder of Before Brands, Alladapt, Latitude, and IgGenix; National Scientific Committee member at Immune Tolerance Network (ITN) and National Institutes of Health (NIH) clinical research centers; and DSMB member for NHLBI. US patents for basophil testing, multifood immunotherapy and prevention, monoclonal antibody from plasmoblasts, and device for diagnostics. The other authors have nothing to disclose.

REFERENCES

1. Turner PJ, Jerschow E, Umasunthar T, et al. Fatal anaphylaxis: mortality rate and risk factors. J Allergy Clin Immunol Pract 2017;5(5):1169–78.
2. Gupta RS, Warren CM, Smith BM, et al. The public health impact of parent-reported childhood food allergies in the United States. Pediatrics 2018;142(6): e20181235.
3. Gupta RS, Warren CM, Smith BM, et al. Prevalence and severity of food allergies among US Adults. JAMA Netw Open 2019;2(1):e185630.
4. Keet CA, Savage JH, Seopaul S, et al. Temporal trends and racial/ethnic disparity in self-reported pediatric food allergy in the United States. Ann Allergy Asthma Immunol 2014;112(3):222–229 e223.
5. Lieberman JA. Severity of peanut allergy and the unmet gaps in care: a call to action. Am J Manag Care 2018;24(19 Suppl):S412–8.
6. Branum AM, Lukacs SL. Food allergy among children in the United States. Pediatrics 2009;124(6):1549–55.
7. Motosue MS, Bellolio MF, Van Houten HK, et al. National trends in emergency department visits and hospitalizations for food-induced anaphylaxis in US children. Pediatr Allergy Immunol 2018;29(5):538–44.
8. Rudders SA, Arias SA, Camargo CA Jr. Trends in hospitalizations for food-induced anaphylaxis in US children, 2000-2009. J Allergy Clin Immunol 2014; 134(4):960–962 e963.
9. Warren CM, Otto AK, Walkner MM, et al. Quality of life among food allergic patients and their caregivers. Curr Allergy Asthma Rep 2016;16(5):38.
10. Allen CW, Bidarkar MS, vanNunen SA, et al. Factors impacting parental burden in food-allergic children. J Paediatr Child Health 2015;51(7):696–8.
11. Wassenberg J, Cochard MM, Dunngalvin A, et al. Parent perceived quality of life is age-dependent in children with food allergy. Pediatr Allergy Immunol 2012; 23(5):412–9.
12. Howe L, Franxman T, Teich E, et al. What affects quality of life among caregivers of food-allergic children? Ann Allergy Asthma Immunol 2014;113(1):69–74.e2.
13. Ward CE, Greenhawt MJ. Treatment of allergic reactions and quality of life among caregivers of food-allergic children. Ann Allergy Asthma Immunol 2015;114(4):312–8.e2.
14. Warren CM, Gupta RS, Sohn MW, et al. Differences in empowerment and quality of life among parents of children with food allergy. Ann Allergy Asthma Immunol 2015;114(2):117–25.

15. Chow C, Pincus DB, Comer JS. Pediatric food allergies and psychosocial functioning: examining the potential moderating roles of maternal distress and overprotection. J Pediatr Psychol 2015;40(10):1065–74.

16. Gupta R, Holdford D, Bilaver L, et al. The economic impact of childhood food allergy in the United States. JAMA Pediatr 2013;167(11):1026–31.

17. Bilaver LA, Chadha AS, Doshi P, et al. Economic burden of food allergy: A systematic review. Ann Allergy Asthma Immunol 2019;122(4):373–80.e1.

18. Chinthrajah RS, Hernandez JD, Boyd SD, et al. Molecular and cellular mechanisms of food allergy and food tolerance. J Allergy Clin Immunol 2016;137(4):984–97.

19. Du Toit G, Roberts G, Sayre PH, et al. Randomized trial of peanut consumption in infants at risk for peanut allergy. N Engl J Med 2015;372(9):803–13.

20. Perkin MR, Logan K, Tseng A, et al. Randomized trial of introduction of allergenic foods in breast-fed infants. N Engl J Med 2016;374(18):1733–43.

21. Turcanu V, Brough HA, Du Toit G, et al. Immune mechanisms of food allergy and its prevention by early intervention. Curr Opin Immunol 2017;48:92–8.

22. Togias A, Cooper SF, Acebal ML, et al. Addendum guidelines for the prevention of peanut allergy in the United States: Report of the National Institute of Allergy and Infectious Diseases-sponsored expert panel. J Allergy Clin Immunol 2017;139(1):29–44.

23. Tham EH, Leung DY. Mechanisms by which atopic dermatitis predisposes to food allergy and the atopic march. Allergy Asthma Immunol Res 2019;11(1):4–15.

24. Lowe AJ, Leung DYM, Tang MLK, et al. The skin as a target for prevention of the atopic march. Ann Allergy Asthma Immunol 2018;120(2):145–51.

25. Lee KH, Song Y, Wu W, et al. The gut microbiota, environmental factors, and links to the development of food allergy. Clin Mol Allergy 2020;18:5.

26. Health NIo. Transforming translational science fact sheet. Bethesda (MD): (NCATS) NCfATS; 2019.

27. Dekruyff RH, Zhang W, Nadeau KC, et al. Summary of the Keystone Symposium "Origins of allergic disease: Microbial, epithelial and immune interactions," March 24-27, Tahoe City, California. J Allergy Clin Immunol 2020;145(4):1072–81.e1.

28. Krempski JW, Dant C, Nadeau KC. The origins of allergy from a systems approach. Ann Allergy Asthma Immunol 2020;125(5):507–16.

29. Shu S-A, Yuen AWT, Woo E, et al. Microbiota and food allergy. Clin Rev Allergy Immunol 2019;57(1):83–97.

30. Stefka AT, Feehley T, Tripathi P, et al. Commensal bacteria protect against food allergen sensitization. Proc Natl Acad Sci U S A 2014;111(36):13145–50.

31. Cao S, Feehley TJ, Nagler CR. The role of commensal bacteria in the regulation of sensitization to food allergens. FEBS Lett 2014;588(22):4258–66.

32. Rodriguez B, Prioult G, Hacini-Rachinel F, et al. Infant gut microbiota is protective against cow's milk allergy in mice despite immature ileal T-cell response. FEMS Microbiol Ecol 2012;79(1):192–202.

33. Noval Rivas M, Burton OT, Wise P, et al. A microbiota signature associated with experimental food allergy promotes allergic sensitization and anaphylaxis. J Allergy Clin Immunol 2013;131(1):201–12.

34. Du Toit G, Tsakok T, Lack S, et al. Prevention of food allergy. J Allergy Clin Immunol 2016;137(4):998–1010.

35. Tordesillas L, Goswami R, Benedé S, et al. Skin exposure promotes a Th2-dependent sensitization to peanut allergens. J Clin Invest 2014;124(11):4965–75.
36. Iijima K, Kobayashi T, Krempski JW, et al. Exposure to peanut flour through disturbed skin initiates peanut allergy via the T follicular helper T (Tfh) cell-dependent pathway in mice. J Allergy Clin Immunol 2018;141(2):AB281.
37. Dolence JJ, Kobayashi T, Iijima K, et al. Airway exposure initiates peanut allergy by involving the IL-1 pathway and T follicular helper cells in mice. J Allergy Clin Immunol 2018;142(4):1144–58.e8.
38. Crotty ST. Follicular helper cell biology: a decade of discovery and diseases. Immunity 2019;50(5):1132–48.
39. Krempski JW, Kobayashi T, Iijima K, et al. Group 2 Innate Lymphoid Cells Promote Development of T follicular helper cells and initiate allergic sensitization to peanuts. J Immunol 2020;204(12):3086–96.
40. Rosenau MJ, Anderson JF. A review of anaphylaxis, with especial reference to immunity. The journal of infectious diseases 1908;5(1):85–105.
41. Wells HG, Osborne TB. The biological reactions of the vegetable proteins. J Infect Dis 1911;8(1):66–124.
42. van Halteren AG, van der Cammen MJ, Cooper D, et al. Regulation of antigen-specific IgE, IgG1, and mast cell responses to ingested allergen by mucosal tolerance induction. J Immunol 1997;159(6):3009–15.
43. Fowler S, Powrie F. CTLA-4 expression on antigen-specific cells but not IL-10 secretion is required for oral tolerance. Eur J Immunol 2002;32(10):2997–3006.
44. Faria AMC, Weiner HL. Oral tolerance. Immunological Rev 2005;206(1):232–59.
45. Mucida D. Oral tolerance in the absence of naturally occurring Tregs. J Clin Invest 2005;115(7):1923–33.
46. Kim AR, Kim HS, Kim DK, et al. Mesenteric IL-10-producing CD5+ regulatory B cells suppress cow's milk casein-induced allergic responses in mice. Sci Rep 2016;6(1):19685.
47. Krempski JW, Iijima K, Kobayshi T, et al. Oral tolerance to peanut allergy is mediated by CTLA-4-positive regulatory T cells. J Immunol 2019;202(1 Supplement):52–5.
48. Greer FR, Sicherer SH, Burks AW. Effects of early nutritional interventions on the development of atopic disease in infants and children: the role of maternal dietary restriction, breastfeeding, timing of introduction of complementary foods, and hydrolyzed formulas. Pediatrics 2008;121(1):183–91.
49. Ierodiakonou D, Garcia-Larsen V, Logan A, et al. Timing of allergenic food introduction to the infant diet and risk of allergic or autoimmune disease: a systematic review and meta-analysis. JAMA 2016;316(11):1181–92.
50. Mikhail IJ. Implementation of early peanut introduction guidelines: it takes a village. Immunol Allergy Clin North Am 2019;39(4):459–67.
51. Santos AF, James LK, Bahnson HT, et al. IgG4 inhibits peanut-induced basophil and mast cell activation in peanut-tolerant children sensitized to peanut major allergens. J Allergy Clin Immunol 2015;135(5):1249–56.
52. Hong X, Caruso D, Kumar R, et al. IgE, but not IgG4, antibodies to Ara h 2 distinguish peanut allergy from asymptomatic peanut sensitization. Allergy 2012;67(12):1538–46.
53. Tsai M, Mukai K, Chinthrajah RS, et al. Sustained successful peanut oral immunotherapy associated with low basophil activation and peanut-specific IgE. J Allergy Clin Immunol 2020;145(3):885–896 e886.

54. Chinthrajah RS, Purington N, Andorf S, et al. Sustained outcomes in oral immunotherapy for peanut allergy (POISED study): a large, randomised, double-blind, placebo-controlled, phase 2 study. Lancet 2019;394(10207):1437–49.
55. Bedoret D, Singh AK, Shaw V, et al. Changes in antigen-specific T-cell number and function during oral desensitization in cow's milk allergy enabled with omalizumab. Mucosal Immunol 2012;5(3):267–76.
56. Abdel-Gadir A, Schneider L, Casini A, et al. Oral immunotherapy with omalizumab reverses the Th2 cell-like programme of regulatory T cells and restores their function. Clin Exp Allergy 2018;48(7):825–36.
57. Abernathy-Carver KJ, Sampson HA, Picker LJ, et al. Milk-induced eczema is associated with the expansion of T cells expressing cutaneous lymphocyte antigen. J Clin Invest 1995;95(2):913–8.
58. Eigenmann PA, Tropia L, Hauser C. The mucosal adhesion receptor alpha4-beta7 integrin is selectively increased in lymphocytes stimulated with beta-lactoglobulin in children allergic to cow's milk. J Allergy Clin Immunol 1999;103(5 Pt 1):931–6.
59. Feehley T, Plunkett CH, Bao R, et al. Healthy infants harbor intestinal bacteria that protect against food allergy. Nat Med 2019;25(3):448–53.
60. He Z, Vadali VG, Szabady RL, et al. Increased diversity of gut microbiota during active oral immunotherapy in peanut-allergic adults. Allergy 2020. https://doi.org/10.1111/all.14540.
61. Gomes-Belo J, Hannachi F, Swan K, et al. Advances in food allergy diagnosis. Curr Pediatr Rev 2018;14(3):139–49.
62. Eigenmann PA. Do we still need oral food challenges for the diagnosis of food allergy? Pediatr Allergy Immunol 2018;29(3):239–42.
63. Cox AL, Nowak-Wegrzyn A. Innovation in food challenge tests for food allergy. Curr Allergy Asthma Rep 2018;18(12):74.
64. Arasi S, Mennini M, Valluzzi R, et al. Precision medicine in food allergy. Curr Opin Allergy Clin Immunol 2018;18(5):438–43.
65. Pettersson ME, Koppelman GH, Flokstra-de Blok BMJ, et al. Prediction of the severity of allergic reactions to foods. Allergy 2018;73(7):1532–40.
66. Chinthrajah RS, Purington N, Andorf S, et al. Development of a tool predicting severity of allergic reaction during peanut challenge. Ann Allergy Asthma Immunol 2018;121(1):69–76 e62.
67. Flores Kim J, McCleary N, Nwaru BI, et al. Diagnostic accuracy, risk assessment, and cost-effectiveness of component-resolved diagnostics for food allergy: A systematic review. Allergy 2018;73(8):1609–21.
68. Jappe U, Breiteneder H. Peanut allergy-Individual molecules as a key to precision medicine. Allergy 2019;74(2):216–9.
69. Saleem R, Keymer C, Patel D, et al. UK NEQAS survey of allergen component testing across the United Kingdom and other European countries. Clin Exp Immunol 2017;188(3):387–93.
70. Nilsson C, Berthold M, Mascialino B, et al. Accuracy of component-resolved diagnostics in peanut allergy: Systematic literature review and meta-analysis. Pediatr Allergy Immunol 2020;31(3):303–14.
71. Datema MR, van Ree R, Asero R, et al. Component-resolved diagnosis and beyond: Multivariable regression models to predict severity of hazelnut allergy. Allergy 2018;73(3):549–59.
72. Heffler E, Puggioni F, Peveri S, et al. Extended IgE profile based on an allergen macroarray: a novel tool for precision medicine in allergy diagnosis. World Allergy Organ J 2018;11(1):7.

73. Di Fraia M, Arasi S, Castelli S, et al. A new molecular multiplex IgE assay for the diagnosis of pollen allergy in Mediterranean countries: A validation study. Clin Exp Allergy 2019;49(3):341–9.

74. Hemmings O, Kwok M, McKendry R, et al. Basophil activation test: old and new applications in allergy. Curr Allergy Asthma Rep 2018;18(12):77.

75. Hung L, Obernolte H, Sewald K, et al. Human ex vivo and in vitro disease models to study food allergy. Asia Pac Allergy 2019;9(1):e4.

76. Larsen LF, Juel-Berg N, Hansen KS, et al. A comparative study on basophil activation test, histamine release assay, and passive sensitization histamine release assay in the diagnosis of peanut allergy. Allergy 2018;73(1):137–44.

77. Santos AF, Couto-Francisco N, Becares N, et al. A novel human mast cell activation test for peanut allergy. J Allergy Clin Immunol 2018;142(2):689–91.e9.

78. Bahri R, Custovic A, Korosec P, et al. Mast cell activation test in the diagnosis of allergic disease and anaphylaxis. J Allergy Clin Immunol 2018;142(2): 485–96.e6.

79. Davis MM, Tato CM, Furman D. Systems immunology: just getting started. Nat Immunol 2017;18(7):725–32.

80. Patil SU, Bunyavanich S, Berin MC. Emerging Food Allergy Biomarkers. J Allergy Clin Immunol Pract 2020;8(8):2516–24.

81. Dhondalay GK, Rael E, Acharya S, et al. Food allergy and omics. J Allergy Clin Immunol 2018;141(1):20–9.

82. Bønnelykke K, Sparks R, Waage J, et al. Genetics of allergy and allergic sensitization: common variants, rare mutations. Curr Opin Immunol 2015;36:115–26.

83. Hong X, Hao K, Ladd-Acosta C, et al. Genome-wide association study identifies peanut allergy-specific loci and evidence of epigenetic mediation in US children. Nat Commun 2015;6:6304.

84. Noguchi E, Akiyama M, Yagami A, et al. HLA-DQ and RBFOX1 as susceptibility genes for an outbreak of hydrolyzed wheat allergy. J Allergy Clin Immunol 2019; 144(5):1354–63.

85. Croote D, Darmanis S, Nadeau KC, et al. High-affinity allergen-specific human antibodies cloned from single IgE B cell transcriptomes. Science 2018; 362(6420):1306–9.

86. Hoh RA, Joshi SA, Lee JY, et al. Origins and clonal convergence of gastrointestinal IgE(+) B cells in human peanut allergy. Sci Immunol 2020;5(45):eaay4209.

87. Ruiter B, Smith NP, Monian B, et al. Expansion of the CD4(+) effector T-cell repertoire characterizes peanut-allergic patients with heightened clinical sensitivity. J Allergy Clin Immunol 2020;145(1):270–82.

88. Portela A, Esteller M. Epigenetic modifications and human disease. Nat Biotechnol 2010;28(10):1057–68.

89. Petrus NCM, Henneman P, Venema A, et al. Cow's milk allergy in Dutch children: an epigenetic pilot survey. Clin Transl Allergy 2016;6:16.

90. Syed A, Garcia MA, Lyu SC, et al. Peanut oral immunotherapy results in increased antigen-induced regulatory T-cell function and hypomethylation of forkhead box protein 3 (FOXP3). J Allergy Clin Immunol 2014;133(2):500–10.

91. Watson CT, Cohain AT, Griffin RS, et al. Integrative transcriptomic analysis reveals key drivers of acute peanut allergic reactions. Nat Commun 2017;8(1): 1943.

92. Wang W, Lyu SC, Ji X, et al. Transcriptional changes in peanut-specific CD4+ T cells over the course of oral immunotherapy. Clin Immunol 2020;219:108568.

93. Spitzer MH, Nolan GP. Mass cytometry: single cells, many features. Cell 2016; 165(4):780–91.

94. Neeland MR, Andorf S, Manohar M, et al. Mass cytometry reveals cellular fingerprint associated with IgE+ peanut tolerance and allergy in early life. Nat Commun 2020;11(1):1091.
95. Di Girolamo F, Muraca M, Mazzina O, et al. Proteomic applications in food allergy: food allergenomics. Curr Opin Allergy Clin Immunol 2015;15(3):259–66.
96. Crestani E, Harb H, Charbonnier LM, et al. Untargeted metabolomic profiling identifies disease-specific signatures in food allergy and asthma. J Allergy Clin Immunol 2020;145(3):897–906.
97. Hill DA, Spergel JM. The atopic march: Critical evidence and clinical relevance. Ann Allergy Asthma Immunol 2018;120(2):131–7.
98. Han H, Roan F, Ziegler SF. The atopic march: current insights into skin barrier dysfunction and epithelial cell-derived cytokines. Immunol Rev 2017;278(1):116–30.
99. Nadeau K. Approach to the patient with allergic or immunologic disease. In: Sciences EH, editor. Goldman-cecil medicine. 26th edition. Lee Goldman, Andrew I. Schafer; 2019.
100. Gupta M, Cox A, Nowak-Węgrzyn A, et al. Diagnosis of food allergy. Immunol Allergy Clin North Am 2018;38(1):39–52.
101. Osborne NJ, Koplin JJ, Martin PE, et al. Prevalence of challenge-proven IgE-mediated food allergy using population-based sampling and predetermined challenge criteria in infants. J Allergy Clin Immunol 2011;127(3):668–76.e2.
102. Sicherer SH, Sampson HA. Food allergy: Epidemiology, pathogenesis, diagnosis, and treatment. J Allergy Clin Immunol 2014;133(2):291–308.
103. Rael E, Sampath V, Nadeau KC. Diagnosis and differential diagnosis of food allergy. In: Gupta RS, editor. Pediatric food allergy : a clinical guide. Cham (Switzerland): Springer International Publishing; 2020. p. 31–44.
104. Pouessel G, Beaudouin E, Tanno LK, et al. Food-related anaphylaxis fatalities: Analysis of the Allergy Vigilance Network(®) database. Allergy 2019;74(6):1193–6.
105. Wilson JM, Schuyler AJ, Schroeder N, et al. Galactose-α-1,3-Galactose: Atypical Food Allergen or Model IgE Hypersensitivity? Curr Allergy Asthma Rep 2017;17(1):8.
106. Blanchard C, Simon D, Schoepfer A, et al. Eosinophilic esophagitis: unclear roles of IgE and eosinophils. J Intern Med 2017;281(5):448–57.
107. Komlósi ZI, Kovács N, Sokolowska M, et al. Mechanisms of Subcutaneous and Sublingual Aeroallergen Immunotherapy: What Is New? Immunol Allergy Clin North Am 2020;40(1):1–14.
108. Yu W, Freeland DMH, Nadeau KC. Food allergy: immune mechanisms, diagnosis and immunotherapy. Nat Rev Immunol 2016;16(12):751–65.
109. Li L, Han Z, Niu X, et al. Probiotic supplementation for prevention of atopic dermatitis in infants and children: a systematic review and meta-analysis. Am J Clin Dermatol 2019;20(3):367–77.

The Phenotype of the Food-Allergic Patient

Amy A. Eapen, MD, MS*, Haejin Kim, MD

KEYWORDS

- Birth cohorts • Food allergy • Food sensitization • Atopic march

KEY POINTS

- Food allergy presents with different phenotypes that are adjusted based on genetic risk, racial background, and environmental factors.
- Sensitization patterns exist in food allergy, and these patterns can give light to the phenotype of food allergy the child may have.
- Food allergy and sensitization is a risk factor for asthma, independent of whether the food allergy is outgrown.
- Assessing the food allergy phenotype of a child can allow physicians to provide the appropriate medical management of their food allergy as well as anticipatory guidance on the presence of other allergic diseases.

BACKGROUND

The prevalence of food allergy among children has been steadily increasing over the past several decades. Published studies have reported a prevalence among children as high as 10%.[1] The National Health and Nutrition Examination, a population-based survey conducted in the United States, reported that self-reported food allergy among children in 2007 to 2010 was 6.53%, with the most common foods being reported as milk (1.94%), peanut (1.16%), and shellfish (0.87%).[2,3]

Among this group of food-allergic children, there is a wide range of phenotypes present. These phenotypes can be divided into several subcategories, not only by specific food but also by race and presence of other atopic manifestations. There is growing evidence that there are significant racial disparities present in food allergy, among other allergic diseases. There are also differences in the phenotype of food allergy among children who have coexistence of eczema, asthma, and allergic rhinitis compared with those who have food allergy alone. Investigating these phenotypes allow us to decipher the multiple risk factors that predispose children to have food

Division of Allergy and Clinical Immunology, Henry Ford Health System, 1 Ford Place, Detroit, MI 48202, USA
* Corresponding author.
E-mail address: aeapen1@hfhs.org

Immunol Allergy Clin N Am 41 (2021) 165–175
https://doi.org/10.1016/j.iac.2021.01.001   immunology.theclinics.com
0889-8561/21/© 2021 Elsevier Inc. All rights reserved.

allergy, as well as those that increase the risk for other allergic diseases. The purpose of this article is to detail the phenotypes of the food allergic patient, with emphasis on published data from significant longitudinal birth cohorts both here in the United States as well as across the globe.

EVALUATION
Familial Inheritance

Previous studies looking at familial aggregation and twin studies have found a strong genetic component in food allergy, with heritability rates ranging from 15% to 82%.[4–7] Two twin studies currently exist looking at these rates among monozygotic and dizygotic twin pairs. Sicherer and colleagues looked at the rates of peanut allergy among 58 twin pairs. Among the monozygotic twin pairs (n = 14), there was a concordance rate of 64.3% (n = 9) for peanut allergy compared with 6.8% (n = 3) among dizygotic twins (n = 44).[8] Second, a study looking at Chinese twins reported the sensitization rates for 9 foods and 5 aeroallergens among 472 monozygotic and 354 dizygotic twins aged 12 to 28 years. They found that there was a higher concordance rate for sensitization among monozygotic than dizygotic twins. However, there were differences in which allergens the twins were sensitized to, relaying a role of environmental factors in the allergic phenotype. Monozygotic twins sensitized to peanut and shellfish had the highest concordance rate at 58%.[9,10] These 2 studies demonstrate the strong genetic component in food allergy, specifically of peanut. There is a need for further twin studies to delineate the heritability patterns among other food allergens and the role of genetic risk with compounding environmental factors.

A common question in the office among parents with food allergy is how likely is their child to also develop food allergy? Liu and colleagues investigated the maternal genotypic and parent-of-origin effects among 588 Caucasian food allergy trios from the Chicago Food Allergy Study. They identified 1 single nucleotide polymorphism (rs423235) with significant maternal effect of any food allergy located in a noncoding RNA (LOC101927947). In addition, they identified 3 other loci with maternal genetic effects: 1 for any food allergy (rs976078 on 13q31.1) and 2 for egg allergy (rs1343795 and rs4572450 in ZNF652 gene). Interestingly, they further demonstrated specific loci that showed significant parent-of-origin effects in boys only: 1 for peanut allergy (rs4896888 in the ADGB gene) and 2 for any food allergy (rs1036504 and rs2917750 in IQCE gene).[4] These findings support a strong parent-to-child inheritance pattern in the food allergy phenotype and a specific strong inheritance pattern from mother to child. Further investigations are needed to identify possible interventions that could protect an infant from these genetic patterns and prevent the onset of food allergy.

Atopic March

The atopic march has been used to signify the progression of allergic diseases through childhood with different ages of mean onset. This progression has identified atopic dermatitis as the predisposing ailment that can lead to other allergic diseases, including food allergy. Atopic dermatitis is thought to provide a break in the skin barrier, that allows sensitization to foods with progression to clinical allergy later on in childhood. However, food allergy can also follow atopic dermatitis, signifying the different endotypes and pathways of the disease. In general, atopic dermatitis has an earlier age of onset with a peak at 6 months,[11] and food sensitization starting shortly after.[12] Although atopic dermatitis can signify the start of a phenotype for food allergy, there is insufficient evidence to recommend routine panel food allergy testing to all infants with atopic dermatitis. Current guidelines do recommend testing for specific foods, such as peanut, to risk stratify infants with specific risk factors and promote early introduction when appropriate.[13] A similar relationship is seen with the incidence of food allergy with asthma and allergic rhinitis. Several birth cohorts have identified these different "food allergic phenotypes," signifying that the allergic disease progression may not truly be a "march" per se in being sequential, but instead dependent on key allergic disease risk factors and characteristics. **Table 1** details key highlights with respect to food allergy phenotypes from 4 specific birth cohorts: WHEALS, CCAAPS, HEALTHNUT, and PASTURE. The remainder of this article will go into details specific on these studies.

LONGITUDINAL BIRTH COHORT DATA
Wayne County Health, Environment, Allergy and Asthma Longitudinal Study Cohort

The Wayne County Health, Environment, Allergy and Asthma Longitudinal Study (WHEALS), a birth cohort from southeastern Michigan, recruited pregnant women between the ages of 21 and 49 years in predefined cluster of zip codes in Detroit and surrounding suburbs from August 2003 to November 2007.[14] Follow-up occurred at 1, 6, 12, 24, and 48 months after the child's birth. Total immunoglobulin E (IgE) and serum-specific IgE was collected from children's blood at 2 years of age for the following 10 allergens: Der f, dog, cat, Timothy grass, ragweed, Alternaria alternata, egg, peanut, cow's milk, and German cockroach.

A latent class analysis was performed, which was described as "an unsupervised statistical method that simultaneously considers a number of variables to identify homogenous, mutually exclusive groups or classes within a heterogenous population".[15] This analysis was used to determine if children could be grouped together based on their patterns of sensitization. The 594 of the 1258 women-children pairs (that had blood samples available) were clustered into 4 groups: class I (n = 457)—low to no sensitization, class 2 (n = 16)—highly sensitized, class 3 (n = 91)—milk and egg dominated, and class 4 (n = 30)—peanut and inhalant/no milk. Class 1 children were characterized as no sensitization (67.8%, n = 310) or monosensitized to either egg (17.2%, n = 23), Alternaria (16.4%, n = 22), Der f (7.5%, n = 10), dog (4.5%, n = 6), cat (1.5%, n = 2), or Timothy grass (0.8%, n = 1). Class 2 children were all sensitized to at least 4 of the following allergens: milk, egg, peanut, and Timothy grass.

In regard to food allergy, class 3 and 4 had the most striking patterns. Class 3 children predominated (94.5%, n = 86) with milk and egg sensitization; 27.9% of these children (n = 24) were sensitized to milk, egg, and peanut. Eighty percent of class 4 was sensitized to peanut (n = 24). Egg sensitization occurred in 43.3% of the individuals (n = 13).

This study also reported interesting findings regarding race. Class 3 (milk and egg dominated) was statistically significantly associated with the Black race, whereas classes 2 and 3 were associated but not statistically significant. In terms of the occurrence of wheezing, class 4 were 2.9 times more likely to have wheezed than those in class 1, but this pattern was not seen in the other 2 classes. Cord blood had also been collected in this cohort. Cord blood total IgE level was significantly higher (P<.01) in both class 2 (highly sensitized) and class 3 (milk and egg dominated) but not in class 4 (peanut and inhalants).

This study demonstrated phenotypes of allergic disease based on allergen-specific IgE patterns. Although the atopic march refers to a stepwise direction in allergic disease onset, it does not address the possibility of different phenotypes in the allergic group.

Table 1
Longitudinal birth cohorts and food allergy

Birth Cohort	WHEALS	CCAPS	HEALTHNUTS	PASTURE
Geographic location	Southeast Michigan, USA	Greater Cincinnati area, Ohio, USA	Melbourne, Australia	Rural areas of 5 European nations: Austria, Finland, France, Germany, and Switzerland
Unique characteristics of cohort	Racially diverse with 62% Black race	Higher risk cohort with at least one atopic parent	Used challenge-proven outcomes to assess the role of infantile food allergy in development of asthma	Assessed role of farm animals on allergic disease presence
Times of follow-up postnatally	1, 6, 12, 24, and 48-months of age	1, 2, 3, 4, and 7 y	11 or 15 mo, 1 y, 4 y	1, 4, and 6 y
Total recruited	1258	762	5276	1133
Food allergens tested	Egg, peanut, cow's milk	Cow's milk, egg	Egg, peanut, sesame, and cow's milk or shrimp	Cow's milk, hen's egg, cow's milk, peanut, hazelnut, carrot, and wheat
Key food allergy phenotype finding	Black race was a significant risk factor for milk and egg allergy	Food sensitization in the presence of *KIF3A* mutations poses a significant risk for asthma, independent of aeroallergen sensitization	Asthma at 4 years of age is twice as common in children with food allergy, irrespective of whether child outgrows allergy	Farm exposure can alter sensitization patterns
PMIDs for key food allergy articles	24636082	30830718, 19759553	29153880, 20608942	28531273

Key highlights

- The "highly sensitized" group class 2 was the most likely to ever have atopic dermatitis and more likely to ever have wheeze and doctor diagnosis of asthma than the "low to no sensitization" class 1.
- Associations between class and asthma diagnosis were similar in class 3 and class 4, suggesting that food allergens are not as strongly associated with asthma as being highly sensitized.
- There seems to be a cosensitization pattern, with peanut sensitization being equally likely to be paired with at least 1 inhalant sensitization as with 2 other food sensitizations.
- Milk and egg cosensitization was the most common pairing, with this pairing consistently associated with the lowest rate of allergic disease outcomes among the 3 higher risk groups (Class 2, 3, 4).
- There are racial differences in which allergic diseases predominate in the Black race, with milk and egg food allergies having a statistically significant association.
- Race was the most obvious risk factor across the classes. The investigators propose that the racial differences observed could play a role in the racial disparities seen in asthma if early life food allergen sensitization is more strongly associated with asthma than with other types of sensitizations.

Cincinnati Childhood Allergy and Air Pollution Study Cohort

The Cincinnati Childhood Allergy and Air Pollution Study (CCAAPS) is a birth cohort of 762 infants born to atopic parents between 2001 and 2003.[16] Follow-up evaluations occurred at 1, 2, 3, 4, and 7 years of age where skin prick testing (SPT) to milk, egg, and 15 aeroallergens was performed. Because only 2 food allergens were tested, they did not examine the pattern of cosensitization of foods but did examine the presence of food sensitization and timing of asthma and eczema onset compared with aeroallergen sensitization. As previous data had shown, of the children who had food and aeroallergen sensitization, 70% were food sensitized by their first birthday, and food sensitization preceded aeroallergen sensitization in 52% of cosensitized children. In the presence of early eczema, the odds of having food sensitization (OR = 3) compared with aeroallergen sensitization (OR = 1.9) was higher in the food-sensitized group. Forty-three percent of their food-sensitized children did not have eczema compared with 58% of the aeroallergen group, which signifies that eczema or atopic dermatitis is not a mandatory precursor to food sensitization.

In regard to presence of asthma risk compared with sensitization patterns, a multivariate model revealed that aeroallergen sensitization load, but not food sensitization load, was associated with asthma among children without a history of early eczema.[17] Among those with early eczema, neither aeroallergen sensitization nor food sensitization was significantly associated with asthma risk. However, being African American was associated with asthma risk among children without early eczema but not among those with early eczema.

This study revealed significant genotype patterns with other allergic disease as well. They specifically looked at the role of a coding subunit of the kinesin-2 motor complex, *KIF3A*, which plays a role in the formation and/or function of primary and motile cilia.[18] In children with early eczema, genotype *KIF3A rs12186803* and food sensitization interacted to significantly increase the risk of asthma at 7 years of age, whereas neither variable on its own was associated with asthma risk. This pattern did not depend on the presence of early aeroallergen sensitization. This signified the role of food sensitization in altering the allergic disease progression to asthma in specific geno-types of children with early eczema onset.

Another analysis focused on the Caucasian children in the group (76.6%, 583) demonstrated food sensitization to be the highest risk factor for development of eczema by age 1 to 3 years.[19] They reported that children with positive SPT (this included foods and/or aeroallergens) by age 3 years were 3 times more likely to have a specific genotype in *CD14* and *IL4α* compared with children without eczema who had negative SPT. This further portrayed the role of genetic susceptibility to allergic disease, such as food allergy and eczema.

Key highlights

- Although eczema predisposes a child to food sensitization, there is a significant number of children (47% in this cohort) who have food sensitization in the absence of eczema.
- Food sensitization in the presence of early eczema posed a significant increase in asthma risk for those with genotype *KIF3A rs12186803*, independent of the presence of early aeroallergen sensitization.
- Food sensitization in Caucasian children were found to be the highest risk factor for development of eczema by age 1 to 3 years.

HEALTHNUTS Cohort

The HEALTHNUTS cohort is a longitudinal population-based cohort study of allergic disease in Melbourne, Australia.[20] Five thousand two hundred seventy-six infants between 11 and 15 months were recruited from immunization clinics around Melbourne with a 74% participation rate. These participants underwent SPT to egg, peanut, sesame, cow's milk, or shrimp and were examined for eczema. If the SPT was positive to egg, peanut, or sesame, the child was invited for an oral food challenge (OFC) to that food. At 4 years of age, the parents were given a questionnaire about their allergic outcomes (asthma, eczema, and allergic rhinitis). The aim of this study was to determine the relationship between the presence and number of food allergies at age 1 years and asthma at age 4 years.

They reported that asthma at 4 years of age was twice as common in those with challenge-proven food allergy. Egg allergy alone was associated with higher risk of asthma, but peanut allergy alone was not. Children with 2 or more food allergies and coexistent eczema were almost 3 times more likely to develop asthma compared with children without food allergy and those with a single food allergy.[21] Interestingly, asymptomatic food sensitization and OFC-proven food allergy in infancy were associated with an increased risk of asthma by 4 years of age. Furthermore, the increased risk of asthma was similarly high among food allergic infants who outgrew and did not outgrow their food allergy. This study further demonstrates the risk that sensitization to foods in addition to challenge-proven food allergy contributes to childhood asthma and defining the food allergy phenotypes.

They performed a latent class analysis, similar to the WHEALS cohort, to identify phenotypes of food allergy.[22] From their analysis, they defined 5 classes: class 1—no allergic disease (70%); class 2—non–food-sensitized eczema (16%); class 3—single egg allergy (9%); class 4—multiple food allergies, predominately peanut (3%); and class 5—multiple food allergies, predominately egg (2%).

They further investigated the risk factors for the different phenotypes. For all phenotypes, males were at increased risk of belonging to non–food-sensitized eczema and multiple food allergy phenotypes (classes 2, 4, and 5). As far as environmental risk factors are concerned, exposure to pet dogs in the home was associated with reduced risk of membership in non–food-sensitized eczema and multiple food allergies—peanut phenotypes but the difference was not statistically significant. Presence of siblings reduced the risk of single egg allergy and non–food-sensitized eczema but not multiple food allergies.

They also noted that filaggrin gene mutations were associated with a higher risk for the non–food-sensitized eczema and egg allergy phenotypes, with an odds ratio of 2.37 but interestingly was not associated with either multiple food allergy phenotypes. There has also been research investigating the role of vitamin D insufficiency in the risk of food allergy. The HEALTHNUTS study group found that the association between vitamin D insufficiency and allergy phenotypes was modified by parent's country of birth. Vitamin D insufficiency was a risk factor for the 3 food allergy phenotypes (class 3–5) only among those infants with both parents born in Australia.

Similar to WHEALS, HEALTHNUTS also identified race as a risk factor for food allergy phenotypes. HEALTHNUTS reported that infants with one or both parents born in Asia, compared with those with both parents born in Australia, were at an increased risk of all 3 food allergy phenotypes. This further emphasizes the role of race and genetic background in the different phenotypes of food allergy. Together, this cohort further identified different food allergy phenotypes and risk factors associated with these classes. It emphasizes that a "one-size-fits-all" approach in both preventive medicine in averting food allergy as well as treatment options would not address the needs and risk factors for each phenotype.

Key highlights

- Asthma at 4 years of age was twice as common in those with challenge-proven food allergy, irrespective of whether the child outgrew the food allergy.
- Those with 2 or more food allergies and coexistent eczema were almost 3 times more likely to develop asthma compared with those children without food allergy and those with a single food allergy.
- Vitamin D insufficiency was a risk factor for the 3 food allergy phenotypes (class 3–5) only among those infants with both parents born in Australia.
- Infants with one or both parents born in Asia, compared with those with both parents born in Australia, were at an increased risk of all 3 food allergy phenotypes.

Protection Against Allergy Study in Rural Environments Study

The Protection Against Allergy Study in Rural Environments (PASTURE) birth cohort included children from rural areas in 5 European countries: Austria, Finland, France, Germany, and Switzerland.[23] It was designed to evaluate risk and preventive factors for atopic diseases. Pregnant women recruited between 2001 and 2005 were divided into 2 groups: those living on family-run farms where livestock was kept (farm group) and those not living on a farm from those same rural areas (reference group). Altogether, 1133 children were included.

A latent class analysis was performed on 1038 of the children.[24] Consistent with other birth cohorts, they identified that early phenotypes of atopic dermatitis (onset before age 2 years) were strongly associated with food allergy, but late phenotypes were not. They also assessed IgE sensitization patterns within the first 12 months of life and maternal and environmental influences. Sensitization to foods was assessed by cord blood (infancy) and peripheral blood (ages 1, 4, and 6 years) to 6 foods. Food sensitization was more common in the farm group only at lower specific IgE levels. This study portrayed the influence of environmental factors on sensitization patterns and the possible alterations due to a modified immune response on production of specific IgE.[25]

Key highlights

- Environmental factors, such as being on a farm, can alter food sensitization patterns through a modified immune response.

DISCUSSION

Food allergy presents in different phenotypes in children, with each phenotype carrying varying risks for future allergic diseases. There are several birth cohorts that have tried to delineate these risks, including those risk factors predisposing infants to become allergic to begin with (**Fig. 1**). In this article, the authors detail 4 studies that highlight a portion of identified food allergy phenotypes. Each cohort is unique and significant in the field of allergy in its own way, contributing to different aspects from racial background to genetic risks and environmental factors. Together, they identify that food allergy and sensitization poses a risk for future allergic diseases but that it may not be in the pattern of the traditional atopic march as previously described.

A meta-analysis and systemic review aimed to assess the association of food sensitization and subsequent allergic diseases in birth cohort studies.[26] Their search

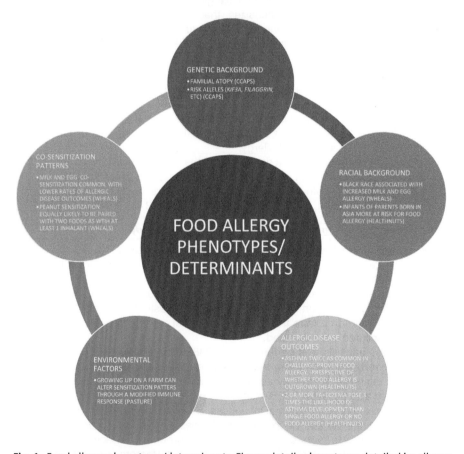

Fig. 1. Food allergy phenotypes/determinants. Figure details phenotypes detailed by allergy birth cohort data from 4 cohorts: WEHALS, CCAPS, HEALTHNUTS, and PASTURE. FA, food allergy.

revealed 13 cohorts across the globe. A common theme among these cohorts was that food sensitization in the first 2 years of life was related to eczema in late infancy, wheeze/asthma, eczema, or allergic rhinitis in childhood and asthma in young adults. Identifying sensitization patterns such as foods sensitized to, as well as predisposing factors such as family atopy, racial background, and living conditions can allow physicians to assess the predisposing factors for each patient and allow more personalized management of each child's food allergy. It can also allow physicians to provide anticipatory guidance to families on the possibilities of other allergic diseases such as asthma that may appear in their child.

Additional birth cohorts are needed to further detail these risks and possible role of interventions in preventing allergy in not only different ethnicities and genetic backgrounds but also varying living conditions to tie in the role of environmental factors with genetics. Overall, food allergy changes quality of life in and of itself and, with the addition of other allergic diseases, poses different risks in different groups of children.[27] It is imperative that physicians assess the role of food allergy in each infant and the different phenotypes in which it may present as to properly counsel each patient.

SUMMARY

Longitudinal birth cohorts have identified previously undescribed food allergy phenotypes that pose different risks for future allergic diseases in children. They characterize different factors that place infant at risk for food allergies. Identifying these phenotypes allows physicians to risk assess each child who comes into the allergy office and also provide a management plan that is best fit for each different phenotype.

CLINICS CARE POINTS

- Food allergy has several different phenotypes; identifying these phenotypes can allow physicians to provide better patient-focused care.
- Food sensitization patterns can identify which infants are at risk for future allergic disease, even in children who outgrow their clinical food allergy.
- Food allergy and sensitization is a strong risk factor for asthma, and physicians should consider counseling both groups of this risk.
- Racial disparities occur in food allergy, and it is important to consider a patient's racial background when assessing management protocols for not only their food allergy but also other allergic diseases.
- Identifying infants early on with risk factors such as food sensitization and atopic dermatitis can help give anticipatory guidance to parents on management of their child's care.
- Determining single food versus multiple food sensitizations can lead to better counseling for parents.

ACKNOWLEDGEMENTS

This study was supported by the National Institute of Allergy and Infectious Diseases awards (grant no. 1UM1AI114271-01, R01AI110450, UM2AI130836-01/UM2AI117870, 2 P01 AI089473-06 to H.K).

DISCLOSURE

The authors have nothing to disclose.

REFERENCES

1. Sicherer SH, Sampson HA. Food allergy: A review and update on epidemiology, pathogenesis, diagnosis, prevention, and management. J Allergy Clin Immunol 2018;141(1):41–58.
2. McGowan EC, Keet CA. Prevalence of self-reported food allergy in the National Health and Nutrition Examination Survey (NHANES) 2007-2010. J Allergy Clin Immunol 2013;132(5):1216–9.e5.
3. Savage J, Johns CB. Food allergy: epidemiology and natural history. Immunol Allergy Clin North Am 2015;35(1):45–59.
4. Liu X, Hong X, Tsai HJ, et al. Genome-wide association study of maternal genetic effects and parent-of-origin effects on food allergy. Medicine (Baltimore) 2018; 97(9):e0043.
5. Tsai HJ, Kumar R, Pongracic J, et al. Familial aggregation of food allergy and sensitization to food allergens: a family-based study. Clin Exp Allergy 2009; 39(1):101–9.
6. Hong X, Tsai HJ, Wang X. Genetics of food allergy. Curr Opin Pediatr 2009;21(6): 770–6.
7. Hourihane JO, Dean TP, Warner JO. Peanut allergy in relation to heredity, maternal diet, and other atopic diseases: results of a questionnaire survey, skin prick testing, and food challenges. BMJ 1996;313(7056):518–21.
8. Sicherer SH, Furlong TJ, Maes HH, et al. Genetics of peanut allergy: a twin study. J Allergy Clin Immunol 2000;106(1 Pt 1):53–6.
9. Liu X, Zhang S, Tsai HJ, et al. Genetic and environmental contributions to allergen sensitization in a Chinese twin study. Clin Exp Allergy 2009;39(7):991–8.
10. Carter CA, Frischmeyer-Guerrerio PA. The Genetics of Food Allergy. Curr Allergy Asthma Rep 2018;18(1):2.
11. National Collaborating Centre for Women's and Children's Health (UK). Atopic Eczema in Children: Management of Atopic Eczema in Children from Birth up to the Age of 12 Years. London: RCOG Press; 2007. (NICE Clinical Guidelines, No. 57.)
12. Burks AW, Jones SM, Boyce JA, et al. NIAID-sponsored 2010 guidelines for managing food allergy: applications in the pediatric population. Pediatrics 2011; 128(5):955–65.
13. Randomized trial of peanut consumption in infants at risk for peanut allergy. N Engl J Med 2016;375(4):398.
14. Havstad S, Wegienka G, Zoratti EM, et al. Effect of prenatal indoor pet exposure on the trajectory of total IgE levels in early childhood. J Allergy Clin Immunol 2011;128(4):880–5.e4.
15. Havstad S, Johnson CC, Kim H, et al. Atopic phenotypes identified with latent class analyses at age 2 years. J Allergy Clin Immunol 2014;134(3):722–7.e2.
16. LeMasters GK, Wilson K, Levin L, et al. High prevalence of aeroallergen sensitization among infants of atopic parents. J Pediatr 2006;149(4):505–11.
17. Johansson E, Biagini Myers JM, Martin LJ, et al. Identification of two early life eczema and non-eczema phenotypes with high risk for asthma development. Clin Exp Allergy 2019;49(6):829–37.
18. Malicki J. Who drives the ciliary highway? Bioarchitecture 2012;2(4):111–7.
19. Biagini Myers JM, Wang N, LeMasters GK, et al. Genetic and environmental risk factors for childhood eczema development and allergic sensitization in the CCAAPS cohort. J Invest Dermatol 2010;130(2):430–7.

20. Osborne NJ, Koplin JJ, Martin PE, et al. The HealthNuts population-based study of paediatric food allergy: validity, safety and acceptability. Clin Exp Allergy 2010; 40(10):1516–22.
21. Vermeulen EM, Koplin JJ, Dharmage SC, et al. Food allergy is an important risk factor for childhood asthma, irrespective of whether it resolves. J Allergy Clin Immunol Pract 2018;6(4):1336–41.e3.
22. Peters RL, Allen KJ, Dharmage SC, et al. Differential factors associated with challenge-proven food allergy phenotypes in a population cohort of infants: a latent class analysis. Clin Exp Allergy 2015;45(5):953–63.
23. Loss G, Bitter S, Wohlgensinger J, et al. Prenatal and early-life exposures alter expression of innate immunity genes: the PASTURE cohort study. J Allergy Clin Immunol 2012;130(2):523–30.e9.
24. Roduit C, Frei R, Depner M, et al. Phenotypes of atopic dermatitis depending on the timing of onset and progression in childhood. JAMA Pediatr 2017;171(7): 655–62.
25. Hose AJ, Depner M, Illi S, et al. Latent class analysis reveals clinically relevant atopy phenotypes in 2 birth cohorts. J Allergy Clin Immunol 2017;139(6): 1935–45.e2.
26. Alduraywish SA, Lodge CJ, Campbell B, et al. The march from early life food sensitization to allergic disease: a systematic review and meta-analyses of birth cohort studies. Allergy 2016;71(1):77–89.
27. Shaker MS, Schwartz J, Ferguson M. An update on the impact of food allergy on anxiety and quality of life. Curr Opin Pediatr 2017;29(4):497–502.

Psychosocial Aspects of Food Allergy
Resiliency, Challenges and Opportunities

Christine J. Rubeiz, MD[a],*, Michelle M. Ernst, PhD[b,c]

KEYWORDS

- Food allergy • Quality of life • Psychosocial • Resilience • Development • Anxiety

KEY POINTS

- Food allergy has many psychosocial impacts and can worsen quality of life in affected patients and their families.
- The psychosocial impacts of food allergy vary by age group and developmental stage.
- Resilience may improve quality of life in food allergy. Allergists can promote resilience through encouraging education, problem-solving, self-efficacy, enhancing social support, engagement in school, and meaning making.

Food allergy (FA) is a public health concern, affecting approximately 8% of US children and 10.8% of adults, and has been growing in prevalence.[1,2] The constant vigilance to avoid allergen exposure can lead to distress and decreased quality of life (QOL).[3] In addition, specific FA treatment, such as oral food challenges and allergen immunotherapy (eg, OIT), which may promote QOL and adjustment in the long-run, are often anxiety-producing while occurring.[4–6] Certainly, the experience of anaphylaxis and the prospect of epinephrine administration by autoinjection (EAI) is often accompanied by heightened anxiety, impacting patients and caregivers.[6,7] Research in other chronic medical diseases has found that a focus on resilience can decrease the burden and improve the experience of living with chronic medical conditions.[8] This article highlights recent (within the past 10 years) research on psychosocial aspects related to FA within a developmental framework. Clinical recommendations are provided, contextualized within the construct of resilience.

DEVELOPMENT AND RESILIENCE

Contextual changes and evolving performance demands interact with brain and hormonal changes to move children through development.[9] Developmental tasks vary

[a] Department of Pediatrics, Cincinnati Children's Hospital Medical Center, 3333 Burnet Avenue, Cincinnati, OH 45229, USA; [b] Department of Pediatrics, University of Cincinnati College of Medicine, Cincinnati, OH, USA; [c] Division of Behavioral Medicine and Clinical Psychology, Cincinnati Children's Hospital Medical Center, 3333 Burnet Avenue, Cincinnati, OH 45229, USA
* Corresponding author.
E-mail address: Christine.Rubeiz@cchmc.org

Immunol Allergy Clin N Am 41 (2021) 177–188
https://doi.org/10.1016/j.iac.2021.01.006   immunology.theclinics.com
0889-8561/21/© 2021 Elsevier Inc. All rights reserved.

greatly by age, but involve growth and maturation in broad areas, such as emotion-behavioral regulation, social connection, and executive functioning.[9] Key microsystem contexts influencing child development include families, early care settings, schools, and peers, whereas macrosystem factors include poverty and racism.[9]

Resilience is characterized by the ability to maintain a positive developmental trajectory, or even flourish, in the face of adversity,[10,11] and has been studied in other chronic pediatric conditions (**Box 1**).[8] A limited view of resilience as a character trait that resides in an individual undervalues the power of systemic processes in promoting healthy outcomes; thus, resilience reflects the systemic influences that an individual accesses across time when managing adversity.[10] Adversity is, of course, not uniformly bad for children; with proper support, navigating challenges can set the stage for the development of adaptive skills,[10] and adaptations in one context can be transferred to other contexts.[9] Factors that are frequently associated with childhood resilience across cultures include family factors (eg, nurturing caregivers), problem-solving skills, self-efficacy, emotion regulation, belief systems (eg, optimism, meaning making), positive engagement in school, and connection within communities.[10] The construct of resilience has been extended to the family itself; key family resilience factors include belief systems, organizational processes (connectedness, flexibility), and communication/problem-solving (eg, open and positive emotional sharing, collaborative problem-solving, clear and consistent information).[11] Importantly, resilience is bolstered by boosting resources or assets and mobilizing systems. Allergists working with individuals with an FA are in an optimal position to enhance resilience by identifying individual and family strengths and providing resources to bolster important resiliency variables.

FOOD ALLERGY THROUGHOUT THE LIFESPAN
Infancy, Toddlerhood, and Preschoolers

Early childhood is marked by the development of interpersonal attachment, executive function, and cognitive-emotional and behavioral integration, setting the stage for later successful self-regulation.[9] These skills are largely dependent on a child's ability to actively engage with their environment. This age group has the highest prevalence of FA[1] and management of FA differs from older developmental stages in that the burden of responsibility falls solely on parents and caregivers.[12,13] Young children, such as toddlers, may require extra oversight because they may independently grab food or introduce oral exposure through thumb sucking or putting toys in their mouths.[14,15] Identifying a food-allergic reaction is particularly difficult because language skills are still being acquired through infancy and toddlerhood, and the child may not be able to communicate a reaction.[13] Parents must balance the difficult FA-related tasks with encouragement of typical development and exploration; constant monitoring of the child may decrease the child's sense of autonomy and increase the risk of separation anxiety.[12,16] As point of fact, mothers of preschool children with FA are more likely to intervene needlessly with general tasks (eg, puzzle solving) than mothers of children without FA.[16]

Box 1
Definition of resilience

Resilience is the ability to maintain a positive developmental trajectory in the face of adversity. The quality of life of children with food allergy and their caregivers is optimized by health care providers bolstering resiliency factors during routine clinical care.

Childcare (eg, day care facilities, babysitters, and/or extended family) may be among the first instances where the child is fed outside the home.[13] One study in anaphylaxis in infants less than 12 months old found that anaphylaxis occurred in the care of the mother 65.2% of the time; the babysitter was present in 30.4% of cases, and the grandmother in 4.3% of cases.[17] Parents with allergic children report worry surrounding the choice of a safe day care, even electing to forgo out-of-home employment,[18] and may limit participation in social activities, such as eating at restaurants, attending preschool, or having playdates.[12]

School-Age Children

Middle childhood is characterized by increasing independence, developing self-regulation, academic knowledge acquisition and deepening interpersonal skills, with relationships to caregivers moving from proximity to availability.[9] FA in school-age children in the United States is common, affecting an estimated 8% of 6- to 10-year-old children, and 7.5% of 11- to 13-year-old children.[1] As children with FA age, their growing awareness of the FA may coincide with a growing sense of uncertainty on how to manage it.[19]

FA may pose challenges for increasing the breadth and depth of interpersonal relationships, critical developmental tasks for school-aged children. Honing social skills and expanding social networks often involve activities outside the home, such as dining at restaurants, participation in sports, and sleeping over at friends' houses. Many of these social activities involve eating without parental oversight; children aged 7 to 12 have worse parent-reported FA-related QOL compared with younger children, which has been related to the perception of a higher risk of accidental ingestion while away from family.[20] The self-reported psychosocial experience of school-aged children with FA has not been well-studied, but existing research suggests generally similar levels of anxiety between children with and without FA,[21] although children with FA may be at increased risk for post-traumatic stress symptoms, particularly if they have experienced an anaphylaxis episode.[22]

One transition that is particularly important for this age group is the increased time spent at school. School is a place where children spend a significant amount of time, and consume meals; several recent reviews highlight important FA school-related considerations, guidelines, and legislation.[23,24] Nearly 40% of schools reported having at least one food-allergic reaction within the past 2 years.[24] Nearly half of all children with FA report the experience of being bullied, which can include teasing, criticism, and even being threatened with the allergen.[3,25]

Adolescents

Adolescence is a period of dramatic brain growth, intentional skill development, emotion intensity, expanding decision-making skills, social cognition, autonomy, self-awareness, and identity formation.[9] It is marked by reliance on the peer group. It is also the developmental stage where the impact of FA is notably potent; adolescents have the highest risk of anaphylactic reactions from FA and the highest risk of death.[26,27] Although there are conflicting results as to whether adolescents with FA have a higher incidence of psychological difficulties compared with healthy peers, some studies do note increased risk of mental health concerns[28,29]; risk factors include gender (eg, boys with FA may be at particular risk for social anxiety) and maternal anxiety.[30] Youth with FA also report greater dating anxiety and fear of negative peer evaluation.[31]

The increased autonomy in adolescence sets the stage for a pivotal transition in FA: the transition of management from the parent to the patient.[12] This increased responsibility has been shown to also increase anxiety for some adolescents with FA.[26,32] Because most fatal food-allergic reactions during adolescence occur when away from home,[12] supporting adolescents in safely navigating new situations and relationships is imperative. Adolescent FA risk-taking behaviors include decreased adherence to carrying epinephrine, eating foods that may contain an allergen, and not speaking up if a reaction is suspected.[19,33] In one study, only 42% of adolescents with FA asked about food ingredients at restaurants, and only 35% asked at friends' houses.[32] Supportive family, peers, and teachers have been shown to be related to less risk-taking behavior, as has having a school 504 plan.[26] Although decreasing risky behaviors is important for successful FA management, there is a downside: youth with FA with less risky behavior also report greater barriers to normal socialization (eg, going to restaurants or to other people's homes) than do youth with more risky behavior, which may put them at risk for greater isolation.[26]

Adults

Developmental tasks of emerging adulthood may include navigating a period of notable instability (eg, multiple job changes, series of intimate relationships), whereas established adulthood often includes commitments in romantic relationships and careers, and the stressors associated with parenthood.[34] Adults with FA have previously been a topic of little attention, with few published studies; however, the prevalence of FA in adults is increasing, estimated to affect approximately 1 in 10 adults.[2,35] One in four adults with FA report developing the allergy as an adult.[36] Only a few psychosocial areas related to adulthood have been studied in FA (eg, college, work); many important areas, such as the experience of pregnancy for a person with FA, cohabitating with friends, the impact on significant partners, or parenting as an adult with FA, remain unexamined.

Literature pertaining specifically to the young adult population with FA is sparse, and young adult samples are often integrated with adolescent samples. Many studies in this age range center on college experiences. Twenty-five percent of FA-related deaths occur in 18 to 22 year olds; approximately 50% of these deaths occurred on college campuses.[37,38] Among students who have had a reaction while at college, 62% of reactions occurred on campus, and 21% occurred at restaurants.[39] College students with FA report generally avoiding foods with known allergens and paying attention to posted ingredients of foods prepared on campus.[40] However, they often do not specifically ask about ingredients in foods prepared by others. Other risky behavior of college students with FA includes inappropriate use of an EAI: 16.4% of college students with an EAI always carry it; 17.9% report never carrying it.[40] There are a variety of factors that contribute to the decision on whether to carry epinephrine, including the concern of informing peers about the FA.[19,41,42] The psychological health of young adults with FA has been understudied, but a greater risk for anxiety or depression has been associated with FA in college students.[43] However, in a study using the National Health and Nutrition Examination Survey data to examine the mental health of adolescents and adults with FA, no association between mental health and FA was found for adults.[29] This may indicate that patients develop their own coping strategies with their FA with time.

Studies examining the daily experience of FA in adults highlight the significant burden associated with FA. In a study collecting daily reports of the experience of more than 100 adults with FA (average age, 40.2 years; range, 18–87), participants reported experiencing an FA-issue on nearly 50% of days, with incidence of FA-issue associated with heightened stress; most common issues were related to availability and cost of allergen-free food, allergic reactions, and the stress of navigating social situations.[44] Studies of FA-specific QOL in adults highlight the negative impact of allergen restriction, fear of FA worsening, uncertainty and anxiety about the diagnosis, and anxiety about an allergic reaction.[45,46]

Because adults are generally autonomous in their management of FA, they also carry the tremendous economic burden of FA,[47] which can include direct (eg, food, medical care) and indirect costs (eg, lost labor productivity, time spent information seeking, time spent on FA-related household tasks).[48,49] More than 25% of adolescents and young adults with FA reported FA as a barrier to obtaining employment.[26] Costs may be one of the contributors to the low rate of EAI access in adults.[36] Only one in three adults with FA have one at age 50, and even less by age 60.[2,14] In addition to life-saving, having an EAI may improve FA QOL.[36]

FAMILY ADJUSTMENT

Parents experience significant challenges caring for a child with FA, including maintaining vigilance and managing uncertainty related to accidental exposures, advocating for their child across systems (eg, school, camps), and managing treatment tasks (eg, OIT or EAI use). Parents must provide ongoing FA education (at the appropriate developmental level), navigate the tension of allowing their child increasing autonomy while maintaining appropriate supervision, and provide emotional support to their child.[6,50] This burden has been found to increase parental anxiety surrounding FA.[12] Mothers specifically have been found to have increased stress and anxiety compared with other family members.[3] Child FA can also exert a financial toll on families, with parents reporting diminished work productivity or job loss related to managing their child's FA.[48] Not surprisingly, parents of children with FA report higher levels of stress, anxiety, and depression compared with parents of healthy children, and fluctuating patterns of parental distress have been found, such as anxiety worsening after an anaphylaxis even.[6,50] Parental distress is related to the psychosocial functioning of their child with the FA.[30] Parenting practices are impacted by FA, with youth who have experienced anaphylaxis reporting greater parental protection,[51] and parents who report high levels of parental overprotection note poorer child functioning.[52] Of course, with FA in particular, families must balance the need for vigilance with promoting child autonomy. In a recent study of family coping patterns, about half of the families fell into the "Balanced Responder" category, characterized by appropriate vigilance, moderate anxiety, the ability to integrate the FA into daily lives, and children with FA having good FA management skills.[53] In addition to impacting child psychosocial functioning, parent anxiety may impact FA knowledge acquisition or retention.[54] Although understudied, siblings of children with FA also report considerable worry about FA, and involvement in FA management, including anaphylaxis events.[55]

PSYCHOSOCIAL TREATMENT

There is a dearth of outcome studies examining the impact of psychosocial interventions for patients with FA. A study of an FA sleep-way camp for 11- to 12-year-old children that focused on education and confidence-boosting physical activities reported improvements in several aspects of anxiety and QOL at 6-month follow-up.[56] A group-based half-day workshop for children 5 to 7 years old that involved medical play, social, and emotion-based activities was rated positively by children (pre and post psychosocial variables were not assessed).[57] Two studies have targeted specific FA anxieties. A prospective randomized trial targeted anxiety about casual allergen exposure in youth 9 to 17.5 years of age; everyone received education about the minimal risk of casual allergen contact, and youth randomized to the intervention were asked to hold a cup with a nut kernel then instructed to touch the nut in a step-wise fashion (followed by hand-washing). All participants reported decreased worry 1 month later.[58] Another randomized trial targeted EAI-related anxiety. Thirty adolescents were coached in the self-injection of a sterile 25-gauge needle, whereas the control group were provided education and demonstration of self-injection on a dummy. All youth in the intervention were able to self-inject, and the group reported improved comfort with self-injection relative to the control subjects.[59]

More research has investigated psychosocial interventions developed to support caregivers. A systematic review conducted in 2020 identified 15 interventions (involving 6511 participants).[50] Of note, only two studies were randomized controlled trials, and most studies scored poorly on the standardized quality assessment tool used for the review. Educational interventions were most common (in 7/15 studies), involved face-to-face and online delivery of material, and consistently improved FA knowledge and caregiver confidence in managing FA. Psychological interventions included components, such as psychoeducation, self-regulation, problem-solving, and cognitive-behavioral therapy, and corresponded with improvements in psychosocial outcomes. Of note, dose of intervention varied widely (eg, one session cognitive behavioral therapy, 12 sessions cognitive behavioral therapy, three 25-minute telephone calls). Two parent support groups were reviewed, with reported decreases in social isolation and anxiety and increased confidence in talking with allergy providers (in a support group including an allergist).

CLINICAL IMPLICATIONS

Pediatric psychosocial preventive health models highlight the importance of assessing risk and resiliency factors, and providing preventive and intervention efforts to optimize child and family biopsychosocial outcomes.[60] Some patients with an FA present with obvious and significant risk factors that require referral to appropriate psychosocial or community services. Signs of significant risk may include (but are not limited to) significant economic hardship; heightened and/or persistent psychological distress; patient struggling to meet developmental milestones; and patient/family inadequately managing FA, such as evidenced by heightened risk of allergen exposure or inability to complete FA treatment tasks (eg, OIT, EAI use). However, all patients with FA benefit from interventions that enhance known resiliency factors. Resiliency factors that dovetail closely with the experience and demands of FA include education, problem-solving, self-efficacy, enhancing social support, engagement in school, and meaning making (eg, coming to understand one's life events in a way that fosters positive adjustment, such as enhancing a personal sense of purpose or growth). FA provides opportunities to the treating clinician to enhance these factors across the developmental span (**Box 2**).

Box 2
Resilience-building clinic activities

Activities that can occur during clinic visits to strengthen resiliency include:
- Education
- Problem-solving
- Enhancing self-efficacy
- Social support
- Meaning making

Education

Education is the cornerstone of successful navigation of any health condition. Families deserve up-to-date information about the true risks related to allergen exposure. FAs, by definition, are restrictive; when people overestimate the risk of exposure and subsequently narrow their experiences beyond what is reasonable or necessary, QOL suffers. Education related to symptoms of allergen exposure should be initiated early; by age 9 to 11, children should be able to recognize signs of anaphylaxis.[61] Education on appropriate use of EAI is also essential, and is life-saving, yet many FA sufferers identify problems with the training that was provided.[36,49] The mandate for high-quality information provided by knowledgeable health care providers is clear; a recent review of the quality of FA publicly available videos (on YouTube) demonstrated poor-quality information, including blatantly misleading information.[62]

Problem-Solving

Problem-solving is a skill set characterized by active engagement in addressing challenges, delineating a challenge into concrete and actionable goals, generation of ideas, selecting a possible solution, and evaluating the result after implementation; training in these skills has been shown to enhance positive adjustment in health conditions.[63,64] Clinicians should regularly ask patients and families the problems they encounter in managing the FA, and can be framed in terms of important activities not occurring ("What are the things you wish you could do but do not, because of your FA"), or lapses in management ("I know it is important to you to not have an allergic reaction – what got in the way of you asking about the ingredients")? Brainstorming solutions means generating a variety of ideas for addressing the problem; clinicians can offer possible solutions from their expertise and experience talking to hundreds of patients/families, but eliciting ideas from the patient/family themselves is critical because these ideas are generated within their own context and values. Importantly, individuals and families may choose a solution that is okay, but not optimal from the perspective of the clinician; a solution that is grounded in a family's values and context is most likely to be used.

A critical caveat that clinicians must be sensitive to is that real health disparities exist among patients and families with FA (discussed elsewhere in this issue). Families should not feel the burden of solving systemic barriers to managing health; allergists must be knowledgeable of community resources available to address disparities, and consider their own role in advocating for equitable health care.

Self-Efficacy

Self-efficacy involves the belief a person has about their ability to perform specific tasks, and their belief that performing the task will have a positive outcome. A person's self-efficacy is enhanced by mastery experiences (personal and observing others) and by the assurances of others that the person can be successful, and has been associated with improved health outcomes, positive psychological adjustment, and improved QOL.[65] Parents with greater self-efficacy in managing FA reported better QOL, particularly in social settings.[66] For young children, general self-efficacy is promoted by parents allowing exploration and highlighting successes in skill acquisition; allergists can discuss with even young children the positive ways they take care of their bodies ("You are learning to brush your teeth! Good for you!"). As children age, allergists can encourage increasingly shared FA responsibilities between the parent and child, such as informing adults about their allergy and symptoms of a reaction, avoidance of sharing food, reading ingredient labels, informing restaurant staff of the allergy, and carriage of medications.[14] For instance, allergists can encourage children to describe their FA during the clinic visit, and reinforce positive communication. Innovative technologies can be used to improve FA self-concept. For example, a mobile application specific to FA anaphylaxis management has been found to improve teenagers' belief in their ability to manage their FA, thereby increasing self-efficacy.[67] In addition, behavioral practice of important skills (eg, self-injection for EAIs) can be conducted within the clinic setting to provide mastery experiences.[59] To build self-efficacy during transition into greater independence as a young adult, allergists can work with patients in mastering important transition steps, such as establishing care with a physician or allergist, becoming familiar with the school clinic, gathering information regarding dining options, and creating an FA action plan.[12,40]

Social Support

Enhancing social support involves optimizing peer and family support for the person with FA. Allergists can promote opportunities for children and adolescents to engage in age-appropriate social activities. In addition, adolescents and young adults with FA would prefer their peers and the public be educated on FA[41,42,68]; allergists can provide this information to their patients for distribution among their social networks to decrease isolation and facilitate engagement. Given that children with FA who reported bullying at school had improved QOL after disclosing the bullying to their parents,[59] allergists can also model for families how to have supportive, nonreactive conversations with youth about their social relationships to enhance the family's ability to provide support.

Safe School Environment

Ensuring a safe school environment for the child with FA involves having clear communication between families and schools.[24] These conversations may also include the allergist, teacher, and school nurse. A written emergency plan should be developed and given to the school, including symptoms of a reaction and instructions of treatment, and should be updated at least every school year.[24] People of all ages with FA must be able to advocate for themselves, whether it is primary or secondary school, higher education, or at work; these conversations can be practiced at the clinic to increase self-efficacy. Certainly, allergists should ask about FA-related victimization, and provide support in enhancing safety.

Meaning-Making

Finally, engaging patients and families in conversations about their strengths and values promotes adaptive meaning-making. A curious, patient/family-centered approach about the experience of managing FA may initially elicit discussion of FA challenges and struggles. Noting adaptive responses that families have made and asking about the strengths and values that are accessed during successful navigation of challenges can shift the conversation toward an affirming and invigorating dialogue about what is most important to patients/families and how their positive responses to FA challenges reflect these attributes. Both adolescents and young adults with FA have reported that their FA made them more responsible, better advocates for themselves and others, and more likely to offer help to those with special needs.[26] Allergists can and should acknowledge the significant adversity that FA poses, and allergists can and should drive conversations that highlight the positive growth and strengths that rising to the challenge of FA has afforded for the patients they serve.

CLINICS CARE POINTS

- Education for patients and families should be developmentally appropriate, and should include accurate estimates of risk for allergen exposure.

- To enhance self-efficacy, have patients and caregivers practice in clinic critical allergy-related health behaviors, such as anaphylactic symptom communication, assertiveness about allergen-avoidance, and use of autoinjector (if it includes a practice device).

- Assess for social concerns, including any incidence of bullying by peers or minimizing of risk by adults who may be involved in gatekeeping patient's food. If these are present, problem-solve with patients and families and provide written or verbal communication to escalate concerns.

- Intentionally assess for barriers to full engagement in developmentally important activities and problem-solve with families to determine solutions.

- Solicit from and reflect to patients and families the strengths that help them navigate the challenges of food allergy.

DISCLOSURE

The authors have nothing to disclose.

REFERENCES

1. Gupta RS, Warren CM, Smith BM, et al. The public health impact of parent-reported childhood food allergies in the United States. Pediatrics 2018;142(6): e20181235.
2. Gupta RS, Warren CM, Smith BM, et al. Prevalence and severity of food allergies among US adults. JAMA Netw Open 2019;2(1):e185630.
3. Feng C, Kim J-H. Beyond avoidance: the psychosocial impact of food allergies. Clin Rev Allergy Immunol 2019;57(1):74–82.
4. Hsu E, Soller L, Abrams EM, et al. Oral food challenge implementation: the first mixed-methods study exploring barriers and solution. J Allergy Clin Immunol Pract 2020;8(1):149–56.e1.
5. Kansen HM, Le TM, Meijer Y, et al. The impact of oral food challenges for food allergy on quality of life: a systematic review. Pediatr Allergy Immunol 2018; 29(5):527–37.
6. Polloni L, Muraro A. Anxiety and food allergy: a review of the last two decades. Clin Exp Allergy 2020;50(4):420–41.
7. Dahlsgaard KK, Lewis MO, Spergel JM. New issue of food allergy: phobia of anaphylaxis in pediatric patients. J Allergy Clin Immunol 2020;146(4):780–2.
8. Hilliard ME, McQuaid EL, Nabors L, et al. Resilience in youth and families living with pediatric health and developmental conditions: introduction to the special issue on resilience. Oxford University Press; 2015.
9. Osher D, Cantor P, Berg J, et al. Drivers of human development: how relationships and context shape learning and development1. Appl Dev Sci 2020; 24(1):6–36.
10. Masten AS, Barnes AJ. Resilience in children: developmental perspectives. Children 2018;5(7):98.
11. Walsh F. Family resilience: a developmental systems framework. Eur J Dev Psychol 2016;13(3):313–24.
12. Herbert L, Shemesh E, Bender B. Clinical management of psychosocial concerns related to food allergy. J Allergy Clin Immunol Pract 2016;4(2):205–13.

13. Houle CR, Leo HL, Clark NM. A developmental, community, and psychosocial approach to food allergies in children. Curr Allergy Asthma Rep 2010;10(5): 381–6.

14. Sicherer SH, Warren CM, Dant C, et al. Food allergy from infancy through adulthood. J Allergy Clin Immunol Pract 2020;8(6):1854–64.

15. Tsuang A, Wang J. Childcare and school management issues in food allergy. Curr Allergy Asthma Rep 2016;16(12):83.

16. Dahlquist LM, Power TG, Hahn AL, et al. Parenting and independent problem-solving in preschool children with food allergy. J Pediatr Psychol 2015;40(1): 96–108.

17. Topal E, Bakirtas A, Yilmaz O, et al. Anaphylaxis in infancy compared with older children. Paper presented at: Allergy & Asthma Proceedings. 2013.

18. Alanne S, Laitinen K, Paavilainen E. Living ordinary family life with an allergic child: the Mother's perspective. J Pediatr Nurs 2014;29(6):679–87.

19. DunnGalvin A, Polloni L, Le Bovidge J, et al. Preliminary development of the food allergy coping and emotions questionnaires for children, adolescents, and young people: qualitative analysis of data on IgE-mediated food allergy from five countries. J Allergy Clin Immunol Pract 2018;6(2):506–13.e1.

20. Wassenberg J, Cochard MM, DunnGalvin A, et al. Parent perceived quality of life is age-dependent in children with food allergy. Pediatr Allergy Immunol 2012; 23(5):412–9.

21. Petrovic-Dovat L, Fausnight T, White AM, et al. Degree of anxiety in food allergic children in a tertiary care center. Ann Allergy Asthma Immunol 2016;116(6): 528–32.

22. Weiss D, Marsac ML. Coping and posttraumatic stress symptoms in children with food allergies. Ann Allergy Asthma Immunol 2016;117(5):561–2.

23. Hui JW, Copeland M, Lanser BJ. Food allergy management at school in the era of immunotherapy. Curr Allergy Asthma Rep 2020;20(8):32.

24. Wang J, Bingemann T, Russell AF, et al. The allergist's role in anaphylaxis and food allergy management in the school and childcare setting. J Allergy Clin Immunol Pract 2018;6(2):427–35.

25. Bingemann T, Herbert LJ, Young MC, et al. Deficits and opportunities in allergists' approaches to food allergy–related bullying. J Allergy Clin Immunol Pract 2020; 8(1):343–5.e2.

26. Warren CM, Dyer AA, Otto AK, et al. Food allergy–related risk-taking and management behaviors among adolescents and young adults. J Allergy Clin Immunol Pract 2017;5(2):381–90.e3.

27. Newman K, Knibb R. The psychosocial impact of adolescent food allergy: a review of the literature. EMJ Allergy Immunol 2020;5(1):54–60.

28. Ferro M, Van Lieshout R, Ohayon J, et al. Emotional and behavioral problems in adolescents and young adults with food allergy. Allergy 2016;71(4):532–40.

29. Dantzer JA, Keet CA. Anxiety associated with food allergy in adults and adolescents: an analysis of data from the National Health and Nutrition Examination Survey (NHANES) 2007-2010. J Allergy Clin Immunol Pract 2020;8(5):1743–6.e5.

30. Fox JK, Masia Warner C. Food allergy and social anxiety in a community sample of adolescents. Children's Health Care 2017;46(1):93–107.

31. Hullmann SE, Molzon ES, Eddington AR, et al. Dating anxiety in adolescents and young adults with food allergies: a comparison to healthy peers. Journal of Asthma & Allergy Educators 2012;3(4):172–7.

32. Jones CJ, Llewellyn CD, Frew AJ, et al. Factors associated with good adherence to self-care behaviours amongst adolescents with food allergy. Pediatr Allergy Immunol 2015;26(2):111–8.

33. Marrs T, Lack G. Why do few food-allergic adolescents treat anaphylaxis with adrenaline? Reviewing a pressing issue. Pediatr Allergy Immunol 2013;24(3):222–9.

34. Mehta CM, Arnett JJ, Palmer CG, et al. Established adulthood: a new conception of ages 30 to 45. Am Psychol 2020;75(4):431.

35. Warren CM, Jiang J, Gupta RS. Epidemiology and burden of food allergy. Curr Allergy Asthma Rep 2020;20(2):1–9.

36. Warren C, Stankey C, Jiang J, et al. Prevalence, severity, and distribution of adult-onset food allergy. Ann Allergy Asthma Immunol 2018;121(5):S14.

37. Bock SA, Muñoz-Furlong A, Sampson HA. Fatalities due to anaphylactic reactions to foods. J Allergy Clin Immunol 2001;107(1):191–3.

38. Bock SA, Muñoz-Furlong A, Sampson HA. Further fatalities caused by anaphylactic reactions to food, 2001-2006. J Allergy Clin Immunol 2007;119(4):1016.

39. Greenhawt MJ, Singer AM, Baptist AP. Food allergy and food allergy attitudes among college students. J Allergy Clin Immunol 2009;124(2):323–7.

40. Duncan SE, Annunziato RA. Barriers to self-management behaviors in college students with food allergies. J Am Coll Health 2018;66(5):331–9.

41. Dyer AA, O'Keefe A, Kanaley MK, et al. Leaving the nest: improving food allergy management on college campuses. Ann Allergy Asthma Immunol 2018;121(1):82–9.e5.

42. Walkner M, Warren C, Gupta RS. Quality of life in food allergy patients and their families. Pediatr Clin 2015;62(6):1453–61.

43. Chen J, Spleen A, Adkins AE, et al. Self-reported food allergy and intolerance among college undergraduates: associations with anxiety and depressive symptoms. J Coll Student Psychother 2020;1–22.

44. Peniamina RL, Mirosa M, Bremer P, et al. The stress of food allergy issues in daily life. Psychol Health 2016;31(6):750–67.

45. Jansson S-A, Heibert-Arnlind M, Middelveld RJ, et al. Health-related quality of life, assessed with a disease-specific questionnaire, in Swedish adults suffering from well-diagnosed food allergy to staple foods. Clin Transl Allergy 2013;3(1):21.

46. Goossens NJ, Flokstra-de Blok BM, van der Meulen GN, et al. Health-related quality of life in food-allergic adults from eight European countries. Ann Allergy Asthma Immunol 2014;113(1):63–8.e1.

47. Dyer AA, Negris OR, Gupta RS, et al. Food allergy: how expensive are they? Curr Opin Allergy Clin Immunol 2020;20(2):188–93.

48. Bilaver LA, Chadha AS, Doshi P, et al. Economic burden of food allergy: a systematic review. Ann Allergy Asthma Immunol 2019;122(4):373–80.e1.

49. Blumchen K, DunnGalvin A, Timmermans F, et al. APPEAL-1: a pan-European survey of patient/caregiver perceptions of peanut allergy management. Allergy 2020;75(11):2920–35.

50. Sugunasingha N, Jones FW, Jones CJ. Interventions for caregivers of children with food allergy: a systematic review. Pediatr Allergy Immunol 2020;31(7):805–12.

51. Herbert LJ, Dahlquist LM. Perceived history of anaphylaxis and parental overprotection, autonomy, anxiety, and depression in food allergic young adults. J Clin Psychol Med Settings 2008;15(4):261–9.

52. Chow C, Pincus DB, Comer JS. Pediatric food allergies and psychosocial functioning: examining the potential moderating roles of maternal distress and overprotection. J Pediatr Psychol 2015;40(10):1065–74.

53. Fedele DA, Kirk K, Wolfe-Christensen C, et al. Primary caregivers of children affected by disorders of sex development: mental health and caregiver characteristics in the context of genital ambiguity and genitoplasty. Int J Pediatr Endocrinol 2010;2010(1):690674.

54. Luke AK, Flessner CA. Examining differences in parent knowledge about pediatric food allergies. J Pediatr Psychol 2020;45(1):101–9.

55. Stensgaard A, Bindslev-Jensen C, Nielsen D. Peanut allergy as a family project: social relations and transitions in adolescence. J Clin Nurs 2017;26(21–22): 3371–81.

56. Knibb RC, Hourihane JOB. The psychosocial impact of an activity holiday for young children with severe food allergy: a longitudinal study. Pediatr Allergy Immunol 2013;24(4):368–75.

57. LeBovidge JS, Timmons K, Rich C, et al. Evaluation of a group intervention for children with food allergy and their parents. Ann Allergy Asthma Immunol 2008; 101(2):160–5.

58. Weinberger T, Annunziato R, Riklin E, et al. A randomized controlled trial to reduce food allergy anxiety about casual exposure by holding the allergen: TOUCH study. J Allergy Clin Immunol Pract 2019;7(6):2039–42.e4.

59. Shemesh E, D'Urso C, Knight C, et al. Food-allergic adolescents at risk for anaphylaxis: a randomized controlled study of supervised injection to improve comfort with epinephrine self-injection. J Allergy Clin Immunol Pract 2017;5(2):391–7.e4.

60. Kazak AE. Pediatric Psychosocial Preventative Health Model (PPPHM): research, practice, and collaboration in pediatric family systems medicine. Families, Systems, & Health 2006;24(4):381.

61. Simons E, Sicherer SH, Weiss C, et al. Caregivers' perspectives on timing the transfer of responsibilities for anaphylaxis recognition and treatment from adults to children and teenagers. J Allergy Clin Immunol Pract 2013;1(3):309–11.

62. Reddy K, Kearns M, Alvarez-Arango S, et al. YouTube and food allergy: an appraisal of the educational quality of information. Pediatr Allergy Immunol 2018;29(4):410–6.

63. Sahler OJZ, Dolgin MJ, Phipps S, et al. Specificity of problem-solving skills training in mothers of children newly diagnosed with cancer: results of a multisite randomized clinical trial. J Clin Oncol 2013;31(10):1329.

64. Rivera PA, Elliott TR, Berry JW, et al. Problem-solving training for family caregivers of persons with traumatic brain injuries: a randomized controlled trial. Arch Phys Med Rehabil 2008;89(5):931–41.

65. Lorig KR, Ritter P, Stewart AL, et al. Chronic disease self-management program: 2-year health status and health care utilization outcomes. Med Care 2001;39(11): 1217–23.

66. Knibb RC, Barnes C, Stalker C. Parental self-efficacy in managing food allergy and mental health predicts food allergy-related quality of life. Pediatr Allergy Immunol 2016;27(5):459–64.

67. Davidson N, Vines J, Bartindale T, et al. Supporting self-care of adolescents with nut allergy through video and mobile educational tools. Paper presented at: Proceedings of the 2017 CHI Conference on Human Factors in Computing Systems. 2017.

68. Monks H, Gowland M, MacKenzie H, et al. How do teenagers manage their food allergies? Clin Exp Allergy 2010;40(10):1533–40.

Racial/Ethnic Differences in Food Allergy

Christopher M. Warren, PhD[a], Audrey G. Brewer, MD, MPH[a,b,c,d],
Benjamin Grobman[a], Jialing Jiang, BA[a], Ruchi S. Gupta, MD, MPH[a,b,c,d],*

KEYWORDS

- Food allergy • Racial and ethnic differences • Prevalence • Disparities

KEY POINTS

- Food allergy prevalence varies by race and ethnicity in North America, with increasing evidence of racial differences in food allergy outcomes from the United States.
- Racial and ethnic differences in food allergy–related psychosocial outcomes, economic burden, and knowledge/education also exist.
- Because the concept of race is socially constructed, it is important also to consider the impact of socioeconomic status in studying differences in food allergy outcomes.

INTRODUCTION

In recent decades, immunoglobulin E (IgE)-mediated food allergy (FA) increasingly has been acknowledged as a major public health concern across the globe.[1] In the United States, the most recent epidemiologic data indicate that FA affects approximately 1 in 13 children[2] and 1 in 10 adults,[3] resulting in substantial physical, psychosocial, and economic burden. Previous research has indicated, however, that the impact of FA is remarkably heterogeneous, varying substantially by age,[4] sex,[5,6] geography,[7,8] and race/ethnicity.[9,10] This review aims to describe what currently is known about the differential burden of FAs among different racial/ethnic groups in North America, particularly in the United States and Canada.

Race is defined as a sociopolitically constructed, nonbiological categorization system based on a combination of personal identity and phenotypical indicators. Ethnicity is a separate but related social construct, which refers to a shared cultural origin.[11] The US Census Bureau separates Hispanic/Latino ethnicity from race, defining Hispanic/Latino origin as the heritage, nationality, lineage, or country of birth of the person or the person's parents or ancestors before arriving in the United States.[12] Individuals who

[a] Center for Food Allergy and Asthma Research, Northwestern University Feinberg School of Medicine, 750 North Lake Shore Drive, Rubloff 6th Floor, Suite 680, Chicago, IL 60611, USA;
[b] Ann and Robert H. Lurie Children's Hospital, 225 E Chicago Ave, Chicago, IL 60611, USA;
[c] Department of Pediatrics, Ann and Robert H. Lurie Children's Hospital of Chicago, 225 E. Chicago Avenue, Box 86, Chicago, IL 60611, USA; [d] Department of Medicine, Northwestern University Feinberg School of Medicine, 420 E Superior St, Chicago, IL 60611, USA
* Corresponding author.
E-mail address: r-gupta@northwestern.edu

Immunol Allergy Clin N Am 41 (2021) 189–203
https://doi.org/10.1016/j.iac.2021.01.007
immunology.theclinics.com
0889-8561/21/© 2021 Elsevier Inc. All rights reserved.

identify as Hispanic/Latino may identify as being from any race.[13] In recent years, Latinx has emerged as a gender-neutral term to identify ethnicity, relating to persons of Latin American origin or descent.[14] When identifying the link between race and health outcomes, race should be viewed in the context of social constructs, because many observed racial differences in health outcomes are reducible to other socioenvironmental factors.[15] In addition, race must not be misconstrued as having a biological or genetic basis, because race is better understood in the context of social factors that drive health outcomes. Race and ethnicity are constructed in a specific way based on national context, and, as such, analyses of racial/ethnic health disparities among specific groups are limited in their applicability across international boundaries.[16] Historical patterns of migration, racism and discrimination, however, particularly in the US context, have made race/ethnicity a significant indicator of health outcomes, with significant disparities in numerous health conditions.[15,17]

RACIAL/ETHNIC DIFFERENCES IN FOOD ALLERGY PREVALENCE

A close examination of major US population–based epidemiologic studies conducted over the past 2 decades reveals a consistent pattern of a higher estimated burden of food-allergic disease among black Americans, relative to their white counterparts. The disparate burden FA appears to place on black Americans is consistent with epidemiologic research on other allergic diseases comprising the atopic march (eg, asthma,[18,19] eczema,[20–23] and environmental allergies[24]). These observations, however, which include higher FA prevalence and more frequent health care utilization among particular racial/ethnic groups, run counter to public perception and media narratives that have framed FAs as having a disproportionate impact on white populations.

The first series of US population–based studies designed to estimate national prevalence of specific FAs were conducted by Sicherer and colleagues[25-28] via random-digit telephone dialing in 1997, 2002, and 2008. Although the 1997 survey did not assess race,[25] the 2002 survey of approximately 15,000 Americans found that rates of probable FA to seafood were dramatically higher among black children and adults relative to their white counterparts (3.7% vs 1.9%, respectively), yet the relative frequency of physician-diagnosed shellfish allergy among these probable cases was almost identical (40% vs 38%, respectively).[26,27] This suggested that the observed differences in prevalence may not entirely be attributable to systematic racial differences in health care access—a well-known phenomenon in other chronic conditions, such as asthma.[29] Updated prevalence estimates from more recent random-digit dial telephone surveys have identified similar disparities and are suggestive of a growing burden of FAs among black Americans. For example, the reported prevalence of probable peanut and/or tree nut allergies rose from 0.7% to 1.9% among black Americans from 2002 to 2008, versus a rise from 1.2% to 1.4% among white Americans.[26,28] Again, similar rates of physician diagnoses were reported (41% of black patients and 44% of white patients with probable FA).[26] These surveys, however, did not assess other common top 8 allergens, including cow's milk, egg, wheat, and soy.

In a 2011 survey, parents of a nationally representative sample of approximately 40,000 US children demonstrated that the odds of any probable FA were approximately double among black children relative to white children, adjusting for gender, age, household income, census region, and multiple FAs.[30] Additionally, black children with reported FA, as well as children with reported FA from families earning less than $50,000/y, were significantly less likely to report receiving a physician diagnosis—highlighting a possible disparity in access to specialist allergy care, discussed later.

A 2014 analysis of previously published FA prevalence data sets,[31] which presented stratified prevalence estimates, including the aforementioned national surveys conducted by Sicherer[25-28] and Gupta[30], calculated that overall FA prevalence among the general US population had increased by 1.2 percentage points during the prior 2 decades, and by 2.1 percentage points each decade among black Americans.[31] More recent data from national population-based surveys have reported that current FA prevalence is now higher among black Americans compared with white Americans. These data suggest that this is the case for each of the top 8 FAs besides wheat and soy and also is the case for sesame allergy.[32] On a somewhat promising note, these recent US epidemiologic data indicate that on average black children no longer are less likely to report receiving a physician diagnosis for parent-reported "convincing" FA than they were in the 2011 survey. Socioeconomic disparities remain, however, with families earning less than $50,000/y significantly less likely to report obtaining a physician diagnosis.

FOOD ALLERGY OUTCOMES AMONG HISPANIC POPULATIONS IN THE UNITED STATES

Recent epidemiologic data also suggest that FAs may disproportionately affect other racial/ethnic minority groups as well. An estimated 8.4% of the US Hispanic pediatric population are food-allergic, compared with 7% of white children.[2] Similarly, an estimated 11.6% of the US Hispanic adult population is food-allergic versus 10.1% of the US white adult population.[3] This marks a shift from previous studies, which indicated that Hispanic children may be less likely to report FA relative to their white counterparts.[15,16] In a US multisite clinical study, observed rates of seafood allergy (both shellfish and finned fish) were significantly higher in Hispanic (and non-Hispanic black) children relative to their white peers.[10] As seen in **Fig. 1**, race/ethnicity-stratified prevalence estimates from a recent national US survey also are consistent with this finding of greater risk of seafood allergy risk among black and Hispanic children, a finding that extends to US adults.[2,3] To date, little attention has been paid to the possible heterogeneity in FA status outcomes within the Hispanic population, depending on region of origin. In the related field of asthma, for example, there are differences in asthma prevalence between Hispanic individuals of Puerto Rican descent (16% prevalence per Centers for Disease Control and Prevention [CDC] data)[33] versus Mexican-Americans (5.4% prevalence).[34] Therefore, future epidemiologic studies of FA outcomes among Hispanic/Latinx should strongly consider collecting data regarding country of origin and examining possible interactions. Such work has the potential to identify the racial/ethnic subpopulations who may be at highest risk.

FOOD ALLERGY AMONG NORTH AMERICAN NATIVE AND FIRST NATIONS COMMUNITIES

In the United States, little is known about the prevalence of FA among Native American populations. In contrast, numerous Canadian population–based epidemiologic studies have aimed to determine the burden of disease among First Nations/Aboriginal populations, with equivocal findings. The 2011 Surveying Prevalence of Food Allergy in All Canadian Environments study surveyed 5734 Canadian households and deliberately oversampled vulnerable populations, including those of Aboriginal identity.[35] In contrast to their study hypothesis, however, which posited the existence of environmental factors that would be protective against atopic disease, they found that rates of FA were similar among Aboriginal and non-Aboriginal Canadians. This

US Children

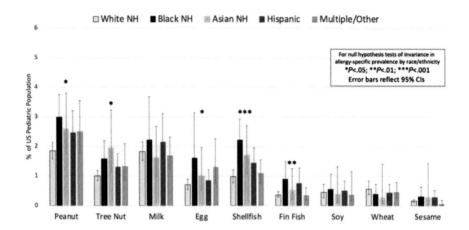

US Adults

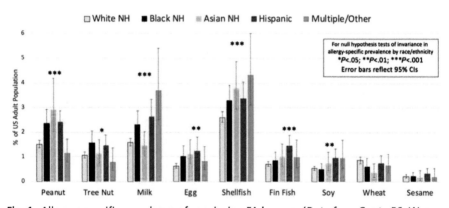

Fig. 1. Allergen-specific prevalence of convincing FA by race. (*Data from* Gupta RS, Warren CM, Smith BM, et al. The Public Health Impact of Parent-Reported Childhood Food Allergies in the United States. Pediatrics 2018;142(6):e20181235; and Gupta RS, Warren CM, Smith BM, et al. Prevalence and Severity of Food Allergies Among US Adults. JAMA Netw Open 2019;2(1):e185630-e185630.)

was in contrast to an earlier analysis of the 2006 Canadian Aboriginal Children's Survey, which found that Aboriginal children living off-reserve were less likely to be food-allergic (2.9% prevalence) than the general Canadian population.[36]

RACIAL/ETHNIC DIFFERENCES IN FOOD-ALLERGIC SENSITIZATION

Recent data from the Boston-area Project Viva prebirth cohort (N = 1148) found that non-Hispanic black adolescents were at increased risk of peanut-allergic symptomatology (odds ratio [OR] 2.41; 95% CI, 1.12–5.17) versus non-Hispanic white adolescents.[37] Non-Hispanic black adolescents also had higher rates of sensitization to peanut, milk, egg, soy, and wheat—all 5 common food allergens evaluated in this study—although these associations were significant only for peanut and wheat after adjustment for maternal education, maternal smoking during pregnancy and infant exposure to environmental tobacco smoke, household income, and census tract median income. In general, inverse associations were identified between maternal education and allergen sensitization, whereas relationships were less clear with respect to household income. Household income was significantly associated only with higher odds of sensitization to soy, and lower maternal educational attainment was associated with higher odds of sensitization to milk and wheat.

These findings are consistent with data from the younger Detroit-area Wayne County Health, Environment, Allergy, and Asthma Longitudinal Study (WHEALS) birth cohort of black and white children, which was established to examine the environmental determinants of childhood atopy. Findings at year 3 of follow-up indicated that sensitization to milk, egg, or peanut was significantly more common among black children relative to their white peers and that household income, Medicaid insurance status, and maternal education were not confounders of this association.[38] Black race, however, was not significantly associated with milk, egg, or peanut allergy status—as determined by a physician panel—at 3 years of age. A previous study reported higher rates of atopic dermatitis, wheeze, and sensitization to a panel of 10 food or environmental allergens and total IgE among black infants in this same cohort versus their white counterparts.[24] At the 10-year follow-up, allergic sensitization still was more common among black versus white children in the WHEALS cohort, even after adjusting for socioeconomic indicators (eg, income, maternal education, and difficulty making housing payments) and a variety of lifestyle variables (eg, presence of pets, siblings, and antibiotic use). Black children also were more likely to have atopic dermatitis and asthma, but FA status was not reported. Because most established racial differences in FA phenotypes between black and white patients are with respect to seafood allergies, in particular, shellfish, it will be interesting to determine if these differences eventually emerge within the WHEALS cohort.

The WHEALS study findings of racial differences in food-allergic sensitization are consistent with previous findings from the CDC National Health and Nutrition Examination Survey (NHANES) III (1991–1994), which found substantial racial heterogeneity between food-allergic sensitization to peanut, egg, milk, and shrimp in a nationally representative sample of greater than 2500 US children ages 6 years to 19 years.[39] The greatest differences in sensitization (specific IgE $\geq$0.35 kU/L) between black and white children were to shrimp (20.6% vs 6.6%, respectively) and milk (12.8% vs 5.6%, respectively), although significant differences in egg sensitization also were present (4.9% vs 3.0%, respectively). Wegienka and colleagues[40] provide a review of previous work in this area.

RACIAL/ETHNIC DIFFERENCES IN INTRODUCTION OF ALLERGENIC SOLIDS

Preliminary analyses of greater than 750 participants from the Food Allergy Management and Outcomes Related to White and African American Racial Differences (FOR-WARD) study have identified racial differences in FA outcomes and disease phenotypes, in addition to mechanistic insights—such as recent reports of substantial delays in the timing of dietary introduction of egg, peanut, and milk among black infants relative to their white counterparts—irrespective of household income strata.[41] This delay in allergenic food introduction among nonwhite populations is consistent with a recent secondary analysis of the Enquiring About Tolerance (EAT) study, which found nonwhite ethnicity to be independently and strongly associated with overall nonadherence to the prescribed "early introduction protocol" among those randomized to the early introduction group.[42] In the EAT study, 85% of participants were white and, due to the low number of black participants, Asian and black participants were pooled together compromising only 6% of the sample comprised only 6% of the sample. Given the disproportionate impact of FAs on black families in the United States, and the evidence for the effectiveness of early introduction of allergenic solids observed among the predominantly white, British Learning Early About Peanut Allergy and EAT trial participants, data from the FORWARD study and other similar efforts will provide valuable context for the generalizability of these approaches to more diverse populations.

RACIAL DIFFERENCES IN FOOD ALLERGY–RELATED HEALTH CARE UTILIZATION

Data indicate that black populations are at increased risk of fatal food-induced anaphylaxis relative to their white peers. An analysis of annual US mortality data from 1999 to 2010 found that rates of fatal food–induced anaphylaxis increased from 0.06 deaths per million (1999–2001) to 0.21 deaths per million (2008–2010) in black boys and men, but were stable among US white, Hispanic, and black girls and women during the same time.[43] Little is known, however, about the extent to which these trends have continued over the past decade.

Data from the CDC 2011 and 2012 National Health Interview Surveys reported significant racial/ethnic disparities in access to health care for food-allergic patients, which persisted after adjusting for income and education.[44] In general, compared with survey respondents without FA, respondents with FA were more likely to report difficulty accessing health care and food. Parents/caregivers of black and/or Hispanic children with FA, however, were significantly more likely to report difficulty affording medical care and medications and low food security compared with parents of white children with FA. Although these associations were somewhat attenuated after adjusting for household income and parental educational attainment, black survey respondents with FA still were significantly more likely to report low food security (OR 2.15; 95% CI, 1.30–3.53), problems affording medical care and prescriptions.

Analysis of more recent national survey data indicate that pediatric black and Hispanic FA patients are more likely to report receiving FA care in the emergency department (ED) than their white peers, with 47.3% of black and 49.2% of Hispanic patients reporting at least 1 FA-related ED visit during their lifetime versus 37.3% of white patients. More dramatic racial differences were found with respect to the reported frequency of FA-related ED visits. Specifically, black and Hispanic patients were at least 40% more likely to report receiving FA treatment in the ED within the past year compared with white patients.

Among US adults, black and Hispanic patients also were more likely to report a history of "severe" food-allergic reaction symptoms (indicated by multiple organ system involvement) and multiple FAs, each of which is likely to contribute to the aforementioned increased rates of ED visits among these racial/ethnic groups. Similarly, rates of reported lifetime epinephrine autoinjector use for food-allergic reaction treatment were greater among black (19.2%) and Hispanic (21.7%) US adults with FAs versus their white peers (17.5%). Rates also were greater among black (28.5%) and Hispanic (25.6%) US children with FAs versus their white peers (23.7%), despite comparable reported rates of current epinephrine prescription possession among black versus white versus Hispanic (38.5% vs 40.7% vs 41.0%, respectively) populations. Aforementioned data are limited, however, by possible bias due to self/parent-proxy report and an inability to validate reported health care utilization against chart review or follow-up allergy testing.[2,45]

Data gleaned from chart reviews of 817 food-allergic patients in Chicago and Cincinnati provide further evidence that black children may be disproportionately burdened by their allergic disease (**Fig. 2**).[10] Specifically, rates of food-induced anaphylaxis and FA-related ED visits were much higher among black relative to white patients (33.9% and 39.7% vs 16.4% and 18.2%, respectively), despite the fact that these populations had similar age distributions and white patients received follow-up allergy care for significantly longer (3.2 years vs 4.3 years, respectively). This multisite study also identified significant racial differences in FA outcomes between Hispanic and white patients, with Hispanic patients approximately 2 times as likely to report food-induced anaphylaxis (35.4% vs 16.4%, respectively) and FA-related ED visits (34.3% vs 18.2%, respectively) versus their white counterparts. Owing to disparities in health care access, however, comparing ED utilization is an imperfect proxy for FA severity, because individuals without access to specialty allergy care may be more likely to receive treatment in the ED even with similar reaction symptomatology.

RACIAL DIFFERENCES IN THE SOCIOECONOMIC BURDEN OF FOOD ALLERGY

In a 2013 study by Gupta and colleagues,[46] the economic burden of FA was estimated to be $24.8 billion annually, exceeding $4000/y per affected child. A follow-up study identified significant socioeconomic disparities in the economic burden of childhood FA, families earning less than $50,000/y spending more than twice as those from higher income families on FA-related ED and hospitalization costs.[47] In contrast, greater household income was associated with greater spending on out-of-pocket medication costs (eg, for epinephrine autoinjectors). This is consistent with previous work, which identified cost as the single most common barrier among adult FA patients of all racial/ethnic backgrounds who reported not filling their prescription for an epinephrine autoinjector.[48] This study, however, did not evaluate the economic burden of FA among adults.

RACIAL DIFFERENCES IN FOOD ALLERGY–RELATED QUALITY OF LIFE AND PSYCHOSOCIAL BURDEN

Even after adjusting for parental income and education, black food-allergic patients are more likely to describe challenges with food insecurity and inability to pay for necessary medication[44]—both likely determinants of greater FA-related psychosocial burden.

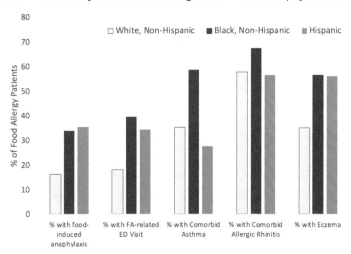

Fig. 2. Burden of food allergy by race and ethnicity. (*Data from* Mahdavinia M, Fox SR, Smith BM, et al. Racial Differences in Food Allergy Phenotype and Health Care Utilization among US Children. J Allergy Clin Immunol Pract 17;5(2):352-357.e351.)

Despite the importance of FA-related quality of life as a patient-reported outcome, there are no published epidemiologic studies that have attempted to systematically compare FA-related psychosocial burden and/or quality of life across major racial/ethnic strata in the United States. For example, the only large (N >1000) published study to date administering a validated instrument (the FA quality of life questionnaire–parent form) to a national sample of US families did not assess participant race.[49]

One notable study of 103 caregivers of food-allergic children recruited from an urban, mid-Atlantic FA clinic did observe remarkable racial/ethnic heterogeneity in FA perceptions and parent-proxy–reported psychosocial burden[50]—with African American caregivers reporting the lowest perceived risk of allergen exposure, but the highest FA-related worry of all racial groups. In contrast, Asian-American caregivers reported the highest perceived risk of allergen exposure and Hispanic caregivers reported the greatest perceived FA severity, while also reporting the lowest perceived burden with respect to the day-to-day management of their child's FA. Another recent study of FA-related quality of life found that Asian patients and parents reported significantly worse pediatric FA-related quality of life relative to their white and black counterparts.[51] At the same time, no differences were observed in patient/parent-reported pediatric FA-related quality of life when comparing patients/parents of children insured through Medicaid compared with privately insured patients. More work is needed, however, to better contextualize these apparent racial differences in patient/caregiver perceptions and determine to what extent they can be generalized to adult patients.

Another study of 80 parent-child dyads found that the children with FA had significantly higher overall scores on the Multidimensional Anxiety Scale for Children as well as on the Humiliation/Rejection and Social Anxiety subscales.[52] FA was not associated, however, with child depression symptoms nor was there a significant difference in anxiety or depression symptoms among caregivers of patients with and without FA. These data suggest that FA appears to be associated with greater social anxiety and greater anxiety overall, but not depressive symptoms, among low socioeconomic status (SES) racial/ethnic minority children. Although the aforementioned studies provide useful information, further research is needed to better characterize psychosocial burden within larger, more nationally representative cohorts of racially diverse FA patients, which can inform future psychosocial interventions. For example, a recent publication from the multisite FORWARD study found that although black children were approximately twice as likely to report bullying victimization for any reason compared with white children (39% vs 18%, respectively), there were no significant racial differences in the overall rates of FA-related bullying and rates of FA-related bullying were higher among white adolescents versus black adolescents greater than or equal to 11 years old. As the FORWARD cohort ages and additional patients are enrolled, including Latinx families, further insights from this National Institutes of Health–supported study are anticipated.[53]

RACIAL DIFFERENCES IN FOOD ALLERGY KNOWLEDGE AND CLINICAL EDUCATION

To help ensure the health and safety of FA patients, it is crucial that they and those around them—especially parents/caregivers—are knowledgeable regarding FA management. Being knowledgeable about allergen avoidance and common routes of accidental exposures as well as signs/symptoms of anaphylaxis and its emergency treatment can empower patients and those around them to engage in more effective advocacy for their well-being, potentially reducing their risk of adverse outcomes. A 2020 qualitative review highlighted work indicating that lower levels of FA knowledge have been associated with poorer FA-related quality of life.[54] Findings from a survey assessing FA knowledge administered in 2009 to members of the general adult public found that black and Hispanic survey respondents were less likely to identify common FA triggers relative to their white counterparts.[55] Black, Hispanic, and Asian adults also were less likely than white adults to identify signs of a milk allergy. Black and Hispanic survey respondents, however, were more likely to note the importance of food allergen avoidance. Additionally, preliminary data from the FORWARD study also suggest that FA knowledge differs by race among parents of children with FA.[56]

A 2020 study by Luke and Flessner[57] surveyed parents of children with FA and found that FA knowledge was significantly lower among parents of racial/ethnic minority FA patients, as well as patients in low-income households. The investigators concluded that parents with low income and/or are of a racial/ethnic minority status may be at risk of FA mismanagement and may benefit from targeted educational interventions.[57]

RACIAL DIFFERENCES IN NON–IMMUNOGLOBULIN E–MEDIATED FOOD ALLERGY

Although racial/ethnic differences in IgE-mediated FA increasingly have been studied, there is a paucity of literature on potential racial/ethnic variations in non–IgE-mediated FAs. Previously, food protein–induced enterocolitis syndrome (FPIES) primarily has been studied in white populations. Racial differences in FPIES phenotypes may exist, however, as suggested by a study of Japanese infants with FPIES.[58,59] These infants presented with symptoms, including vomiting, bloody stool, and/or fever, whereas some also exhibited positive cow's milk–specific IgE antibody levels. Bloody stool and positive food-specific IgE antibodies reportedly are rare among FPIES patients in Western countries but in the aforementioned Japanese sample of infants with FPIES, bloody stool occurred among 47% of patients and milk-specific IgE antibodies were positive among 32% of patients.[59] Although further exploration of racial differences is necessary, a US population–based survey of FA prevalence also suggests that children with FPIES are more likely to be Asian.[60]

Additionally, racial differences can be observed in other non–IgE-mediated FAs besides FPIES. In a prevalence study of celiac disease using data from NHANES from 2009 to 2012, the prevalence of celiac disease was 4-times to 8-times higher among white individuals compared with other races. Differences in eosinophilic esophagitis (EoE) outcomes by race also been have observed; however, there remains a gap in knowledge concerning reasons for these differences and population-level inferences of EoE by race. Previous studies suggest that EoE patients are more likely to be white,[61] although EoE can occur among other racial/ethnic groups and African American children may have a larger EoE burden.[62] EoE symptoms may differ by race because African American children have been previously more likely to report failure to thrive[62,63] whereas dysphagia is more common among whites.[64] These studies note, however, that age of symptom presentation and diagnosis can have an impact on symptoms presented and noted that after accounting for age, racial differences in symptoms were not as apparent. Failure to thrive and vomiting are common among younger children, and African American children may present with EoE onset at a younger age, which could explain the racial differences initially observed.[62]

BEYOND RACIAL/ETHNIC DIFFERENCES—THE IMPORTANCE OF SOCIOECONOMIC STATUS

Although this review is intended to focus on racial/ethnic differences in FA, it is essential to note that the independent effects of ethnicity on the etiology of food-allergic

Table 1
Recommended practices for assessment of socioeconomic status in health research

Socioeconomic Status Indicator	How to Assess
Education	• Measure in single years completed up to 5 or more years of college and also should include collection of information on whether the individual obtained a high school diploma or equivalent. • Surveys also should collect information on degree attainment.
Income	• Income should be asked for the individual survey respondent and for the respondent's entire family as well as household income. • Collected income information should include the measurement of total income, earned or unearned, from specific sources (wages and salaries, dividends and interest, Social Security, unemployment insurance, disability income, etc.)
Occupation	• Occupation should be measured at a minimum by a set of 2 standardized questions: 1 question to collect occupation and 1 question to collect industry. • Additional information about work tasks and employer also should be considered.
Family size and relationships	• Given that family size and household composition are required to calculate poverty, survey measures should collect information on family size and household composition in compliance with official federal poverty guidelines as issued and published each year.

Data from Statistics NCoVaH. Development of Standards for the Collection of Socioeconomic Status in Health Surveys Conducted by the Department of Health and Human Services. 2012; https://www.ncvhs.hhs.gov/wp-content/uploads/2014/05/120622lt.pdf.

disease are difficult to disentangle from other frequently associated socioenvironmental factors. These include the putative environmental determinants of childhood atopy assessed by the aforementioned cohort studies (eg, environmental tobacco smoke, diet, air pollution, dust mite, and cockroach exposure) as well as SES, which is an important determinant of health care access and quality. SES also is highly correlated with the presence of both chronic and acute stressors (eg, adverse childhood experiences[42,65]), which can have profound health effects including proinflammatory immunologic effects.[66]

The National Committee on Vital and Health Statistics has issued a set of recommendations aiming to standardize the assessment of the following key indicators of SES: education, income, occupation, and family size/relationships. These recommendations are summarized in **Table 1**.

Although education, income, and occupation are core elements of SES assessment, there are other complementary domains that also should be considered. The American Psychological Association Stop Skipping Class initiative has highlighted the potential importance of considering subjective social status, occupational prestige, absolute poverty, relative poverty, and additional resource-based SES measures beyond household income when assessing SES. Further detail regarding each of these is provided in a review by Diemer and colleagues[67] as well as resources available at the MacArthur Research Network on SES and Health.[68]

SUMMARY

By improving and expanding assessment of SES in FA research, the social context of study participants can be contextualized better and therefore understanding improved of the complex role of race/ethnicity as a determinant of FA outcomes. In this way, insights can be gained into the most promising and effective strategies for reducing the disproportionate burden that FA places on specific racial/ethnic minority communities.

CLINICS CARE POINTS

- This synthesis of the latest epidemiologic data suggests that the burden of FA falls disproportionately on North American racial/ethnic minority populations.

- Further research should focus on better characterizing psychosocial burden among larger nationally representative racial/ethnically diverse FA patient populations to inform interventions to improve FA management and outcomes among vulnerable populations.

- It is crucial that future epidemiologic and clinical research studies incorporate more rigorous, standardized assessment of SES—in addition to race/ethnicity—to inform interventions that can advance equity in FA management and outcomes.

DISCLOSURE

Dr R.S. Gupta received grants from the National Institutes of Health (NIH) during the conduct of the study and from Stanford Sean N. Parker Center for Allergy Research, UnitedHealth Group, Thermo Fisher Scientific, Genentech, and the National Confectioners Association as well as personal fees from Before Brands, Kaléo Inc, Genentech, Institute for Clinical and Economic Review, Food Allergy Research & Education, Aimmune Therapeutics, and DBV Technologies outside the submitted work. No other disclosures are reported.

REFERENCES

1. Warren CM, Jiang J, Gupta RS. Epidemiology and Burden of Food Allergy. Curr Allergy asthma Rep 2020;20(2):6.
2. Gupta RS, Warren CM, Smith BM, et al. The public health impact of parent-reported childhood food allergies in the United States. Pediatrics 2018;142(6): e20181235.
3. Gupta RS, Warren CM, Smith BM, et al. Prevalence and severity of food allergies among US adults. JAMA Netw Open 2019;2(1):e185630.
4. Sicherer SH, Warren CM, Dant C, et al. Food allergy from infancy through adulthood. J Allergy Clin Immunol Pract 2020;8(6):1854–64.
5. Pali-Schöll I, Jensen-Jarolim E. Gender aspects in food allergy. Curr Opin Allergy Clin Immunol 2019;19(3):249–55.
6. Kelly C, Gangur V. Sex disparity in food allergy: evidence from the pubmed database. J Allergy 2009;2009:159845.
7. Gupta RS, Springston EE, Smith B, et al. Geographic variability of childhood food allergy in the United States. Clin Pediatr 2012;51(9):856–61.
8. Goossens NJ, Flokstra-de Blok BM, van der Meulen GN, et al. Health-related quality of life in food-allergic adults from eight European countries. Ann Allergy Asthma Immunol 2014;113(1):63–8.e61.
9. Kumar R, Tsai HJ, Hong X, et al. Race, ancestry, and development of food-allergen sensitization in early childhood. Pediatrics 2011;128(4):e821–9.

10. Mahdavinia M, Fox SR, Smith BM, et al. Racial differences in food allergy pheno-type and health care utilization among US children. J Allergy Clin Immunol Pract 2017;5(2):352–7.e1.

11. Ford ME, Kelly PA. Conceptualizing and categorizing race and ethnicity in health services research. Health Serv Res 2005;40(5 Pt 2):1658–75.

12. Bureau USC. Hispanic origin. 2020. Available at: https://www.census.gov/topics/population/hispanic-origin.html. Accessed September 22, 2020.

13. Khanna N, Harris CA. Teaching race as a social construction: two interactive class exercises. Teach Sociol 2009;37(4):369–78.

14. Noe-Bustamante L, Mora L, Lopez MH. About one-in-four U.S. Hispanics have heard of Latinx, but just 3% use it. Washington, DC: Pew Research Center; 2020.

15. Egede LE. Race, ethnicity, culture, and disparities in health care. J Gen Intern Med 2006;21(6):667–9.

16. Pickett REM, Saperstein A, Penner AM. Placing racial classification in context. Socius 2019;5. https://doi.org/10.1177/2378023119851016.

17. Oppenheimer GM. Paradigm lost: race, ethnicity, and the search for a new pop-ulation taxonomy. Am J Public Health 2001;91(7):1049–55.

18. Akinbami LJ, Simon AE, Rossen LM. Changing trends in asthma prevalence among children. Pediatrics 2016;137(1):1–7.

19. Canino G, McQuaid EL, Rand CS. Addressing asthma health disparities: a multi-level challenge. J Allergy Clin Immunol 2009;123(6):1209–17 [quiz: 1218–9].

20. Kim Y, Blomberg M, Rifas-Shiman SL, et al. Racial/ethnic differences in incidence and persistence of childhood atopic dermatitis. J Invest Dermatol 2019;139(4): 827–34.

21. Brunner PM, Guttman-Yassky E. Racial differences in atopic dermatitis. Ann Al-lergy Asthma Immunol 2019;122(5):449–55.

22. Silverberg JI. Racial and ethnic disparities in atopic dermatitis. Curr Dermatol Rep 2015;4(1):44–8.

23. Shaw TE, Currie GP, Koudelka CW, et al. Eczema prevalence in the United States: data from the 2003 National Survey of Children's Health. J Invest Dermatol 2011; 131(1):67–73.

24. Wegienka G, Havstad S, Joseph CL, et al. Racial disparities in allergic outcomes in African Americans emerge as early as age 2 years. Clin Exp Allergy 2012; 42(6):909–17.

25. Sicherer SH, Muñoz-Furlong A, Burks AW, et al. Prevalence of peanut and tree nut allergy in the US determined by a random digit dial telephone survey. J Allergy Clin Immunol 1999;103(4):559–62.

26. Sicherer SH, Muñoz-Furlong A, Godbold JH, et al. US prevalence of self-reported peanut, tree nut, and sesame allergy: 11-year follow-up. J Allergy Clin Immunol 2010;125(6):1322–6.

27. Sicherer SH, Muñoz-Furlong A, Sampson HA. Prevalence of seafood allergy in the United States determined by a random telephone survey. J Allergy Clin Immu-nol 2004;114(1):159–65.

28. Sicherer SH, Muñoz-Furlong A, Sampson HA. Prevalence of peanut and tree nut allergy in the United States determined by means of a random digit dial tele-phone survey: a 5-year follow-up study. J Allergy Clin Immunol 2003;112(6): 1203–7.

29. Council TAaAFoAaTNP. Ethnic Disparities in the Burden and Treatment of Asthma. 2005.

30. Gupta RS, Springston EE, Warrier MR, et al. The prevalence, severity, and distribution of childhood food allergy in the United States. Pediatrics 2011;128(1): e9–17.

31. Keet CA, Savage JH, Seopaul S, et al. Temporal trends and racial/ethnic disparity in self-reported pediatric food allergy in the United States. Ann Allergy Asthma Immunol 2014;112(3):222–9.e3.

32. Warren CM, Chadha AS, Sicherer SH, et al. Prevalence and Severity of Sesame Allergy in the United States. JAMA Netw Open 2019;2(8):e199144.

33. Akinbami LJ, Moorman JE, Bailey C, et al. Trends in asthma prevalence, health care use, and mortality in the United States, 2001-2010. NCHS Data Brief 2012;(94):1–8.

34. Szentpetery SE, Forno E, Canino G, et al. Asthma in Puerto Ricans: Lessons from a high-risk population. J Allergy Clin Immunol 2016;138(6):1556–8.

35. Soller L, Ben-Shoshan M, Harrington DW, et al. Prevalence and predictors of food allergy in Canada: a focus on vulnerable populations. J Allergy Clin Immunol Pract 2015;3(1):42–9.

36. Harrington DW, Wilson K, Elliott SJ, et al. Diagnosis and treatment of food allergies in off-reserve Aboriginal children in Canada. Can Geographer/Le Géographe canadien 2013;57(4):431–40.

37. Coulson E, Rifas-Shiman SL, Sordillo J, et al. Racial, ethnic, and socioeconomic differences in adolescent food allergy. J Allergy Clin Immunol Pract 2020;8(1): 336–8.e3.

38. Joseph CL, Zoratti EM, Ownby DR, et al. Exploring racial differences in IgE-mediated food allergy in the WHEALS birth cohort. Ann Allergy Asthma Immunol 2016;116(3):219–24.e1.

39. McGowan EC, Matsui EC, Peng R, et al. Racial/ethnic and socioeconomic differences in self-reported food allergy among food-sensitized children in National Health and Nutrition Examination Survey III. Ann Allergy Asthma Immunol 2016; 117(5):570–2.e3.

40. Wegienka G, Johnson CC, Zoratti E, et al. Racial differences in allergic sensitization: recent findings and future directions. Curr Allergy asthma Rep 2013;13(3): 255–61.

41. Jiang J, Dinakar C, Fierstein JL, et al. Food allergy among Asian Indian immigrants in the United States. J Allergy Clin Immunol Pract 2020;8(5):1740–2.

42. Perkin MR, Bahnson HT, Logan K, et al. Factors influencing adherence in a trial of early introduction of allergenic food. J Allergy Clin Immunol 2019;144(6): 1595–605.

43. Jerschow E, Lin RY, Scaperotti MM, et al. Fatal anaphylaxis in the United States, 1999-2010: temporal patterns and demographic associations. J Allergy Clin Immunol 2014;134(6):1318–28.e7.

44. Johns CB, Savage JH. Access to health care and food in children with food allergy. J Allergy Clin Immunol 2014;133(2):582–5.

45. Wang HT, Warren CM, Gupta RS, et al. Prevalence and characteristics of shellfish allergy in the pediatric population of the United States. J Allergy Clin Immunol Pract 2020;8(4):1359–70.e2.

46. Gupta R, Holdford D, Bilaver L, et al. The economic impact of childhood food allergy in the United States. JAMA Pediatr 2013;167(11):1026–31.

47. Bilaver LA, Kester KM, Smith BM, et al. Socioeconomic disparities in the economic impact of childhood food allergy. Pediatrics 2016;137(5):e20153678.

48. Warren CM, Zaslavsky JM, Kan K, et al. Epinephrine auto-injector carriage and use practices among US children, adolescents, and adults. Ann Allergy Asthma Immunol 2018;121(4):479–89.e2.

49. DunnGalvin A, Koman E, Raver E, et al. An examination of the food allergy quality of life questionnaire performance in a countrywide american sample of children: cross-cultural differences in age and impact in the United States and Europe. J Allergy Clin Immunol Pract 2017;5(2):363–8.e2.

50. Widge AT, Flory E, Sharma H, et al. Food allergy perceptions and health-related quality of life in a racially diverse sample. Children (Basel, Switzerland) 2018; 5(6):70.

51. Rubeiz C, Siddiqui J, Ernst M, et al. A041 race/ethnicity and socioeconomic status effect on food allergy-related quality of life in children and caregivers. Ann Allergy Asthma Immunol 2020;125(5):S8.

52. Goodwin RD, Rodgin S, Goldman R, et al. Food allergy and anxiety and depression among ethnic minority children and their caregivers. J Pediatr 2017;187: 258–64.e1.

53. Brown D, Negris O, Gupta R, et al. Food allergy-related bullying and associated peer dynamics among Black and White children in the FORWARD study. Ann Allergy Asthma Immunol 2020. https://doi.org/10.1016/j.anai.2020.10.013.

54. Moen ØL, Opheim E, Trollvik A. Parents experiences raising a child with food allergy; a qualitative review. J Pediatr Nurs 2019;46:e52–63.

55. Gupta RS, Kim JS, Springston EE, et al. Food allergy knowledge, attitudes, and beliefs in the United States. Ann Allergy Asthma Immunol 2009;103(1):43–50.

56. Jiang J, Bilaver L, Warren C, et al. A305 differences in food allergy knowledge between black and white parents in the forward study. Ann Allergy Asthma Immunol 2019;123(5, Supplement):S10–1.

57. Luke AK, Flessner CA. Examining differences in parent knowledge about pediatric food allergies. J Pediatr Psychol 2020;45(1):101–9.

58. Nowak-Węgrzyn A, Chehade M, Groetch ME, et al. International consensus guidelines for the diagnosis and management of food protein–induced enterocolitis syndrome: Executive summary—Workgroup Report of the Adverse Reactions to Foods Committee, American Academy of Allergy, Asthma & Immunology. J Allergy Clin Immunol 2017;139(4):1111–26.e4.

59. Nomura I, Morita H, Ohya Y, et al. Non–IgE-mediated gastrointestinal food allergies: distinct differences in clinical phenotype between Western Countries and Japan. Curr Allergy asthma Rep 2012;12(4):297–303.

60. Nowak-Wegrzyn A, Warren CM, Brown-Whitehorn T, et al. Food protein-induced enterocolitis syndrome in the US population-based study. J Allergy Clin Immunol 2019;144(4):1128–30.

61. Liacouras CA, Furuta GT, Hirano I, et al. Eosinophilic esophagitis: updated consensus recommendations for children and adults. J Allergy Clin Immunol 2011;128(1):3–20.e26 [quiz: 21–2].

62. Weiler T, Mikhail I, Singal A, et al. Racial differences in the clinical presentation of pediatric eosinophilic esophagitis. J Allergy Clin Immunol Pract 2014;2(3):320–5.

63. Sperry SL, Woosley JT, Shaheen NJ, et al. Influence of race and gender on the presentation of eosinophilic esophagitis. Am J Gastroenterol 2012;107(2): 215–21.

64. Moawad FJ, Dellon ES, Achem SR, et al. Effects of Race and Sex on Features of Eosinophilic Esophagitis. Clin Gastroenterol Hepatol 2016;14(1):23–30.

65. Walsh D, McCartney G, Smith M, et al. Relationship between childhood socioeconomic position and adverse childhood experiences (ACEs): a systematic review. J Epidemiol Community Health 2019;73(12):1087.
66. John-Henderson NA, Henderson-Matthews B, Ollinger SR, et al. Adverse childhood experiences and immune system inflammation in adults residing on the blackfeet reservation: the moderating role of sense of belonging to the community. Ann Behav Med 2020;54(2):87–93.
67. Diemer MA, Mistry RS, Wadsworth ME, et al. Best practices in conceptualizing and measuring social class in psychological research. Analyses Social Issues Public Policy 2013;13(1):77–113.
68. Network TMRf. MacArthur Foundation Research Network on Socioeconomic Status and Health. 2008. Available at: https://macses.ucsf.edu/default.php. Accessed September 22, 2020.

Tackling Food Allergy in Infancy

Ashley Lynn Devonshire, MD, MPH[a],*, Adora A. Lin, MD, PhD[b]

KEYWORDS

- Food allergy • Infancy • Atopic dermatitis • Prevention • Oral food challenge

KEY POINTS

- Adverse food reactions, including immunoglobulin E (IgE)-mediated and non-IgE-mediated food allergy, are common in infancy.
- IgE-mediated food allergy diagnosis is based on clinical history and confirmed with skin prick or serum-specific IgE testing. US guidelines currently only recommend proactive screening for peanut sensitization prior to oral introduction in infants with severe atopic dermatitis and/or egg allergy.
- Unless an infant has experienced symptoms after breastfeeding, there are no recommendations regarding maternal dietary modification for the treatment or prevention of food allergy.
- Evidence suggests that IgE-mediated food allergy is preventable through the earlier introduction of allergenic food; however, this is not yet a broad recommendation for all foods and populations of infants.

INTRODUCTION

Adverse food reactions are a common concern in infancy. Nonimmune-mediated susceptibilities are referred to as food intolerances.[1,2] Food allergies are defined as adverse health effects arising from a specific immune response that occurs reproducibly upon exposure to a specific food.[2,3] These immune responses can be categorized based on the immune system components involved: non-immunoglobulin E (IgE)-mediated and IgE-mediated food allergies.[3,4]

With recent changes to infant feeding recommendations, attention has shifted to IgE-mediated food allergy in the infant population. Infancy is often defined as 0 to 12 months of age, a time of tremendous change both clinically and with respect to the immune system. Now, allergists are frequently seeing infants in their clinics for

[a] Department of Pediatrics, Division of Allergy and Immunology, Cincinnati Children's Hospital Medical Center, 3333 Burnet Avenue, MLC 2000, Cincinnati, OH 45229, USA; [b] Department of Pediatrics, Division of Allergy and Immunology, Children's National Hospital, Room 5225, 111 Michigan Avenue Northwest, Washington, DC 20010, USA
* Corresponding author.
E-mail address: ashley.devonshire@cchmc.org

Immunol Allergy Clin N Am 41 (2021) 205–219
https://doi.org/10.1016/j.iac.2021.01.008
0889-8561/21/© 2021 Elsevier Inc. All rights reserved.
immunology.theclinics.com

food allergy evaluation, either for suspected allergic reactions or proactively in the context of atopic dermatitis (AD) or a positive family history.

The following case will be referred to throughout this article to address the assessment and management of infants with suspected food allergy. A 4 month-old male infant with AD was referred to allergy prior to solid food introduction. His AD began around 2 months of age and has been visible daily with intermittent flares. He is bathed 1 to 2 times per day, applying a petroleum-based emollient several times per day, and using prescribed topical steroids twice per day to flares throughout the week. He has had a superinfection requiring oral antibiotics and has disrupted sleep because of pruritus. He spits up frequently and used to cry for an hour every evening, but is now only intermittently fussy. He is gaining weight normally and overall has a happy disposition. He is exclusively breastfed, and the maternal diet has been unrestricted. On examination, his AD affects greater than 50% of his body surface area, and appears erythematous, lichenified, and excoriated. The parents wonder if his regurgitation and fussiness are caused by a particular food his mother is consuming. In addition, the parents have heard about associations between AD and food allergy and are concerned he may already have a food allergy.

DISCUSSION
Non-IgE-mediated Food Allergy

Commonly encountered non-IgE-mediated food allergies in infancy include food protein-induced allergic proctocolitis (FPIAP), food protein-induced enterocolitis syndrome (FPIES), and food protein-induced enteropathy (FPE) (**Table 1**).[5-9] Other non-IgE-mediated adverse food reactions include eosinophilic esophagitis (EoE), celiac

Table 1 Characteristics of non-immunoglobulin E-mediated food allergies			
	FPIAP	**FPIES**	**FPE**
Typical age of onset	Days to 6 months	Days to 12 months	2–24 months
Typical symptoms	Painless, bloody and/or mucous-containing stools in an otherwise healthy infant	• Acute: severe vomiting, pallor, and lethargy; sometimes diarrhea • Chronic: chronic diarrhea and/or vomiting that can lead to nutritional deficiencies and failure to thrive (FTT)	Chronic diarrhea, malabsorption, anemia, hypoproteinemia, FTT
Timing of symptoms in relation to food ingestion	6–72 h	• Acute: vomiting in 1–4 h; diarrhea within 5–10 h	40–72 h
Most common culprit foods	Cow's milk (CM), soy, egg, wheat	CM, soy, rice, oat	CM, soy, egg, wheat
Natural history	Usually resolves by age 1 y	Varies by allergen, but generally resolves by age 3–4 y	Usually resolves by age 1–2 y

Data from Refs.[7-9,14]

disease, and lactose intolerance; these have been reviewed elsewhere.[10–12] Symptoms of non-IgE-mediated allergies typically involve the gastrointestinal system and are usually delayed in onset and/or chronic.[5–8] Diagnosis is based on history, without any role for skin prick testing (SPT) or serum-specific IgE (sIgE) testing, given their non-IgE-mediated pathogenesis.[5–8] Diagnosis is aided by a trial elimination diet with improvement in symptoms, with oral food challenge (OFC) acting to confirm the diagnosis following symptom resolution or to determine if tolerance has been achieved.[7,8] Management of non-IgE-mediated food allergies (ie, FPIAP, FPIES, and FPE) is through strict elimination of the culprit food(s); although foods with precautionary allergen labeling (eg, "may contain trace," "processed in a facility," etc.) may still be consumed.[8] Breastfeeding may continue if the mother is willing to eliminate the food(s) from her diet.[8] Elimination of multiple foods from the maternal diet may not only affect the nutritional health of the mother, but also may impact the nutritional profile of her breastmilk.[13] Thus, strong consideration should be made prior to recommending a multiple food elimination diet for a breastfeeding mother, and, if it is deemed necessary, involvement of a nutritionist is recommended.

Gastroesophageal reflux (GER) and colic are common pediatric disorders that may be seen in the allergist's office, although the role of food allergy in their pathogenesis is less clear. GER is the physiologic passage of gastric contents into the esophagus, and may occur at least 30 times a day in healthy infants, decreasing with age.[15,16] Symptoms include intermittent vomiting, spitting up, coughing, and food aversion.[17] Most infants with GER have a normal examination and do not require treatment.[18] CM sensitivity or intolerance has been implicated in 40% to 50% of infants with GER, based on elimination of CM and OFC.[19,20] For infants with frequent and/or severe regurgitation, food aversion, and FTT, a few week trial elimination of CM can aid in diagnosis of food-related GER, especially if subsequent reintroduction is performed confirming the diagnosis.

Infantile colic is described as unexplained episodes of inconsolable crying early in life.[21] Colic has largely been attributed to intestinal immaturity, hypermotility, alterations in the fecal microbiome, and faulty feeding techniques.[22] Although studies have shown benefits from hydrolyzed formula, soy formula, and low-allergenic maternal diets in breastfed infants with colic, the transient nature and spontaneous improvement of colic render true confirmation of the effect of food elimination difficult.[23] The history of the infant presented previously is consistent with colic, now resolved, and normal GER, which does not require intervention.

IgE-Mediated Food Allergy

IgE-mediated food allergy is a type I hypersensitivity reaction.[5] During sensitization, B cells are directed to produce allergen-specific IgE, which binds to high-affinity FcεRI receptors on mast cells and basophils. Upon re-exposure to the allergen, surface-bound IgE is cross-linked, resulting in mast cell and basophil degranulation and the release of preformed mediators, including histamine and tryptase. There is also rapid synthesis of cytokines and lipid mediators.[24,25] This swift response leads to onset of clinical symptoms within minutes. Signs and symptoms of IgE-mediated reactions have variable severity and affect multiple organ systems (**Table 2**). These signs and symptoms may be more subjective and subtle in the infant population. Anaphylaxis is a "severe, potentially fatal, systemic allergic reaction that occurs suddenly after contact with an allergy-causing substance," and may result in death if not treated appropriately.[26] Clinical criteria center around symptoms in more than 1 organ system and/or hypotension following ingestion of an allergen.[26]

The prevalence of IgE-mediated food allergy among children ages 0 to 2 years in the United States is 6.3%.[27] Allergy to CM is the most common (2.0%) in this age group,

Table 2 Systems-based manifestations of immunoglobulin E-mediated food allergies in infants	
Organ System	**Manifestations**
Skin/mucous membranes	• Erythema • Pruritus • Urticaria • Angioedema • Ear picking or rubbing • Sticking out and rubbing tongue or putting a hand in the mouth
Gastrointestinal	• Emesis • Diarrhea
Respiratory	• Rhinorrhea and/or congestion • Sneezing • Stridor • Cough • Increased work of breathing • Wheezing
Cardiovascular	• Syncope • Hypotension/tachycardia
Neurologic/behavior	• Change in demeanor (ie, irritability, clinging to parent, or inconsolable crying) • Change in mental status or somnolence • Food refusal and/or aversion

followed by peanut (1.4%), egg (1.0%), shellfish (0.5%), fish (0.3%), soy (0.3%), wheat (0.3%), and tree nut (0.2%).[27] IgE-mediated allergy to food appears within the first 2 years of life and may increase or decrease, with decreases associated with tolerance of the food.[28] The likelihood of resolution depends on the allergen. Approximately 70% to 80% of milk, egg, wheat, and soy allergies are outgrown by adolescence,[29–32] with roughly 50% of milk and egg allergies resolved by age 6.[33] Peanut and tree nut allergies are often life-long, with only 20% and 10% resolving, respectively.[34–36]

Diagnosis of IgE-mediated food allergy is driven by clinical history, which informs testing based on the suspected trigger, symptoms experienced, and timing.[5,6] Testing can involve SPT, in vitro serum sIgE testing, and OFC. Skin prick and sIgE testing are used to confirm diagnosis, but alone, these cannot be considered diagnostic for food allergy.[5,6] Specific IgE-based testing using allergen extracts, whether by skin prick or serum, is highly sensitive for food allergy but poorly specific; the presence of food sIgE merely indicates sensitization and cannot predict individuals at risk for clinical reactivity. Prior studies in infants and children show that only 30% to 70% of sensitized patients will display symptoms following exposure to the food in question.[37–40] For patients sensitized to a particular food, size of the SPT wheal or magnitude of the sIgE cannot be used to predict reaction severity and can only serve to determine the likelihood a reaction will occur.[36,39–45] However, most reference values for these purposes have not been standardized for infants.[46,47] In addition, variability in testing results can occur because of differences in SPT technique, biologic composition and quality of extracts, and laboratory methods.[48–50]

Infants are often subjected to indiscriminate testing for food sIgE in an attempt to catch food allergy prior to initial exposure for various reasons, including AD, family history of food allergy, and caregiver anxiety.[51] Unfortunately, indiscriminate testing often leads to further testing, unnecessary food avoidance, and concern for adequate nutrition and growth.[5,52–54] In turn, these consequences can dramatically impact an infant's development and cause undue family stress.[55–60]

Oral Food Challenges in Infants

OFC remains the most accurate tool to diagnose food allergy.[5,6,61,62] However, OFCs require time, trained personnel, and access to emergency resources; additionally, they impart significant risk to the patient. OFCs in infants carry unique concerns. Infants are unable to use words to express discomfort or symptoms, and instead develop changes in demeanor or behavior that may be interpreted as a reaction or normal behavior.[57,63,64] Increased vigilance from the providers administering the OFC is needed to perceive subtle signs of a reaction (see **Table 2**).[65] Another challenge is that infants who are still developing feeding skills can have difficulty consuming standard OFC doses,[57,64,66] either because of satiety or time constraints. An infant who does not react to 50% of the OFC dose but does not consume the complete dose may be still be advised to avoid the food in question, leading some to propose supervised challenges with lower, age-appropriate doses, with continued incorporation of the food into the diet and further dose increases at home, or arbitrarily determining that the infant has eaten enough to rule out the diagnosis of IgE-mediated food allergy.[64,66]

Despite these obstacles, infant OFCs are safe and can be used to diagnose food allergy or determine tolerance. Infants appear to have a low rate of anaphylaxis, with most reactions being mild and cutaneous.[38,39,66–71] Efforts should be made to create an infant-friendly environment including the use of high chairs, the child's own cups and/or utensils, as well as books, toys, and other entertainment. The dose should be age-appropriate and the vehicle, food form, and food texture should be familiar and should not pose a choking hazard. Ample time (eg, 4–6 hours) should be planned for feeding and observation. Ideally, the OFC should be scheduled for a time of day when the infant is usually awake, to avoid complications with feeding or interpretation of the results. The infant should be without signs of illness that could interfere with interpreting signs and symptoms of a reaction and/or could increase the risk of reaction. Infant OFCs should be performed in a monitored setting, with emergency medications available, and by providers familiar with infant vital signs and with clear indications for stopping the OFC, administering treatment, and transferring the patient to more advanced care.[57,61,63,64] If OFC is tolerated, guidance should be given to aim for an age-appropriate serving size of the food at a regular frequency in the diet.[57,64,68,70] If OFC is not tolerated, the infant should be managed in accordance with established food allergy treatment guidelines[72] and the family given counseling to help maintain a healthy perspective on the infant's diagnosis.[64]

Atopic Dermatitis and IgE-Mediated Food Allergy

AD is among the most common pediatric dermatologic conditions, with a reported prevalence in infants and toddlers of 14%.[73] AD is often a reason for referral to an allergist, particularly in the infant population.[74] Among infants with moderate to severe AD, up to a third may have IgE-mediated food allergy.[75] Although acute reactions (see **Table 2**) can be seen with exposure to a suspected allergen, individuals with food-triggered AD may also describe nonimmediate AD flares associated with ingestion of the suspected allergen.

If the infant's history is consistent with an IgE-mediated food allergy, targeted testing should proceed as already reviewed. SPT is typically pursued first given its high negative predictive value and tolerability; however, serum sIgE testing may be required in the case of extensive and severe AD.[75] Both testing modalities are limited by a high rate of false positives, particularly among individuals with AD.[76] In a clinical trial studying infants with AD, sIgE levels to common food allergens were measured, and, based on clinical history, were found to have poor positive predictive value ($\leq$30%).[77] Up to 50% of infants with AD will have evidence of sensitization to food allergens, despite consumption of the food without a history of a reaction or no history of oral exposure, with highest sIgE found among those with early onset AD and more severe AD.[78] If a patient is found to have positive testing, but the history is inconsistent or unclear, an OFC should occur. Of 364 OFCs performed for the diagnosis of food allergy at a tertiary care center among 125 children (96% with AD), 89% were negative.[79] Forty-four children in this study were avoiding 111 foods because of positive testing results, and 93% of OFCs performed in this context were negative.[79]

Data describing OFC-proven delayed AD flares triggered by food are limited. In a retrospective study of 106 OFCs conducted in 64 children with AD, 6 OFCs resulted in isolated delayed AD flares (>24 hours), and 50% of these were triggered by wheat consumption.[80] However, of 364 OFCs performed among 125 children (120 with AD), there were no AD flares in the 24 hours following the OFC.[79] If the patient's history is consistent with a delayed AD flare following consumption of a particular food, it is of utmost importance that the patient's AD regimen be optimized prior to proceeding with any diagnostic tests or diets (**Fig. 1**).

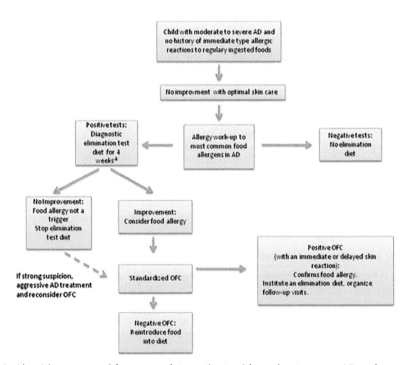

Fig. 1. Algorithm proposed for approach to patients with moderate-severe AD and concern about potential food trigger. [a] (see additional comments in text). (*From* Bergmann MM et al. Evaluation of food allergy in patients with atopic dermatitis. *J Allergy Clin Immunol Pract.* 2013;1(1):25; with permission.)

The decision to prescribe an elimination diet for AD in an infant is challenging, particularly amidst evidence for earlier introduction of allergenic foods as a means of primary food allergy prevention. Elimination diets are not without risk. Among 183 subjects diagnosed with food-triggered AD, nearly 19% developed an immediate reaction to a food without having a previous history of such, and most reactions were triggered by foods being actively avoided.[81] If an elimination diet is prescribed to assess the role of a food in the patient's AD, this should be considered only for a few weeks and, if there is no improvement, the food should be readily reintroduced.[75] If there is improvement in the patient's AD, an OFC should be considered and a conversation about the risks and benefits of an avoidance diet should ensue. The infant presented earlier is at high risk for an IgE-mediated food allergy given the onset and severity of his AD. Prior to evaluating the role of food in his AD, an aggressive skin care regimen should be prescribed and compliance with the regimen emphasized.

Management of IgE-Mediated Food Allergy in Infants

Once an IgE-mediated food allergy has been diagnosed, strict avoidance of the implicated food is of utmost importance. For breastfed infants, questions arise regarding modification of the maternal diet during lactation. Allergenic protein is detectable in the breastmilk of some nursing mothers; however, the quantity and timing are variable.[82,83] The allergenic protein content of breast milk seems to correlate with maternal dietary ingestion[74] and may be immunologically functional; peanut protein found in breast milk can bind peanut-specific IgE and elicit effector cell responses.[84] Among breastfed infants with IgE-mediated food allergy, some may react when exposed to their allergen through maternal milk, whereas others may be tolerant.[85] The reason behind this discrepancy has not been thoroughly studied. Thus, guidelines for maternal dietary avoidance in the setting of a breastfed infant with an IgE-mediated food allergy have not been developed, and recommendations regarding maternal dietary adjustment should be made on a case-by-case basis by a provider familiar with this evolving literature base (**Fig. 2**). The effect of ongoing exposure to allergenic protein through maternal milk on tolerance and sensitization is unclear. An analysis of data from the Canadian Asthma Primary Prevention Study found peanut sensitization at 7 years of age was lower in children whose mothers consumed peanut during lactation and who were orally exposed to peanut before 1 year of age, suggesting the combination of peanut consumption by both the mother and young children may prevent sensitization.[86]

Although a peanut oral immunotherapy (OIT) product has been US Food and Drug Administration (FDA)-approved for peanut allergic individuals aged 4 years and older in the United States, these products have not been thoroughly studied in the infant population. A study of peanut OIT in 9 -to 36-month-old peanut-allergic subjects found that the OIT promoted tolerance to peanut in 80% of the subjects, resulting in their ability to freely introduce peanut-containing foods into the diet 4 weeks after the cessation of therapy. The effect of OIT on long-term peanut tolerance in this age group is not yet known.[87]

Primary Prevention of IgE-Mediated Food Allergy

Given the increased incidence of food allergy, recent research has focused on strategies for primary prevention. After the discovery that peanut allergy rates were lower in communities whose children consumed peanut earlier in life, the Learning Early About Peanut Allergy (LEAP) trial was conducted.[68,88] This clinical trial of early peanut introduction in a group of infants with AD and/or egg allergy found a significant reduction in the incidence of peanut allergy among infants randomized to early, regular peanut

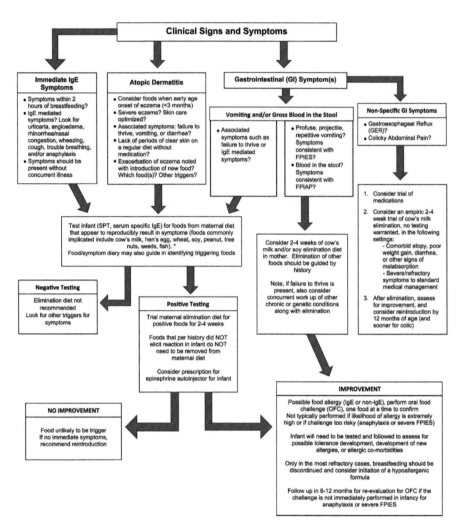

Fig. 2. Algorithm proposed for approach to infants with an adverse food reaction following breastfeeding. (*From* Rajani PS et al. Presentation and Management of Food Allergy in Breastfed Infants and Risks of Maternal Elimination Diets. *J Allergy Clin Immunol Pract.* 2020;8(1):61; with permission.). * Recommend advising against proceeding with panel testing.

consumption.[68] A subsequent trial of 3-month-old, exclusively breastfed infants randomized to early introduction of multiple allergenic foods or standard consumption of allergenic foods after 6 months of age found that among the infants able to comply with the early allergenic food diet, the prevalence of egg and peanut allergy was significantly lower.[70] Follow-up clinical trials of early egg introduction have had variable results; however, a systematic review and meta-analysis of allergenic food introduction did conclude that early egg introduction is beneficial for the prevention of egg allergy (**Fig. 3**).[89] A recent randomized trial of CM-based formula introduction at 1 to 2 months of age while breastfeeding showed a decreased incidence of OFC-proven CM allergy at 6 months of age,[90] providing further evidence that earlier introduction of allergenic foods may prevent the development of food allergy.

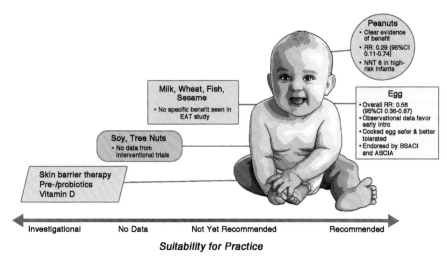

Fig. 3. Status of interventions for the primary prevention of food allergy in infancy. (*From* Bird JA et al. Prevention of food allergy: Beyond peanut. *J Allergy Clin Immunol.* 2019;143(2):546; with permission.)

With these critical findings, professional societies and experts authored guidelines to change infant feeding recommendations. In the United States, it is now recommended that infants with severe AD and/or egg allergy undergo screening for peanut sensitization prior to its oral introduction and, if possible, oral peanut introduction should occur by 4 to 6 months of age.[91] Among infants with mild-moderate AD, oral peanut introduction should occur by 6 months of age.[91] However, these recommendations differ by country. In Australia, experts recommend introduction of allergenic foods within the first year of life, regardless of the presence of atopic diagnoses conveying increased risk.[92] The British Society of Allergy and Clinical Immunology has provided similar recommendations.[93] The infant presented in the previously mentioned clinical vignette should be screened for the presence of peanut-specific IgE with SPT and, if negative, peanut should be introduced and maintained in the diet.

Although the American Academy of Pediatrics (AAP) recommends exclusive breast-feeding as the primary source of nutrition until 6 months of age, breastfeeding has not been shown to prevent food allergy. Modification of the pregnant or lactating mother's diet in an effort to prevent food allergy is not recommended. The AAP previously recommended the use of partially or extensively hydrolyzed formula in infants at high risk for atopy who are unable to be breastfed in an attempt to prevent the development of allergy. Recently, these recommendations were overturned, and hydrolyzed formulas are no longer recommended for the prevention of atopy.[94]

Citing the dual-allergen exposure hypothesis, efforts have ensued attempting to prevent food allergy by targeting the skin.[95] A randomized trial of aggressive emollient application in early life and allergenic food introduction at 3 to 4 months of age found that neither intervention prevented the development of AD by 1 year of age.[96] Similar studies of early emollient application have shown a protective effect against the development of AD[97,98]; however, protective effects against the development of allergic sensitization were not seen.[98]

SUMMARY

Infants may experience IgE-mediated or non-IgE-mediated adverse food reactions. Diagnoses are made based on the clinical history. Signs and symptoms of IgE-mediated food allergy may be different in the infant population, and providers must be aware of subtle manifestations. The epidemiology of food allergy in infancy is likely to change in the coming years, with changes to early life feeding practices and the focus shifting to prevention. Strong evidence supports the early introduction of peanut among infants with AD or egg allergy in attempts to prevent the development of a peanut allergy. There continue to be many unanswered questions regarding food allergy in the infant population, including the effect of breastfeeding and maternal diet on food allergy outcomes, whether early introduction guidelines apply to other allergenic foods, and how current testing modalities utilized for IgE-mediated food allergy perform in the infant population.

CLINICS CARE POINTS

- Both IgE-mediated and non-IgE mediated food allergies can be seen in infancy, and the patient's clinical history is a crucial element in making this distinction.
- The OFC is an important tool for food allergy diagnosis. Providers should be aware of the differences and challenges of conducting these procedures in the infant population.
- Increasing evidence strongly suggests that IgE-mediated food allergy may be preventable with earlier oral introduction of allergenic foods.

DISCLOSURE

A.L. Devonshire does not have any commercial or financial conflicts of interest. A.L. Devonshire is supported by the National Center for Advancing Translational Sciences of the National Institutes of Health (NIH), under Award Number 5KL2TR001426-04. A.A. Lin does not have any commercial or financial conflicts of interest. A.A. Lin is supported by the American Academy of Allergy, Asthma, and Immunology Foundation and the National Institute of Allergy and Infectious Diseases of the National Institutes of Health, under Award Number K23 AI153543-01. The content is solely the responsibility of the authors and does not necessarily represent the official views of the NIH.

REFERENCES

1. Bock SA, Atkins FM. Patterns of food hypersensitivity during sixteen years of double-blind, placebo-controlled food challenges. J Pediatr 1990;117(4):561–7.
2. Bruijnzeel-Koomen C, Ortolani C, Aas K, et al. Adverse reactions to food. European Academy of Allergology and Clinical Immunology Subcommittee. Allergy 1995;50(8):623–35.
3. Johansson SG, Bieber T, Dahl R, et al. Revised nomenclature for allergy for global use: Report of the Nomenclature Review Committee of the World Allergy Organization, October 2003. J Allergy Clin Immunol 2004;113(5):832–6.
4. Sackeyfio A, Senthinathan A, Kandaswamy P, et al. Diagnosis and assessment of food allergy in children and young people: summary of NICE guidance. BMJ 2011;342:d747.
5. Boyce JA, Assa'ad A, Burks AW, et al. Guidelines for the diagnosis and management of food allergy in the United States: Summary of the NIAID-sponsored expert panel report. J Allergy Clin Immunol 2010;126(6):1105–18.
6. Muraro A, Werfel T, Hoffmann-Sommergruber K, et al. EAACI food allergy and anaphylaxis guidelines: diagnosis and management of food allergy. Allergy 2014;69(8):1008–25.

7. Nowak-Wegrzyn A, Katz Y, Mehr SS, et al. Non-IgE-mediated gastrointestinal food allergy. J Allergy Clin Immunol 2015;135(5):1114–24.

8. Caubet JC, Szajewska H, Shamir R, et al. Non-IgE-mediated gastrointestinal food allergies in children. Pediatr Allergy Immunol 2017;28(1):6–17.

9. Lake AM, Whitington PF, Hamilton SR. Dietary protein-induced colitis in breast-fed infants. J Pediatr 1982;101(6):906–10.

10. Caio G, Volta U, Sapone A, et al. Celiac disease: a comprehensive current review. BMC Med 2019;17(1):142.

11. Gonsalves NP, Aceves SS. Diagnosis and treatment of eosinophilic esophagitis. J Allergy Clin Immunol 2020;145(1):1–7.

12. Heine RG, AlRefaee F, Bachina P, et al. Lactose intolerance and gastrointestinal cow's milk allergy in infants and children - common misconceptions revisited. World Allergy Organ J 2017;10(1):41.

13. Rajani PS, Martin H, Groetch M, et al. Presentation and management of food allergy in breastfed infants and risks of maternal elimination diets. J Allergy Clin Immunol Pract 2020;8(1):52–67.

14. Nowak-Wegrzyn A. Food protein-induced enterocolitis syndrome and allergic proctocolitis. Allergy Asthma Proc 2015;36(3):172–84.

15. Campanozzi A, Boccia G, Pensabene L, et al. Prevalence and natural history of gastroesophageal reflux: pediatric prospective survey. Pediatrics 2009;123(3):779–83.

16. Vandenplas Y, Goyvaerts H, Helven R, et al. Gastroesophageal reflux, as measured by 24-hour pH monitoring, in 509 healthy infants screened for risk of sudden infant death syndrome. Pediatrics 1991;88(4):834–40.

17. Lightdale JR, Gremse DA. Section on Gastroenterology H, Nutrition. Gastroesophageal reflux: management guidance for the pediatrician. Pediatrics 2013;131(5):e1684–95.

18. Vandenplas Y, Rudolph CD, Di Lorenzo C, et al. Pediatric gastroesophageal reflux clinical practice guidelines: joint recommendations of the North American Society for Pediatric Gastroenterology, Hepatology, and Nutrition (NASPGHAN) and the European Society for Pediatric Gastroenterology, Hepatology, and Nutrition (ESPGHAN). J Pediatr Gastroenterol Nutr 2009;49(4):498–547.

19. Iacono G, Carroccio A, Cavataio F, et al. Gastroesophageal reflux and cow's milk allergy in infants: a prospective study. J Allergy Clin Immunol 1996;97(3):822–7.

20. Nielsen RG, Bindslev-Jensen C, Kruse-Andersen S, et al. Severe gastroesophageal reflux disease and cow milk hypersensitivity in infants and children: disease association and evaluation of a new challenge procedure. J Pediatr Gastroenterol Nutr 2004;39(4):383–91.

21. Barr RG. Colic and crying syndromes in infants. Pediatrics 1998;102(5 Suppl E):1282–6.

22. Shamir R, St James-Roberts I, Di Lorenzo C, et al. Infant crying, colic, and gastrointestinal discomfort in early childhood: a review of the evidence and most plausible mechanisms. J Pediatr Gastroenterol Nutr 2013;57(Suppl 1):S1–45.

23. Bergmann MM, Caubet JC, McLin V, et al. Common colic, gastroesophageal reflux and constipation in infants under 6 months of age do not necessitate an allergy work-up. Pediatr Allergy Immunol 2014;25(4):410–2.

24. Iweala OI, Burks AW. Food allergy: our evolving understanding of its pathogenesis, prevention, and treatment. Curr Allergy Asthma Rep 2016;16(5):37.

25. Renz H, Allen KJ, Sicherer SH, et al. Food allergy. Nat Rev Dis Primers 2018;4:17098.

26. Sampson HA, Munoz-Furlong A, Campbell RL, et al. Second symposium on the definition and management of anaphylaxis: summary report–Second National Institute of Allergy and Infectious Disease/Food Allergy and Anaphylaxis Network symposium. J Allergy Clin Immunol 2006;117(2):391–7.

27. Gupta RS, Springston EE, Warrier MR, et al. The prevalence, severity, and distribution of childhood food allergy in the United States. Pediatrics 2011;128(1): e9–17.

28. Shek LP, Soderstrom L, Ahlstedt S, et al. Determination of food specific IgE levels over time can predict the development of tolerance in cow's milk and hen's egg allergy. J Allergy Clin Immunol 2004;114(2):387–91.

29. Kattan JD, Cocco RR, Jarvinen KM. Milk and soy allergy. Pediatr Clin North Am 2011;58(2):407–26, x.

30. Keet CA, Matsui EC, Dhillon G, et al. The natural history of wheat allergy. Ann Allergy Asthma Immunol 2009;102(5):410–5.

31. Savage JH, Kaeding AJ, Matsui EC, et al. The natural history of soy allergy. J Allergy Clin Immunol 2010;125(3):683–6.

32. Savage JH, Matsui EC, Skripak JM, et al. The natural history of egg allergy. J Allergy Clin Immunol 2007;120(6):1413–7.

33. Sicherer SH, Wood RA, Vickery BP, et al. The natural history of egg allergy in an observational cohort. J Allergy Clin Immunol 2014;133(2):492–9.

34. Arshad SH, Venter C, Roberts G, et al. The natural history of peanut sensitization and allergy in a birth cohort. J Allergy Clin Immunol 2014;134(6):1462–3.e6.

35. Fleischer DM, Conover-Walker MK, Matsui EC, et al. The natural history of tree nut allergy. J Allergy Clin Immunol 2005;116(5):1087–93.

36. Skolnick HS, Conover-Walker MK, Koerner CB, et al. The natural history of peanut allergy. J Allergy Clin Immunol 2001;107(2):367–74.

37. DunnGalvin A, Daly D, Cullinane C, et al. Highly accurate prediction of food challenge outcome using routinely available clinical data. J Allergy Clin Immunol 2011;127(3):633–9.e1-3.

38. Osborne NJ, Koplin JJ, Martin PE, et al. Prevalence of challenge-proven IgE-mediated food allergy using population-based sampling and predetermined challenge criteria in infants. J Allergy Clin Immunol 2011;127(3):668–76.e1-2.

39. Perry TT, Matsui EC, Kay Conover-Walker M, et al. The relationship of allergen-specific IgE levels and oral food challenge outcome. J Allergy Clin Immunol 2004;114(1):144–9.

40. Sampson HA, Ho DG. Relationship between food-specific IgE concentrations and the risk of positive food challenges in children and adolescents. J Allergy Clin Immunol 1997;100(4):444–51.

41. Celik-Bilgili S, Mehl A, Verstege A, et al. The predictive value of specific immunoglobulin E levels in serum for the outcome of oral food challenges. Clin Exp Allergy 2005;35(3):268–73.

42. Clark AT, Ewan PW. Interpretation of tests for nut allergy in one thousand patients, in relation to allergy or tolerance. Clin Exp Allergy 2003;33(8):1041–5.

43. Fleischer DM, Conover-Walker MK, Christie L, et al. The natural progression of peanut allergy: Resolution and the possibility of recurrence. J Allergy Clin Immunol 2003;112(1):183–9.

44. Sporik R, Hill DJ, Hosking CS. Specificity of allergen skin testing in predicting positive open food challenges to milk, egg and peanut in children. Clin Exp Allergy 2000;30(11):1540–6.

45. Verstege A, Mehl A, Rolinck-Werninghaus C, et al. The predictive value of the skin prick test weal size for the outcome of oral food challenges. Clin Exp Allergy 2005;35(9):1220–6.

46. Hill DJ, Heine RG, Hosking CS. The diagnostic value of skin prick testing in children with food allergy. Pediatr Allergy Immunol 2004;15(5):435–41.

47. Roberts G, Lack G. Diagnosing peanut allergy with skin prick and specific IgE testing. J Allergy Clin Immunol 2005;115(6):1291–6.

48. Bernstein IL, Li JT, Bernstein DI, et al. Allergy diagnostic testing: an updated practice parameter. Ann Allergy Asthma Immunol 2008;100(3 Suppl 3):S1–148.

49. Hamilton RG. Clinical laboratory assessment of immediate-type hypersensitivity. J Allergy Clin Immunol 2010;125(2 Suppl 2):S284–96.

50. Wang J, Godbold JH, Sampson HA. Correlation of serum allergy (IgE) tests performed by different assay systems. J Allergy Clin Immunol 2008;121(5):1219–24.

51. Sampson HA. Food allergy. Part 2: diagnosis and management. J Allergy Clin Immunol 1999;103(6):981–9.

52. Bird JA, Crain M, Varshney P. Food allergen panel testing often results in misdiagnosis of food allergy. J Pediatr 2015;166(1):97–100.

53. Mehta H, Groetch M, Wang J. Growth and nutritional concerns in children with food allergy. Curr Opin Allergy Clin Immunol 2013;13(3):275–9.

54. Skypala IJ, McKenzie R. Nutritional Issues in Food Allergy. Clin Rev Allergy Immunol 2019;57(2):166–78.

55. Beken B, Celik V, Gokmirza Ozdemir P, et al. Maternal anxiety and internet-based food elimination in suspected food allergy. Pediatr Allergy Immunol 2019;30(7):752–9.

56. Cummings AJ, Knibb RC, King RM, et al. The psychosocial impact of food allergy and food hypersensitivity in children, adolescents and their families: a review. Allergy 2010;65(8):933–45.

57. Greiwe J. Oral Food Challenges in Infants and Toddlers. Immunol Allergy Clin North Am 2019;39(4):481–93.

58. Herbert L, Shemesh E, Bender B. Clinical management of psychosocial concerns related to food allergy. J Allergy Clin Immunol Pract 2016;4(2):205–13 [quiz 214].

59. Lieberman JA, Sicherer SH. Quality of life in food allergy. Curr Opin Allergy Clin Immunol 2011;11(3):236–42.

60. Ravid NL, Annunziato RA, Ambrose MA, et al. Mental health and quality-of-life concerns related to the burden of food allergy. Immunol Allergy Clin North Am 2012;32(1):83–95.

61. Nowak-Wegrzyn A, Assa'ad AH, Bahna SL, et al. Work Group report: oral food challenge testing. J Allergy Clin Immunol 2009;123(6 Suppl):S365–83.

62. Sampson HA, Gerth van Wijk R, Bindslev-Jensen C, et al. Standardizing double-blind, placebo-controlled oral food challenges: American Academy of Allergy, Asthma & Immunology-European Academy of Allergy and Clinical Immunology PRACTALL consensus report. J Allergy Clin Immunol 2012;130(6):1260–74.

63. Bird JA, Groetch M, Allen KJ, et al. Conducting an oral food challenge to peanut in an infant. J Allergy Clin Immunol Pract 2017;5(2):301–11.e1.

64. Greenhawt M. Pearls and pitfalls of food challenges in infants. Allergy Asthma Proc 2019;40(1):62–9.

65. Simons FE, Sampson HA. Anaphylaxis: Unique aspects of clinical diagnosis and management in infants (birth to age 2 years). J Allergy Clin Immunol 2015;135(5):1125–31.

66. Lin A, Uygungil B, Robbins K, et al. Low-dose peanut challenges can facilitate infant peanut introduction regardless of skin prick test size. Ann Allergy Asthma Immunol 2020;125(1):97–9.

67. Bellach J, Schwarz V, Ahrens B, et al. Randomized placebo-controlled trial of hen's egg consumption for primary prevention in infants. J Allergy Clin Immunol 2017;139(5):1591–9.e2.

68. Du Toit G, Roberts G, Sayre PH, et al. Randomized trial of peanut consumption in infants at risk for peanut allergy. N Engl J Med 2015;372(9):803–13.

69. Palmer DJ, Sullivan TR, Gold MS, et al. Randomized controlled trial of early regular egg intake to prevent egg allergy. J Allergy Clin Immunol 2017;139(5):1600–7.e2.

70. Perkin MR, Logan K, Tseng A, et al. Randomized trial of introduction of allergenic foods in breast-fed infants. N Engl J Med 2016;374(18):1733–43.

71. Wei-Liang Tan J, Valerio C, Barnes EH, et al. A randomized trial of egg introduction from 4 months of age in infants at risk for egg allergy. J Allergy Clin Immunol 2017;139(5):1621–8.e8.

72. Sampson HA, Aceves S, Bock SA, et al. Food allergy: a practice parameter update-2014. J Allergy Clin Immunol 2014;134(5):1016–25.e3.

73. Silverberg JI. Public health burden and epidemiology of atopic dermatitis. Dermatol Clin 2017;35(3):283–9.

74. Metcalfe JR, Marsh JA, D'Vaz N, et al. Effects of maternal dietary egg intake during early lactation on human milk ovalbumin concentration: a randomized controlled trial. Clin Exp Allergy 2016;46(12):1605–13.

75. Bergmann MM, Caubet JC, Boguniewicz M, et al. Evaluation of food allergy in patients with atopic dermatitis. J Allergy Clin Immunol Pract 2013;1(1):22–8.

76. Sampson HA, Albergo R. Comparison of results of skin tests, RAST, and double-blind, placebo-controlled food challenges in children with atopic dermatitis. J Allergy Clin Immunol 1984;74(1):26–33.

77. Spergel JM, Boguniewicz M, Schneider L, et al. Food allergy in infants with atopic dermatitis: limitations of food-specific IgE measurements. Pediatrics 2015;136(6):e1530–8.

78. Hill DJ, Hosking CS, de Benedictis FM, et al. Confirmation of the association between high levels of immunoglobulin E food sensitization and eczema in infancy: an international study. Clin Exp Allergy 2008;38(1):161–8.

79. Fleischer DM, Bock SA, Spears GC, et al. Oral food challenges in children with a diagnosis of food allergy. J Pediatr 2011;158(4):578–83.e1.

80. Breuer K, Heratizadeh A, Wulf A, et al. Late eczematous reactions to food in children with atopic dermatitis. Clin Exp Allergy 2004;34(5):817–24.

81. Chang A, Robison R, Cai M, et al. Natural history of food-triggered atopic dermatitis and development of immediate reactions in children. J Allergy Clin Immunol Pract 2016;4(2):229–36.e1.

82. Pastor-Vargas C, Maroto AS, Diaz-Perales A, et al. Sensitive detection of major food allergens in breast milk: first gateway for allergenic contact during breastfeeding. Allergy 2015;70(8):1024–7.

83. Schocker F, Baumert J, Kull S, et al. Prospective investigation on the transfer of Ara h 2, the most potent peanut allergen, in human breast milk. Pediatr Allergy Immunol 2016;27(4):348–55.

84. Bernard H, Ah-Leung S, Drumare MF, et al. Peanut allergens are rapidly transferred in human breast milk and can prevent sensitization in mice. Allergy 2014;69(7):888–97.

85. Netting MJ, Allen KJ. Reconciling breast-feeding and early food introduction guidelines in the prevention and management of food allergy. J Allergy Clin Immunol 2019;144(2):397–400.e1.
86. Pitt TJ, Becker AB, Chan-Yeung M, et al. Reduced risk of peanut sensitization following exposure through breast-feeding and early peanut introduction. J Allergy Clin Immunol 2018;141(2):620–5.e1.
87. Vickery BP, Berglund JP, Burk CM, et al. Early oral immunotherapy in peanut-allergic preschool children is safe and highly effective. J Allergy Clin Immunol 2017;139(1):173–81.e8.
88. Du Toit G, Katz Y, Sasieni P, et al. Early consumption of peanuts in infancy is associated with a low prevalence of peanut allergy. J Allergy Clin Immunol 2008; 122(5):984–91.
89. Ierodiakonou D, Garcia-Larsen V, Logan A, et al. Timing of allergenic food introduction to the infant diet and risk of allergic or autoimmune disease: a systematic review and meta-analysis. JAMA 2016;316(11):1181–92.
90. Sakihara T, Otsuji K, Arakaki Y, et al. Randomized trial of early infant formula introduction to prevent cow's milk allergy. J Allergy Clin Immunol 2020;147(1): 224–32.e8.
91. Togias A, Cooper SF, Acebal ML, et al. Addendum guidelines for the prevention of peanut allergy in the United States: Report of the National Institute of Allergy and Infectious Diseases-sponsored expert panel. J Allergy Clin Immunol 2017; 139(1):29–44.
92. Netting MJ, Campbell DE, Koplin JJ, et al. An Australian consensus on infant feeding guidelines to prevent food allergy: outcomes from the Australian Infant Feeding Summit. J Allergy Clin Immunol Pract 2017;5(6):1617–24.
93. Bird JA, Parrish C, Patel K, et al. Prevention of food allergy: Beyond peanut. J Allergy Clin Immunol 2019;143(2):545–7.
94. Greer FR, Sicherer SH, Burks AW, et al. The effects of early nutritional interventions on the development of atopic disease in infants and children: the role of maternal dietary restriction, breastfeeding, hydrolyzed formulas, and timing of introduction of allergenic complementary foods. Pediatrics 2019;143(4): e20190281.
95. Brough HA, Nadeau KC, Sindher SB, et al. Epicutaneous sensitization in the development of food allergy: What is the evidence and how can this be prevented? Allergy 2020;75(9):2185–205.
96. Skjerven HO, Rehbinder EM, Vettukattil R, et al. Skin emollient and early complementary feeding to prevent infant atopic dermatitis (PreventADALL): a factorial, multicentre, cluster-randomised trial. Lancet 2020;395(10228):951–61.
97. Simpson EL, Chalmers JR, Hanifin JM, et al. Emollient enhancement of the skin barrier from birth offers effective atopic dermatitis prevention. J Allergy Clin Immunol 2014;134(4):818–23.
98. Horimukai K, Morita K, Narita M, et al. Application of moisturizer to neonates prevents development of atopic dermatitis. J Allergy Clin Immunol 2014;134(4): 824–30.e6.

Developing National and International Guidelines

Maurizio Mennini, MD, PhD[a],*, Stefania Arasi, MD, PhD[a],
Alessandro Giovanni Fiocchi, MD[a], Amal Assa'ad, MD[b]

KEYWORDS

• Guidelines • Food allergy • Methodology • Evidence-based medicine

KEY POINTS

- Allergic diseases are considered an important public health problem, and the development of guidelines aims to help health care professionals in an accurate diagnosis and management of such diseases in order to match patient's requirements and provide more standardized procedures.
- The management of food allergy may differ among countries.
- Standardization processes are needed to guarantee the quality of the critical analysis of the evidences and the methodology in the implementation of the guidelines.
- World Allergy Organization applied the standardized Grading of Recommendations Assessment, Development and Evaluation methodology for the first time in the field of food allergy.
- As we consider a cost-effective approach to health care, the quality of evidence and tradeoffs between strategies will emerge to provide care tailored to fit each patient and family.

INTRODUCTION

Allergic diseases are considered an emerging public health problem worldwide, mainly because of the increasing prevalence and the risk of severe and even life-threatening reactions with high impact on quality of life and social costs. Globally established scientific allergy societies are investing their efforts into the development of evidence-based guidelines to help health care professionals for an accurate diagnosis and appropriate management. Guidelines may potentially smooth out the variations existing between the different centers in the different countries of the world.

[a] Translational Research in Pediatric Specialities Area, Division of Allergy, Bambino Gesù Children's Hospital, IRCCS, Piazza Sant'Onofrio, 4, Rome 00165, Italy; [b] Division of Allergy and Immunology, Cincinnati Children's Hospital Medical Center, University of Cincinnati, 3333 Burnet Avenue, Cincinnati, OH 45229, USA
* Corresponding author.
E-mail address: Maurizio.mennini@opbg.net

Immunol Allergy Clin N Am 41 (2021) 221–231
https://doi.org/10.1016/j.iac.2021.02.001   immunology.theclinics.com
0889-8561/21/© 2021 The Authors. Published by Elsevier Inc. This is an open access article under the CC BY-NC-ND license (http://creativecommons.org/licenses/by-nc-nd/4.0/).

EPIDEMIOLOGY

The epidemiology of food allergy (FA) paints a contrasting picture across countries worldwide. International studies found that the overall prevalence of oral challenge-proven FA in children younger than 5 years was only 1% in Thailand but as high as 5.3% in Korean infants and 10% in Australian preschoolers.[1–3]

Although milk and eggs are the most common allergens in early childhood in the United Kingdom, United States, Australia, and many parts of Europe and Asia, distinct differences in prevalence are observed even between countries located within the same continent. The EuroPrevall birth cohort, which recruited infants from 9 European centers with different climatic and cultural backgrounds, found that the incidence of challenge-proven cow's milk allergy was lower in southwestern European countries, such as Greece (0%) and Italy (0.3%), but was highest in the United Kingdom (1.24%).[4] The prevalence of egg allergy was also variable—the highest incidence was reported in the United Kingdom (2.18%) and the lowest in Greece (0.07%).[5]

Differences in Food Allergy Around the World

There are differences in the presence of factors that influence FA development and management in the various regions of the world, including the following[6]:

1. *Genetics:* peanut allergy heritability has been demonstrated in western populations in absence of studies in nonwhite populations; associations between filaggrin null mutations and FA risk vary between different populations.
2. *Atopic dermatitis (AD):* AD phenotypes and skin immune responses differ between Asians and Caucasians.
3. *Aeroallergen cross-reactivity:* variable patterns of cross-sensitization between aeroallergens components and food allergens exist in different geographic regions; cross-sensitization with different aeroallergen components confer differential severity of FA symptoms.
4. *Dietary patterns:* food preparation methods may alter food allergenicity.
5. *Meteorologic influences:* climatic factors (eg, latitude, season of birth, vitamin D status, ethnicity-related vitamin D binding protein polymorphisms) confer differential FA risk.

From this perspective, different national guidelines have been created that consider the FA epidemiology of different geographic area with variable local algorithms for diagnosis and specific prevention objectives.

On the other side, it is necessary to encourage standardization processes that have the sole objective of guaranteeing the quality of the critical analysis of the evidences and of the methodology in the implementation of the guidelines.

APPROPRIATE AND UNIVERSAL METHODOLOGY IN DEVELOPING GUIDELINES

Whatever the pathology and the geographic context to which the guidelines are addressed, there are aspects that need to be respected.

The Grading of Recommendations Assessment, Development and Evaluation (GRADE) collaboration compiled a comprehensive checklist of items linked to relevant resources and tools that guideline developers could consider, without the expectation that every guideline would address each item.[7] The items are summarized in **Fig. 1**.

A fundamental role is played by a Coordinating Committee (CC), which has the following main tasks:

a. Oversight of the development of the Guidelines;

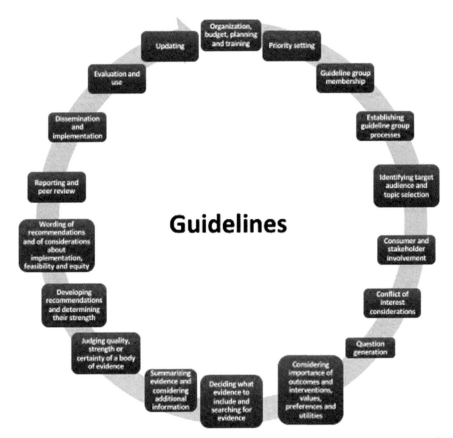

Fig. 1. The items that guideline developers should consider for Grading of Recommendations Assessment, Development and Evaluation (GRADE) collaboration.

b. Review of the Guidelines draft for accuracy, practicality, clarity, and broad utility of the recommendations in clinical practice;
c. Review of the final draft of the Guidelines;
d. Dissemination of the Guidelines.

Along these lines, each guideline is promoted by a CC, who convene an Expert Panel (EP): specialists from a variety of relevant clinical, scientific, and public health areas, with the essential participation of patient representatives.

Every member should be vetted for financial Conflict of Interest (COI) and approved by the CC.

The charge to the EP is to use an independent up-to-date systematic literature review providing a quantitative (when applicable) and/or qualitative synthesis of the scientific evidence, in conjunction with consensus expert opinion and EP-identified supplementary documents, to develop Guidelines that provide a comprehensive approach based on the current state of the science.

A well-recognized Evidence-Based Medicine (EBM) group prepares an independent, systematic literature review and evidence report on the state of the science in FA. The CC and the EP develop an extensive set of key questions, which are further refined in discussions with the EBM group. Literature searches are performed on the most important database (eg, PubMed, Cochrane Database of Systematic Reviews, Cochrane Database of Abstracts of Reviews of Effects, and Cochrane Central Register of Controlled Trials). Inclusion and exclusion criteria are strictly defined in terms of populations, study design, year, and language of publication. After identification of potentially eligible studies, duplicate publications are removed and titles and abstracts of identified studies are checked against the inclusion/exclusion criteria independently by 2 reviewers. Afterward, full-text papers are retrieved if their titles and/or abstracts seemed to meet the eligibility criteria or if the decision could not be made based on the titles and/or abstracts alone. Assessment of the full texts of each retrieved paper is undertaken independently by 2 reviewers using the same criteria. Furthermore, for each key question, in addition to assessing the quality of each of the included studies, the EBM group assesses the quality of the body of evidence. The main tool for this purpose is currently recognized in the GRADE approach, which was developed in 2004.[8] GRADE provides a comprehensive and transparent methodology to develop recommendations for the diagnosis, treatment, and management of patients. In assessing the body of evidence, GRADE considers study design and other factors, such as the precision, consistency, and directness of the data. Using this approach, GRADE then provides a grade for the quality of the body of evidence.

Based on the available scientific literature, the EBM group assesses the overall quality of evidence according to the following criteria[9,10]:

High—further research is very unlikely to have an impact on the quality of the body of evidence, and therefore, the confidence in the recommendation is high and unlikely to change.

Moderate—further research is likely to have an impact on the quality of the body of evidence and may change the recommendation.

Low—further research is very likely to have an important impact on the body of evidence and is likely to change the recommendation.

The EP prepares a draft version of the Guidelines based on EBM group's evidence report and supplementary documents that are identified by the EP but not included in the report.

The EP uses this additional information only to clarify and refine conclusions drawn from sources in the systematic literature review. All the EP members discuss the first written draft version of the Guidelines and their recommendations. Then, the EP incorporates any panel-wide changes to the recommendations within the draft Guidelines. These revised recommendations are then subjected to an initial panel-wide vote to identify whether there is any panel disagreement. Controversial recommendations are discussed to achieve group consensus.

Following discussion and revision as necessary, a second vote is held. All recommendations that received 90% or higher agreement are included in the draft Guidelines for public review and comment.

FROM NATIONAL ALLERGY SOCIETY POSITION PAPERS TO STANDARDIZED INTERNATIONAL GUIDELINES
The DRACMA Experience

Up to 2008, clinical practice parameters for the treatment of cow's milk allergy (CMA) consisted mainly of national allergy society position papers reflecting local views and needs. These were aimed at different treatment strategies and were not always evidence based. For these reasons, it was decided that clinical practice guidelines issued on behalf of WAO would apply the GRADE methodology for the first time in the field of FA.

WAO tried to apply this standardized approach to the management of CMA and developed the Diagnosis and Rationale for Action against Cow's Milk Allergy (DRACMA) guidelines.[11]

Before DRACMA, oral food challenge (OFC) was not part of the diagnostic workup and was indicated only after an elimination period of a few months or on a specialist's advice in more severe cases; this exposed whole populations to overdiagnosis of CMA and excessive use of elimination diets.[12]

DRACMA guidelines strongly recommended OFC for diagnosing CMA to avoid the risk of anaphylactic reactions at home in false-negative sensitization tests, unnecessary treatment for false-positive cases, and inappropriate resource utilization. On the other side, they also indicated that challenge may not be necessary in many cases. Assessing the clinical history, physicians can determine the diagnostic likelihoods estimating the pretest probability of CMA. As examples, the pretest probability will be low in cases of AD or gastroesophageal reflux disease, average in cases of immediate reactions, or high in cases of anaphylaxis. In the latter, physicians reach a highly probable diagnosis using simpler diagnostic tests such as skin prick tests and/or specific immunoglobulin E (IgE) determination.[13]

OFCs remain necessary in all cases of high uncertainty. The search for replacement tests has been very active in the past years. Specific IgE cutoff points, skin prick tests diameters, and/or atopy patch test have been proposed as replacement tests. In DRACMA, the limits of these diagnostic practices are clearly indicated, and their possible use is reevaluated.

The other area in which DRACMA guidelines heavily influenced clinical practice is CMA treatment. Outcomes and their ranking were not arbitrarily chosen but selected from the literature by the expert panel. This method allows the pediatrician to tailor treatment of CMA to changing conditions while observing the recommendations.

The guidelines can affect the market but the reverse should not happen

CC and EP have an enormous responsibility in the realization of guidelines free from conflicts of interest and that reflect a scientific methodology free from any influence.

However, there are factors linked to the geographic context that require the recommendations to be adapted to the population to which the guidelines are addressed.

In the context of CMA, as the cost of the same formula differs substantially from country to country, the implementation of the recommendations may differ. Among DRACMA recommendation, for example, extensively hydrolyzed formula (eHF) is preferred to amino acid formula (AAF), if there is no risk of anaphylaxis. The reason for this approach is mainly the high cost of AAF formula, together with the low palatability of the latter. Based on these considerations, at least an Italian company decided in 2012 to decrease the cost of their AAF by 30%, so that it dropped from 2.4 to 2 times that of eHF. Although the prescription of a specific formula ideally includes economic modeling, the factors in the equation generated in the mind of every single pediatrician is multifold and include the seriousness of the condition, the assessable economic capacity of the family, the psychological readiness of the family to meet with failure of the dietary therapy, and the probability of the refusal of the child due to the low palatability of the formula itself.[14]

The EAACI Guidelines on Food Allergy

The *European Academy of Allergy and Clinical Immunology* (EAACI) plays a crucial role as well in the development of international evidence-based guidelines for different stakeholders in the field of FA. In 2014,[15] the EAACI Food Allergy and Anaphylaxis Group provided evidence-based recommendations for the diagnosis and management of FA based on previous EAACI position papers on adverse reaction to foods and 3 recent systematic reviews on the epidemiology, diagnosis, and management of FA.[16–18] The document offered the current understanding of the manifestations of FA, the role of diagnostic tests, and the effective management of patients with FA of all ages. The acute management of non–life-threatening reactions has been covered in these guidelines,[15] whereas a guidance on the emergency management of anaphylaxis was published in the EAACI Anaphylaxis Guidelines. Evidence level and grade have been provided for each recommendation.[15] An update of the abovementioned EAACI guidelines is ongoing and highly anticipated due mainly to the novelties in the field of FA diagnosis. Recently the updated systematic review on anaphylaxis[19] has been published, and respective guidelines based on GRADE approach are expected soon.

In 2014, EAACI recommended approaches to prevent the development of immediate-onset/IgE-mediated FA in infants and young children.[20] The EAACI Food Allergy Prevention Guideline Task Force has revised the 2014 EAACI guidelines. The guideline has been developed using the AGREE II framework and the GRADE approach. An international Task Force with representatives from 11 countries and different disciplinary and clinical backgrounds systematically reviewed research and considered expert opinion. Recommendations were created by weighing benefits and harms, considering the certainty of evidence and examining values, preferences, and resource implications. The guideline was peer-reviewed by external experts, and feedback was incorporated from public consultation. Key changes from the 2014 guideline include suggesting the following: (1) supporting breast feeding and avoiding supplementation with routine cow's milk formula in the first week of life (low certainty of evidence) and (2) the introduction of peanut and well-cooked egg as part of complementary feeding (moderate certainty of evidence).

Other Relevant International Guidelines

In 2006, an FA practice parameter was published by a task force established by the American College of Allergy, Asthma and Immunology; the American Academy of Allergy, Asthma, and Immunology; and the Joint Council of Allergy, Asthma and Immunology. The document, *"Food Allergy: A Practice Parameter,"* has been an outstanding resource for the allergy and immunology clinical community, but may not have had broad impact outside of this community, and did not use GRADE methodology.[21]

In 2010, because of concerns about different settings for FA diagnosis and the need to distinguish FA and food intolerance, *the National Institute of Allergy and Infectious Diseases (NIAID)*, part of the National Institutes of Health, working with more than 30 professional organizations, federal agencies, and patient advocacy groups, led the development of clinical guidelines for the diagnosis and management of FA in United States.[22]

Based on a comprehensive review and objective evaluation of the scientific and clinical literature on FA, the Guidelines were developed by and designed for allergists/immunologists, clinical researchers, and practitioners in the areas of pediatrics, family medicine, internal medicine, dermatology, gastroenterology, emergency medicine, pulmonary and critical care medicine, and others. The Guidelines included both IgE-mediated and some non–IgE-mediated reactions to food.

The evidences were evaluated through the GRADE approach. US Guidelines were specifically aimed at all health care professionals who cared for adult and pediatric patients with FA and related comorbidities.

Although these guidelines explored the diagnosis and management of FA, the absence of the theme of prevention emerged. The NIAID therefore decided to fill that gap in 2017.[23]

The evidences of a landmark clinical trial and other emerging data suggested that peanut allergy could be prevented through introduction of peanut-containing foods beginning in infancy.

Prompted by these findings, the NIAID facilitated development of addendum guidelines to specifically address the prevention of peanut allergy.

The addendum provided 3 separate guidelines for infants at various risk levels for the development of peanut allergy and is intended for use by a wide variety of health care providers. Topics addressed include the definition of risk categories, appropriate use of testing, and the timing and approaches for introduction of peanut-containing foods in the health care provider's office or at home. The addendum guidelines provided the background, rationale, and strength of evidence for each recommendation.

Other organizations developed, or are currently developing, guidelines for FA. Clinical practice guidelines on FA in children and young people have been developed for use in the National Health Service in England, Wales, and Northern Ireland by the *National Institute for Health and Clinical Excellence* (NICE). These guidelines are intended for use predominantly in primary care and community settings. The model used for development of the NICE guidelines is overall similar to that used to generate some of the EAACI and US Guidelines.[24]

IMPLEMENTATION

The production of clinical practice guidelines alone is not sufficient, and there is a need for implementation strategies for their introduction into daily practice.

The relevance of guidelines is widespread recognized as pivotal. Overall, their dissemination is interpreted as articulating a "standard of care," a standard that has political, sociologic, and even legal ramifications when compared with day-to-day practice. Notwithstanding, guidelines are not always translated to policy or practice.[25] Their limited use contributes to omission of nonbeneficial treatments, preventable harm, suboptimal patient outcomes or experiences, or waste of resources.[26]

The implementation science aims to identify barriers and choose and tailor implementation strategies to optimize their clinical impact.[27,28] Implementation approaches and strategies have been categorized and include characteristics of the recommended practice and patient, provider, institutional, and system-level factors.[29]

There is evidence that many guidelines are implemented using educational approaches, such as workshops, directed at health professionals or patients. Educational approaches are often combined with other more complex interventions such as organizational, financial, or regulatory strategies, which require large-scale change and/or considerable funding.[30] However, the use of single versus multiple implementation approaches and strategies remains controversial, and the choice of the most effective tools should be defined case by case.[31]

CONTROVERSIES

In FA, health-economic models are limited by how health state utilities are derived and generalized. When faced with low-benefit/high-cost care propositions, the role for understanding patient-preference sensitive decision-making, and how this may change over the course of specific diseases, must be clarified. In some population segments such care has higher relative value. This complicates the quest for the "best" practice, which depends on the patient. Today the practicing allergist is part of a complex health care system in a dynamic world. Understanding the broader ramifications of clinical decision-making and appreciating how risks, benefits, and costs become manifest over short- and long-term horizons is key. Providing optimal care incorporates patient preferences at every stage, and these preferences may shift discrete individual values and cost-effectiveness of some interventions. As we consider a cost-effective approach to health care, the quality of evidence and tradeoffs between strategies will emerge to provide care tailored to fit each patient and family.[32]

DISCUSSION

To optimize the clinical management of FA, it is therefore necessary to analyze the state of the art at the national and local level.

From this analysis, the management aspects that need real improvement and implementation can emerge. The questions that need to be answered will therefore arise from these aspects. In this context, the patients' point of view would also be pivotal.

The burden of the disease, the local logistical difficulties, costs, and quality of life are in fact elements that could be affected by the guidelines produced.

The scientific methodological approach described will therefore be the impartial tool that will allow experts to express the best of their knowledge and experience.

Schünemann HJ, describing the work of the GRADE working group based in the field of allergy and asthma, stated that "decisions are like double-edged swords: they always come with benefits and downsides. That is, any decision in life bears desirable and undesirable consequences, even if the latter only involves the time it takes to make or think about the decision, which can be considered the harm of decision making. Therefore, it is impossible to adhere to the Hippocratic Oath's concept of "primum non nocere," which is frequently interpreted as "never do harm." The guiding principle for health care decision making should be to ensure that there is, in summary, more benefit than harm—in other words, "to do no net harm" ("primum non nocere"). Practice guidelines support decision making and, consequently, would require the explicit consideration of both desirable and undesirable consequences, and assigning due considerations depending on the magnitude and importance of the consequences.".[33]

FUTURE DIRECTIONS

The current challenge is to integrate omics into the implementation of guidelines for FA.

Precision medicine aims to empower clinicians to predict the most appropriate course of action for patients with complex diseases.

With a progressive interpretation of the clinical, molecular, and genomic factors at play in diseases, more effective and personalized medical treatments are anticipated for many disorders. Understanding patient's metabolomics and genetic make-up in conjunction with clinical data will significantly lead to determining predisposition, diagnostic, prognostic, and predictive biomarkers and paths, ultimately providing optimal and personalized care for diverse and targeted chronic and acute diseases. In clinical settings, we need to timely model clinical and multiomics data to find statistical patterns across millions of features to identify underlying biological pathways, modifiable risk factors, and actionable information that support early detection and prevention of complex disorders and development of new therapies for better patient care.[34]

SUMMARY

In conclusion, the national and international guidelines for FA should start from an interpretation of the real local and universal needs of patients.

However, the action of the panels of experts should be organized according to a rigorous scientific methodology, capable of bringing out high-quality evidence and therefore universally recognized and applicable conclusions in different clinical contexts.

Guideline statements should be free from conflicts of interest and tested by clinicians in the context of validation workshops. The -omics sciences promise to transform allergy into precision medicine capable of delivering the best for the specific patient.

For now, it is worthwhile to identify what is best for most patients.

CLINICS CARE POINTS

- FA management may differ in various regions of the world based on socioeconomic conditions.
- To standardize FA guidelines, the most effective approach seems to be the "Grading of Recommendations Assessment, Development and Evaluation" (GRADE).
- Guideline statements should be tested by clinicians in the context of validation workshops.

DISCLOSURE

The authors have nothing to disclose.

REFERENCES

1. Lao-araya M, Trakultivakorn M. Prevalence of food allergy among preschool children in northern Thailand. Pediatr Int 2012;54(2):238–43.
2. Kim J, Chang E, Han Y, et al. The incidence and risk factors of immediate type food allergy during the first year of life in Korean infants: a birth cohort study. Pediatr Allergy Immunol 2011;22(7):715–9.
3. Peters RL, Koplin JJ, Gurrin LC, et al. The prevalence of food allergy and other allergic diseases in early childhood in a population-based study: HealthNuts age 4-year follow-up. J Allergy Clin Immunol 2017;140(1):145–53.e8.
4. Schoemaker AA, Sprikkelman AB, Grimshaw KE, et al. Incidence and natural history of challenge-proven cow's milk allergy in European children–EuroPrevall birth cohort. Allergy 2015;70(8):963–72.
5. Xepapadaki P, Fiocchi A, Grabenhenrich L, et al. Incidence and natural history of hen's egg allergy in the first 2 years of life-the EuroPrevall birth cohort study. Allergy 2016;71(3):350–7.
6. Tham EH, Leung DYM. How different parts of the world provide new insights into food allergy. Allergy Asthma Immunol Res 2018;10(4):290–9.
7. Schünemann HJ, Wiercioch W, Etxeandia I, et al. Guidelines 2.0: systematic development of a comprehensive checklist for a successful guideline enterprise. CMAJ 2014;186(3):E123–42.
8. GRADE working group. 2000-present. Internet. Available at: http://www.gradeworkinggroup.org/. Accessed January 9, 2021.
9. Brozek JL, Akl EA, Jaeschke R, et al, GRADE Working Group. Grading quality of evidence and strength of recommendations in clinical practice guidelines: Part 2 of 3. The GRADE approach to grading quality of evidence about diagnostic tests and strategies. Allergy 2009;64(8):1109–16.

10. Schünemann HJ, Oxman AD, Brozek J, et al, GRADE Working Group. Grading quality of evidence and strength of recommendations for diagnostic tests and strategies. BMJ 2008;336(7653):1106–10. Erratum in: BMJ. 2008;336(7654).
11. Fiocchi A, Brozek J, Schünemann H, et al. World Allergy Organization (WAO) Special Committee on Food Allergy. World Allergy Organization (WAO) Diagnosis and Rationale for Action against Cow's Milk Allergy (DRACMA) Guidelines. Pediatr Allergy Immunol 2010;21(Suppl 21):1–125.
12. Fierro V, La Marra F, Fiocchi A. Interpreting the Results of Guideline Implementation: A Long and Winding Road. J Pediatr Gastroenterol Nutr 2016;62:665–6.
13. Fiocchi A, Schunemann H, Terracciano L, et al. DRACMA one year after: Which changes have occurred in diagnosis and treatment of CMA in Italy? Ital J Pediatr 2011;37:53.
14. Vandenplas Y, Alarcon P, Fleischer D, et al. Should partial hydrolysates be used as starter infant formula? a working group consensus. J Pediatr Gastroenterol Nutr 2016;62(1):22–35.
15. Muraro A, Werfel T, Hoffmann-Sommergruber K, et al. EAACI Food Allergy and Anaphylaxis Guidelines Group. EAACI food allergy and anaphylaxis guidelines: diagnosis and management of food allergy. Allergy 2014;69(8):1008–25.
16. Nwaru BI, Hickstein L, Panesar SS, et al. EAACI Food Allergy and Anaphylaxis Guidelines Group. The epidemiology of food allergy in Europe: a systematic review and meta-analysis. Allergy 2014;69(1):62–75.
17. Soares-Weiser K, Takwoingi Y, Panesar SS, et al. EAACI Food Allergy and Anaphylaxis Guidelines Group. The diagnosis of food allergy: a systematic review and meta-analysis. Allergy 2014;69(1):76–86.
18. de Silva D, Geromi M, Panesar SS, et al. EAACI Food Allergy and Anaphylaxis Guidelines Group. Acute and long-term management of food allergy: systematic review. Allergy 2014;69(2):159–67.
19. de Silva D, Singh C, Muraro A, et al. European Academy of Allergy and Clinical Immunology Food Allergy and Anaphylaxis Guidelines Group. Diagnosing, managing and preventing anaphylaxis: Systematic review. Allergy 2020. https://doi.org/10.1111/all.14580.
20. Muraro A, Halken S, Arshad SH, et al. EAACI Food Allergy and Anaphylaxis Guidelines Group. EAACI food allergy and anaphylaxis guidelines. Primary prevention of food allergy. Allergy 2014;69(5):590–601.
21. American College of Allergy, Asthma, & Immunology. Food allergy: a practice parameter. Ann Allergy Asthma Immunol 2006;96(3 Suppl 2):S1–68.
22. NIAID-Sponsored Expert Panel, Boyce JA, Assa'ad A, Burks AW, et al. Guidelines for the diagnosis and management of food allergy in the United States: report of the NIAID-sponsored expert panel. J Allergy Clin Immunol 2010;126(6 Suppl): S1–58.
23. Togias A, Cooper SF, Acebal ML, et al. Addendum guidelines for the prevention of peanut allergy in the United States: Report of the National Institute of Allergy and Infectious Diseases-sponsored expert panel. J Allergy Clin Immunol 2017; 139(1):29–44.
24. Walsh J, O'Flynn N. Diagnosis and assessment of food allergy in children and young people in primary care and community settings: NICE clinical guideline. Br J Gen Pract 2011;61(588):473–5.
25. Gagliardi AR, Alhabib S, members of Guidelines International Network Implementation Working Group. Trends in guideline implementation: a scoping systematic review. Implement Sci 2015;10:54.

26. Pronovost PJ. Enhancing physicians' use of clinical guidelines. JAMA 2013; 310(23):2501–2.
27. Francke AL, Smit MC, de Veer AJ, et al. Factors influencing the implementation of clinical guidelines for health care professionals: a systematic meta-review. BMC Med Inform Decis Mak 2008;8:38.
28. Flottorp SA, Oxman AD, Krause J, et al. A checklist for identifying determinants of practice: a systematic review and synthesis of frameworks and taxonomies of factors that prevent or enable improvements in healthcare professional practice. Implement Sci 2013;8:35.
29. Mazza D, Bairstow P, Buchan H, et al. Refining a taxonomy for guideline implementation: results of an exercise in abstract classification. Implement Sci 2013; 8:32.
30. Gagliardi AR. "More bang for the buck": exploring optimal approaches for guideline implementation through interviews with international developers. BMC Health Serv Res 2012;12:404.
31. Kajermo KN, Boström AM, Thompson DS, et al. The BARRIERS scale – the barriers to research utilization scale: A systematic review. Implement Sci 2010;5:32.
32. Shaker M, Greenhawt M. Providing cost-effective care for food allergy. Ann Allergy Asthma Immunol 2019;123(3):240–8.e1.
33. Schünemann HJ. Guidelines 2.0: do no net harm-the future of practice guideline development in asthma and other diseases. Curr Allergy Asthma Rep 2011;11(3): 261–8.
34. Ahmed Z. Practicing precision medicine with intelligently integrative clinical and multi-omics data analysis. Hum Genomics 2020;14(1):35.

Dietary Management of Food Allergy

Raquel Durban, MS, RDN, LDN[a], Marion Groetch, MS, RDN[b], Rosan Meyer, PhD, RD[c],
Sherry Coleman Collins, MS, RDN, LD[d,1], Wendy Elverson, RD, LDN[e],
Alyssa Friebert, MS, RD[f], Jamie Kabourek, MS, RD[g],
Stephanie M. Marchand, PhD, RD, CNSC, CLC, LDN[h,i], Vicki McWilliam, PhD, AdvAPD[j,k,2],
Merryn Netting, PhD, AdvAPD[l,m,n], Isabel Skypala, PhD, RD[o,p], Taryn Van Brennan, RD[q],
Emillia Vassilopoulou, PhD, RD[r], Berber Vlieg–Boerstra, PhD, RD[s],
Carina Venter, PhD, RD[q,*]

KEYWORDS

• Food allergy • Nutrition • Allergens • Malnutrition • Management

Continued

[a] Carolina Asthma & Allergy Center, 2600 E 7th St unit a, Charlotte, NC 28204, USA; [b] Division of Allergy & Immunology, Icahn School of Medicine at Mount Sinai, 1 Gustave L. Levy Place, Box 1198, New York, NY 10029, USA; [c] Department of Pediatrics, Imperial College, London, UK; [d] Southern Fried Nutrition Services LLC, Marietta, GA, USA; [e] Boston Children's Hospital Center for Nutrition, 333 Longwood Avenue, 4th floor, Boston, MA 02115, USA; [f] Allergy and Immunology Clinic, 13123 East 16th Avenue Box 270, Aurora, CO 80045, USA; [g] University of Nebraska-Lincoln, Food Innovation Center, Room 279c, 1901 North 21 Street, Lincoln, NE 68588, USA; [h] Department of Pediatrics, The Warren Alpert School of Medicine at Brown University, 593 Eddy Street, Providence, RI 02903, USA; [i] Food and Nutrition Services, Hasbro Children's Hospital, 593 Eddy Street, Providence, RI 02903, USA; [j] Department of Allergy and Immunology, Royal Children's Hospital, Melbourne, Australia; [k] Murdoch Children's Research Institute, Melbourne, Australia; [l] Women and Kids Theme, South Australian Health and Medical Research Institute, 72 King William Road, North Adelaide, South Australia 5006, Australia; [m] Department of Pediatrics, University of Adelaide, Adelaide, South Australia, Australia; [n] Nurition Department, Women's and Children's Health Network, North Adelaide 5006, South Australia, Australia; [o] Imperial College, London, UK; [p] Department of Allergy and Clinical Immunology, Royal Brompton & Harefield NHS Foundation Trust, Royal Brompton Hospital, 4th Floor Fulham Wing, Sydney Street, London SW3 6NP, UK; [q] Children's Hospital of Colorado, 13123 East 16th Avenue Box B518 Anschutz Medical Campus, Aurora CO 80045, USA; [r] Department of Nutritional Sciences and Dietetics, International Hellenic University, Thessaloniki 57400, Greece; [s] Department of Pediatrics, OLVG Hospital, PO Box 95500, Amsterdam 1090HM, The Netherlands

[1] Present address: 490 Woodvalley Drive, Marietta, GA 30064.
[2] Present address: Flemington Road, Parkville 3052, Victoria.
* Corresponding author.
E-mail address: Carina.Venter@childrenscolorado.org

Immunol Allergy Clin N Am 41 (2021) 233–270
https://doi.org/10.1016/j.iac.2021.01.009
0889-8561/21/© 2021 Elsevier Inc. All rights reserved.

immunology.theclinics.com

KEY POINTS

- Food allergy management is based on an individualized approach, which includes information on food avoidance and suitable substitutes, equally important to maintain safety and growth.
- To ensure appropriate avoidance and prevention over restriction, up-to-date information is required about label reading, cross-contamination, and allergen cross-reactions.
- The nutritional consultation should also focus on overall nutrition, feeding behavior, and nutritional status.
- The dietitian plays an integral role in providing this information and ensuring that the family's quality of life is maintained.

INTRODUCTION

The World Allergy Organization[1] and the Institute of Medicine[2] state that the prevalence of food allergies is increasing dramatically. This increase is especially problematic in children, who are carrying the greatest disease burden. Worldwide food allergy prevalence ranges from 1.1% to 10.8%. Although prevalence figures differ depending on the country and age studied, the most important prevalent food allergens include milk, egg, peanut and tree nuts, fish and seafood, wheat, soy, and sesame.[2] Adverse reactions to foods are divided into IgE-mediated and non–IgE-mediated food allergies. Although the majority of this article focuses on IgE-mediated food allergies, reflecting current research, where available, data on non–IgE-mediated food allergies is also covered.

The dietary management of food allergies depends on a clear clinical diagnosis and the clinical history is key in obtained the relevant information as outlined in the article by Skypala and colleagues.[3] After the diagnosis, an individualized avoidance strategy includes appropriate avoidance of the trigger food(s), knowledge of suitable alternatives, and ensuring that the diet is nutritionally sound to support optimal growth and oral motor skill development.

FOOD LABELS

The mainstay of safe food allergen avoidance is knowledge regarding label reading. Food allergen labeling laws differ around the world and are summarized in **Table 1**. US food allergen labeling laws are governed by the US Food and Drug Administration's Food Allergen Labeling And Consumer Protection Act (https://www.fda.gov/food/food-allergensgluten-free-guidance-documents-regulatory-information/food-allergen-labeling-and-consumer-protection-act-2004-questions-and-answers), in Canada by the Food and Drugs Act and the Safe Foods for Canadians Act (https://www.inspection.gc.ca/food-safety-for-industry/toolkit-for-food-businesses/sfcr-handbook-for-food-businesses/eng/1481560206153/1481560532540?chap=0), in Europe by the European Commission (https://ec.europa.eu/food/sites/food/files/safety/docs/codex_ccfl_cl-2018-24_ann-02.pdf), and the Food Standards Australia New Zealand (FSANZ) in Australasia (https://www.foodstandards.gov.au/industry/labelling/pages/default.aspx).

Food allergen labeling laws require that food manufacturers clearly identify ingredients considered major allergens using the food allergen's common name. Country or region-specific laws differ regarding which foods are considered major allergens. The US food labeling laws identify the major allergens requiring full disclosure as milk, egg,

Table 1
Food allergen labeling laws in the United States, the EU, Canada, and Australia/New Zealand

		US	EU	Canada	Aust/NZ
Allergens labeled	Celery		✔		
	Crustacean	✔	✔	✔	
	Egg	✔	✔	✔	✔
	Fish	✔	✔	✔	✔
	Cereal containing gluten (excluding wheat)	a	✔	✔	✔
	Lupin		✔		✔
	Milk	✔	✔	✔	✔
	Mollusk		✔	✔	
	Mustard		✔	✔	
	Peanut	✔	✔	✔	✔
	Sesame		✔	✔	✔
	Soybean	✔	✔	✔	✔
	Sulfur dioxide and sulfites [b]	✔	✔	✔	✔
	Tree nut [c]	✔	✔	✔	✔
	Wheat	✔	✔	✔ [d]	✔
Labeling statements allowed	"Contains"	✔		✔	✔
	Allergen emphasized in ingredient list	✔	✔	✔	✔
Precautionary allergen labeling	Voluntary	✔	✔	✔ [e]	✔
	Regulated				
Type of food labeled	Prepacked	✔	✔	✔	✔
	Prepacked for direct sale		✔ [f]		o
	Not prepacked		g		o
Foods covered under allergen labeling laws	Over-the-counter or prescription drugs				
	Cosmetics and beauty products		✔ [h]		
	Meat, poultry, and egg products	i			
	Alcoholic drinks, wine, spirits, beer, and tobacco products		✔ [j]	k	
	Pet foods				
	Fresh fruits and vegetables		i		
	Restaurant foods		i	i	
Exemptions[m]	Highly refined oils	✔		✔	
	Wheat-based glucose syrups		✔		✔ [n]
	Wheat-based maltodextrins		✔		
	Barley-based glucose syrups		✔		
	Cereals used in distillates for spirits		✔		✔
	Lysozyme (from egg) used in wine		✔		
	Albumin (from egg) used as a fining agent in wine and cider		✔		
	Ice structuring protein	✔			
	Fish gelatin used as a carrier for vitamins and flavors		✔		
	Isinglass used as fining agent in beer, cider, and wine		✔		✔
	Fully refined soybean oil and fat		✔		✔
	Tocopherols [l]		✔		✔
	Vegetable oils derived phytosterols and phytosterol esters from soybeans		✔		✔

(continued on next page)

	US	EU	Canada	Aust/NZ
Table 1 *(continued)*				
Plant stanol ester from soybeans		✓		
Soy lecithin used as a release or processing agent	✓			
Whey used in distillates for spirits		✓		✓
Lactitol		✓		
Milk (casein) products used as fining agents in cider and wines		✓		
Nuts used in distillates for spirits		✓		
Nuts used as flavor in spirits		✓		
Celery leaf and seed oil		✓		
Celery seed oleoresin		✓		
Mustard oil		✓		
Mustard seed oil		✓		
Mustard seed oleoresin		✓		

[a] Although gluten does not have to be labeled in the United States, the US Food and Drug Administration defined the term gluten-free for voluntary use. For a product to be gluten-free, it must (1) not contain gluten-containing grains; (2) not be derived from a gluten-containing grain that has not been processed to remove the gluten; and (3) not be derived from a gluten-containing grain that has been processed to remove gluten, but still has ≥ 20 ppm gluten.

[b] Not covered under the Food Allergen Labeling and Consumer Protection Act of 2004 in the United States but must be declared at concentrations of ≥ 10 ppm. In Canada, sulfites also must be labeled when ≥ 10 ppm. In the EU, sulfites must be labeled when in concentrations of >10 ppm.

[c] EU legislation only contains almond, brazil nut, cashew, hazelnut, macadamia nut, pecan, pistachio, and walnut; Canada also includes pine nut. Tree nuts in the United States include all of the above, as well as beech nut, butternut, chestnut, chinquapin, coconut, ginkgo nut, hickory nut, lychee, pili nut, and shea nut.

[d] Also includes triticale.

[e] It is recommended to use "may contain" instead of other precautionary labeling statements.

[f] In effect October 1, 2021.

[g] Allergen information must be supplied to the consumer, but labeling is not required.

[h] There are 26 fragrance allergens that must be labeled if they are present in concentrations greater than 0.01% in rinse-off products or 0.001% in leave-on products. The allergens are alpha-isomethyl ionone, amyl cinnamal, amylcinnamyl alcohol, anise alcohol, benzyl alcohol, benzyl benzoate, benzyl cinnamate, benzyl salicylate, butylphenyl methylpropional, cinnamal, cinnamyl alcohol, citral, citronellol, coumarin, eugenol, farnesol, geraniol, hexyl cinnamal, hydroxycitronnellal, hydroxyisohexyl 3-cyclohexene carboxaldehyde, isoeugenol, limonene, linalool, methyl 2-octynoate, Evernia prunastri, and Evernia furfuracea.

[i] These products are considered nonprepacked foods, and thus do not need to be labeled.

[j] If there is >1.2% alcohol by volume, the product does not need a full ingredient list, but must have a "contains" statement listing the allergens.

[k] Allergens must be declared for beer, but not for other alcoholic drinks.

[l] Natural mixed tocopherols (E306), natural D-alpha tocopherol, natural D-alpha tocopherol acetate, natural D-alpha tocopherol succinate from soybean sources.

[m] No information found for Canadian exemptions besides highly refined oils.

[n] FSANZ Standard 1.2.3: Glucose syrups must have no more than 20 mg/kg detectable gluten to meet the requirements for an exemption from mandatory labeling of wheat.

[o] FSANZ must be able to produce ingredient information, including allergen information if asked.

finfish, crustacean shellfish, peanut, tree nuts, wheat, and soy. Canada covers the same 8 foods and food groups in addition to sesame. In Australia and New Zealand, lupin, a legume, is also required. European food labeling laws identify the most extensive major allergen list including the 8 foods and food groups, lupin and sesame, but also celery, mollusks, and mustard. Sulfur dioxide and sulfites are included by all these countries. Uniquely, though, coconut is considered a tree nut by US food allergen labeling but not by Canada, Australasia, or the EU.

Similarly, food allergens can be indicated in bold or parenthesis in the United States and Canada, but are highlighted by means of a distinguishing typeset, for example, bold or italics, in the EU. In most countries, major allergens must be listed either in the ingredient list or in a "contains statement"; however, the in EU, the use of contains statements are against the law. Labeling laws also differ in terms of which ingredients are being exempted. Irrespective of where the food is being produced, the food labeling should adhere to the labeling laws of the country where it is being sold.

Challenges can arise for families traveling to a country where their allergen is not considered a major food allergen. Only major allergens recognized by the country where sold require full disclosure on product labels. If avoiding an allergen not considered a major allergen, caution is warranted with foods that list natural flavors, colorings, additives, or other vague food descriptions in the ingredient list. The manufacturer should always be contacted if questions arise.

Key points to remember when educating patients about label reading include the following.

- Always check and recheck food labels, because ingredients or recipes may have changed.
- If there is any uncertainty about the allergen content of a food, it is best to call the manufacturer for clarification.
- Useful information about label reading can be obtained from patient and professional organizations.

Precautionary Allergen Labeling (PAL) includes statements such as "May contain…" or "Manufactured on the same equipment as…" or "Produced in the same facility as…." These precautions may follow ingredient lists and contains statements.[4] All PAL indicate that cross-contact with trace amounts of the allergen may have occurred during manufacturing; however, no specific PAL statement indicates a greater exposure risk than the others. PALs are used voluntarily by food manufacturers and are not regulated. The decision to eat or avoid foods with PAL is individualized and should be discussed with the patient and their allergist.

GROWTH AND FEEDING ISSUES IN INDIVIDUALS WITH FOOD ALLERGIES

The onset of food allergies usually occurs in early childhood, a time of rapid growth, cognitive and oral motor development, and a period when feeding patterns are established.[5,6] The mainstay of food allergy management is the elimination of the offending food.[7] Many of the more common allergens contribute essential nutrients during this vulnerable time and inappropriate advice and alternatives may increase risk of growth faltering and nutrient deficiencies with potential long-term effects. Additionally, parental anxiety regarding the food allergy may worsen feeding practices (**Fig. 1**).[8,9]

Faltering growth, in particular low height for age has been reported in children with both IgE- and non–IgE-mediated food allergies.[9,10] The impact on growth is not only seen in young children, but also in young adults with persistent cow's milk allergy,[7] where low final heights were recorded in comparison with nonallergic young adults. There are also cases of more serious malnutrition disorders, including kwashiorkor and marasmus while following an excessive allergen elimination diet, without sufficient dietary support.[11,12] Low intake of crucial micronutrients—particularly calcium, vitamin D, iron, and zinc—can negatively impact normal growth and development.[13–16] Although the impact of nutritional intervention on growth is indisputable,[8,10]

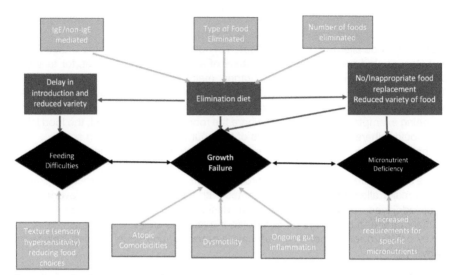

Fig. 1. Interplay between growth failure, micronutrient deficiencies and feeding difficulties. (*Adapted from* Meyer R. Nutritional disorders resulting from food allergy in children. Pediatr Allergy Immunol 2018;29(7):689-704; with permission.)

studies have highlighted the possibility of inflammation, including atopic eczema and gastrointestinal inflammation also playing a role.[17,18]

Feeding difficulties are reported in between 40% and 90% of children with food allergies, depending on the definition used and the population studied.[19,20] Although the majority of the data is produced in non–IgE-mediated allergies where abdominal discomfort plays a role in the origin of the aversive feeding,[21] it is known that dietary elimination changes the modeling around food intake, may heighten anxiety around mealtimes and thereby disrupt the development of a positive association with food.[22–24] There is a clear interplay between dietary elimination, feeding difficulties, dietary adequacy, and growth concerns in food allergy. Parental fear of an allergic reaction with new food introductions, perception of allergic reactions to multiple foods without clinical diagnosis and/or limited dietary education with appropriate substitutes, leads to dietary restrictions, poor feeding skills, and/or maladaptive feeding behaviors that can affect growth.[25] Moreover, studies indicate that having avoided a food for the first year of life owing to an adverse reaction, children continue with aversive eating and limited food choices, even when they overcome the specific food allergy.[6,13]

Optimal nutritional management, therefore, plays a critical role in the avoidance and management of nutritional disorders related to food allergy. Evidence has indicated that dietary input from a registered dietitian improves both growth parameters and nutritional biomarkers as part of a multidisciplinary team.[21,26]

Practical points to consider in the prevention and management of nutritional disorders related to food allergy

1. Ensure that regular and accurate weight, length, height, and where appropriate head circumference measurements are taken and plotted on appropriate growth chart/converted to z-scores using the World Health Organization's Anthro software (https://www.who.int/childgrowth/software/en/).

2. Act early when growth is faltering with optimal dietary management, which includes optimizing protein: energy ratio according to the World Health Organization/Food and Agriculture Organization/United Nations University guidelines outlined in **Table 2**.[27]
3. Assess micronutrient intake of all micronutrients (not only calcium/vitamin D) and perform targeted nutritional blood markers where necessary.[28]
4. Be proactive in feeding advice, to ensure normal oral motor skill development by advising on age-appropriate introduction of tastes and textures.
5. When feeding difficulties are present, in addition to constructive feeding advice,[21] ensure that medical management is optimal and that dietary requirements are met to support growth.

NUTRITIONAL IMPACT OF AVOIDANCE DIETS

Many of the common food allergens are found in core food groups, and the removal of these allergens from the diet will limit essential macronutrients and micronutrients. As such, it is important that appropriate substitutes are included in the diet. **Tables 3** and **4** summarize the main nutrients provided by common food allergens and suitable replacement foods for nutrients lost to the elimination diet. Below follows a detailed discussion of each of the main food allergens: milk, egg, wheat and grains, fish and seafood, peanut and tree nuts, soy, and sesame.

SPECIFIC FOOD ALLERGENS
Cow's Milk Allergy

Cow's milk allergy is one of the first food allergies to manifest in infants because it is the first potential food allergen to which infants are exposed.[29] Worldwide, it is estimated that cow's milk allergy has a prevalence of 1.0% to 4.9%,[30,31] and although cow's milk allergy often resolves during childhood, it may persist into adulthood.[32]

Dietary management of cow's milk allergy
Avoidance of all sources of cow's milk protein underpins the dietary management of cow's milk allergy. **Table 5** outlines the foods that should be avoided, and those that are safe to include in a cow's milk free diet. **Table 1** outlines labeling laws relating to cow's milk protein avoidance.

Cow's milk and cow's milk–containing foods contribute important energy, protein, calcium, phosphorus, and many other vitamins and minerals to the diet, making it essential that a nutritionally equivalent milk substitute is used.[10,31] Cow's milk protein may be found as an ingredient in many foods, including foods one would not expect to find cow's milk (eg, baby teething rusks; tubes of herbs, bread, beef hot dogs, and tomato sauce). Cow's milk protein may also be present in medications, which are not covered by the US Food Allergen Labeling And Consumer Protection Act. Families

Table 2			
Optimal protein: energy ratio according to the World Health Organization/Food and Agriculture Organization/United Nations University guidelines			
Catch-Up Growth	Protein (g/kg/d)	Energy (kcal/kg/d)	Protein/Energy (%)
5 g/kg/d	1.82	105	6.9
10 g/kg/d	2.82	126	8.9
20 g/kg/d	4.82	167	11.5

Table 3
Nutrients provided by food containing common food allergens

Eliminated Food		Nutrients at Risk										
	Protein	Carbo-Hydrate	Fat	Fiber	Calcium	Vitamin D	Vitamin B$_{12}$	Folate	Iodine	Biotin	Iron	Omega −3 Fatty Acids
Milk	x	X	x		x	x	x		x			
Egg	x					x				x	x	
Wheat		x		x				x		x	x	
Soy	x		x	x	x			x		x	x	
Tree nuts and seeds	x		x	x								
Seafood	x		x			x	x		x			x
Peanut			x									

Each food supplies specific nutrients that require attention when the food is eliminated to avoid inadequacies.

Table 4
Substitute foods for nutrients lost to the elimination diet

Calcium	Milk and dairy products, calcium-fortified plant beverages, calcium-set tofu, canned sardine or salmon with bones, fortified breakfast cereals	Children and adults
Vitamin D	Vitamin D fortified foods (in particular, milk and plant-based beverages but also breakfast cereals), Fatty fish, cod liver oil, UV light exposed mushrooms, egg yolk	Children and adults
Iodine	Seaweed, fish, milk, egg, enriched grains, iodized salt	Children and adults
Protein	Meat, fish, poultry, eggs, nuts, seeds, legumes	Children and adults
Fat	Vegetable oils, fatty fish, whole dairy products, meats, nuts, seeds	Children <4 years of age
Vitamin B_{12}	Animal products and fortified foods (breakfast cereals, fortified beverages, fortified nutritional yeast)	Vegan dietary pattern
Omega 3 fatty acids DHA–Docosahexaenoic acid EPA–Eicosapentaenoic acid ALA–Alpha-linolenic acid	DHA and EPA: cold water fatty fish, marine algae-based supplements, algal oil ALA: nuts, (walnuts) seeds (such as chia, flax, etc), canola and soybean oil	Children and adults (especially important for cognitive development in children)
Biotin	Beef liver, salmon, egg, pork, beef, sunflower seeds, sweet potato	Pregnant and breastfeeding
Iron	Fortified breakfast cereals, oysters, beef liver, white beans, lentils, tofu, spinach	Young children, females with menses, pregnant
Folate	Beef liver, spinach, legumes, avocado, dark green vegetables, wheat germ and folic acid in fortified grains	Woman of childbearing years
Fiber	Whole grains, nuts, seeds, legumes, fruits and vegetables	Children and adults

When foods are eliminated, the nutrients lost to the elimination diet should come from other foods and/or dietary supplements.

need to be instructed on how to identify the presence of cow's milk in commercial foods, prepare suitable meals at home (**Table 6**), and avoid the ingestion of cow's milk protein in foods prepared outside of the home, including at school, restaurants, and social gatherings.[33]

Table 5
Foods to choose and foods to avoid in cow's milk free diet

Food/Food Group	Foods to Choose	Ingredient/Foods to Avoid
Milk products and alternatives	The following plant-based milk alternatives: soy, pea, coconut, almond, seed, oat, and rice beverages, plant based cheese, plant based yogurt	The following (fresh, UHT, dried, condensed, or evaporated): cow, goat, sheep, and other animal milks (camel, buffalo), butter, buttermilk, cheese, cream, creme fraiche curds, custard, ghee, half and half, ice cream, milk fat, milk protein, pudding, sour cream, yogurt, cottage cheese
Meats and other protein-rich foods	The following prepared without milk or milk ingredients (fresh, frozen, canned, dried, cured, processed, smoked, or brined): beef, pork, lamb, other meats, poultry, fish, seafood, nut, nut butters, seeds, beans, tofu, eggs (avoid meats sliced on the same equipment as milk containing products such as cheese)	The following prepared with milk or milk ingredients (batters, sauces, toppings, breading): beef, pork, lamb, other meats, poultry, fish, seafood, nut, nut butters, seeds, beans, tofu, eggs (avoid meats sliced on the same equipment that may lead to cross-contact with milk)
Grains	The following prepared without milk or milk ingredients: grains, breads, cold cereals, hot cereals, breads, baked goods, crackers, pasta, pancakes, waffles, chips, pretzels, and tortillas	The following prepared with milk or milk ingredients: grains, breads, cold cereals, hot cereals, baked goods, crackers, pasta, pancakes, waffles, chips, pretzels and tortillas
Fruits	Pure fruits (fresh, frozen, canned, pureed, juiced, and dried)	Fruits prepared with milk and milk ingredients
Vegetables	Pure vegetables (fresh, frozen, canned, pureed, juiced, and dried)	Vegetables prepared with milk and milk ingredients
Fats	Vegetable oils, seed oils; margarine, gravies, sauces and salad dressings made without milk ingredients; canned coconut milk	The following prepared with milk or milk ingredients: butter, butterfat, cream, ghee; margarine, gravies, sauces and salad dressings
Ingredients/miscellaneous	The following ingredients do not contain milk unless otherwise noted: calcium lactate, cocoa butter, cream of tartar, herbs, lactic acid (although lactic acid starter culture may contain milk), pepper, salt, spices	Milk, casein, casein hydrolysates, caseinates, diacetyl, lactalbumin, lactoferrin, lactoglobulin, lactose, lactulose, milk protein hydrolysates, milk protein, recaldent, rennet, casein, simplesse, sour milk solids, tagatose, whey (in all forms)

Table 6
Substitutes for milk in baking and cooking

Ingredient	Substitute
Cow's milk	For recipes calling for 1 cup or less of milk: Substitute equal amounts nondairy, plant-based "milk." For recipes calling for 1 cup or more of milk: Substitute 7 fluid oz. nondairy, plant based "milk "per 8 fluid oz. of dairy milk.
Butter	Allowed margarine, shortening or oil. In baking stick margarine may be preferable to tub margarines
Buttermilk	Add 1 tbsp vinegar (or lemon juice) to 1 cup of alternative, nondairy, plant based "milk."[a]
Cheese	Avocado, bean ,or legume spread, commercially available options
Sour cream	1 cup tofu blended with 1–2 teaspoons lemon juice, commercially available options

[a] Curdling will settle once the item is baked/cooked.

Infants

Cow's milk allergens including β-lactoglobulin have been identified in the breastmilk of some but not all breastfeeding mothers, regardless of the milk content of the maternal diet.[34] For many infants with cow's milk allergy, the maternal diet does not need to be restricted.[35,36] If a maternal elimination diet is required, the maternal diet should be evaluated for nutritional adequacy for maternal and infant health. In cases where infants with cow's milk protein allergy are asymptomatic on an unrestricted maternal diet, unnecessary maternal dietary avoidance should be discouraged.[35–37]

It is essential that infants not breastfeeding are prescribed a suitable substitute formula that is free from cow's milk protein.[37] Hypoallergenic formulas in the United States, must demonstrate that at least 90% of infants with cow's milk protein allergy tolerated them with a 95% confidence interval and extensively hydrolyzed cow's milk protein formulas (casein or whey) and amino acid–based formulas meet this criterion.[38,39] Other potential substitute milk-free formulas are made from soy protein isolate or hydrolyzed rice protein. Infant formula based on partially hydrolyzed cow's milk protein is not recommended for the management of cow's milk allergy.[40]

Toddlers and older children

Children with cow's milk allergy should use a substitute formula or breast milk until 2 years of age,[41] given their extra nutritional needs for growth and development (see section on growth and food allergy). Plant-based fortified beverages can be used in cooking or in cereal for most babies over 6 months of age if there are no concerns about growth. It is important to choose one that has added calcium. A dietitian will be able to advise on the best alternative taking the child's food allergies and nutritional intake into account.[42] However, if there are no growth concerns and/or feeding difficulties, and after a nutritional assessment it is determined that the infant's nutritional needs can be met with a plant-based beverage in combination with the solid food diet, a dietitian may suggest an earlier transition. This point is especially true in light of the proliferation of a wider range of plant-based beverages with better nutritional profiles. Not all of these beverages are nutritionally equivalent to cow's milk; the protein and fat content varies significantly among the various beverages available and the bioavailability of the nutrients may be limited.[33,43] Consultation with a dietitian is strongly recommended to ensure adequate nutrient intake in infants and children with cow's milk protein allergy, especially before a transition from breast milk or formula to a plant-based beverage.

Teens and adults

There is emerging evidence pointing to an increased incidence of cow's milk allergy among teens and young adults.[32,44] The management of cow's milk allergy in this age group becomes more difficult as individuals eat away from home more frequently and become independent in their food choices. It is essential that teenagers and young adults have ongoing education and monitoring with their allergist.[30,31] Alternative sources of calcium can be found in **Table 7**.

Key points regarding cow's milk allergy

- Complete avoidance of cow's milk protein is required unless tolerance to baked milk develops in IgE-mediated allergy. Baked milk can be tolerated by a significant percentage of children with cow's milk allergy and should be introduced timely under allergist recommendations and supervision[45](see section on Baked Milk and Baked Egg).
- Complete avoidance of cow's milk protein is also required in non–IgE-mediated allergy, but a milk ladder may be trialed, if this is local practice, to establish tolerance to baked milk, cheese, yogurt, or other forms of processed milk.
- Plan for adequate micronutrient and macronutrient intake on cow's milk free diet.
- Appropriate formula (in non–breast-fed infant) or plant-based milk substitute (>2 years of age) should be chosen to replace important nutrients and support growth.
- Ongoing management of teens or adults with milk allergy is recommended.

Hen's Egg Allergy

IgE-mediated egg allergy is one of the most common food allergies, with an estimated incidence ranging from 0.5% to up to 8.9%.[46,47] Clinical tolerance to egg is usually acquired by two-thirds of children with egg allergy by 5 years of age; however, recent evidence suggests an increasing persistence of egg allergy with tolerance developing later in childhood.[48,49] Tolerance to well-baked egg (defined as egg mixed thoroughly with a grain creating a matrix, then heated at a temperature >350° F for 30 minutes) is usually achieved before tolerance to partially cooked or raw, unbaked, or less heated

Table 7
Alternative sources of calcium

Category (Serving Size)	Food/Beverage	Calcium (mg)
Beans/Legumes (1 cup or 175 g cooked)	Soybeans (immature)	260
	Navy beans	125
	Black beans	120
Fish (3 oz or 84 g cooked)	Sardines	110
	Perch	85
	Shrimp	75
Nuts and seeds (1 oz or 28 g)	Almond	75
	Chia seeds	180
	Flax seeds	70
Fruits (2 oz or 56 g)	Figs	90
Vegetables (1 cup cooked)	Broccoli	60
	Bok Choy	160
	Collard greens	268

forms of egg.[48,49] However, for IgE-mediated allergy, other forms should not be trialed unsupervised. Eggs contain a wide range of important nutrients including, iron, zinc, protein, and vitamins A, B$_{12}$, and D. **Table 8** provides details on which foods to avoid alongside foods to choose in the management of an egg-free diet.

As an ingredient, eggs are included in many foods to provide binding and aeration. Although commercial egg replacers are available, many other foods can be used in place of egg in recipes. **Table 9** outlines common substitutes for egg in baking and other foods products.

Unexpected sources of egg

Unexpected sources of egg may include the following: pasta, pizza crust, ice cream, candy, and cake frosting. Egg may also be present in craft paints, and children with egg allergy should not be allowed to play with egg cartons owing to the risk of exposure to raw egg. Some traditional cultures use egg white as a topical treatment for burns, which may place the egg-allergic individual at risk of severe reactions.

Key points regarding egg allergy

- The incidence of egg allergy seems to be increasing and has reached almost 10% in some countries.
- Choosing an appropriate egg substitute in baking or cooking depends on whether the egg in the recipe is being used for binding, leavening, or thickening.
- Baked egg tolerance occurs in as many as 70% of children with egg allergy.
- Baked egg or advancement of egg into the diet in IgE-mediated allergy should be introduced under a physician supervised oral food challenge.

Baked Milk and Baked Egg

Heating disrupts the structure of the conformational epitopes in cow's milk and egg proteins, making them less allergenic. Up to 70% children with cow's milk or egg allergies can tolerate baked milk or egg (baked in a flour matrix) before they tolerate unbaked milk or less well-cooked forms of egg.[50] The addition of baked milk or egg in the diet may improve the nutritional profile, reduce avoidance burdens, and promote inclusion in social activities for children.[50]

For children with IgE-mediated cow's milk and egg allergies, the timing and place of introduction to baked milk or baked egg should be discussed with the treating allergist. This is because of the risk of severe allergic reactions.[50] Once baked milk or baked egg is introduced into the diet, it is important that they are consumed regularly to maintain tolerance.[50] **Box 1** gives some examples of recipes for baked milk and baked egg products, as well as suggestions for modification of recipes to include less sugar and more fiber. After a baked egg or milk challenge has been passed, individuals should be educated about nonbaked sources of the allergen that they should continue to avoid, such as the milk in milk chocolate chips, or egg in frosting or egg, and/or milk in less well-cooked cake (eg, mud cake or other cakes with a less-baked center).

Wheat and Other Grain Allergies

The prevalence of reported reactions to wheat is 3.6%, but only 0.1% of those have IgE-mediated wheat allergy confirmed by oral food challenge.[51] Wheat allergy usually manifests in early childhood, with a median age of onset of 7 months, often on first ingestion.[52,53] Barley is also be a relevant allergen in some populations, as are wheat substitutes, such as buckwheat and quinoa.[54–56] Wheat allergy usually resolves in childhood, with most children experiencing resolution by the age of 6 years.[57] In adults, wheat is a common cause of food-dependent exercise-induced

Table 8
Foods to choose and foods to avoid in an egg-free diet

Food Group	Foods to Choose	Foods/Ingredients to Avoid
Meat and other protein-rich foods	The following prepared without egg or egg ingredients (fresh, frozen, canned, dried, cured, processed, smoked, or brined): beef, pork, lamb, other meats, poultry, fish, seafood, nut, nut butters, seeds, beans, tofu, cheese	The following prepared with egg or egg ingredients (batters, sauces, toppings, breading): beef, pork, lamb, other meats, poultry, fish, seafood Egg, dried egg powder, egg substitutes that include egg ingredients
Dairy	The following prepared without egg or egg ingredients: cheese, cream cheese, heavy cream, milk (including condensed, evaporated or dried), yogurt, ice cream, pudding	The following prepared with egg or egg ingredients: ice cream, pudding, custard Eggnog
Grains	The following prepared without egg or egg ingredients: breads, crusts, baked goods (brownies, cakes, cookies, muffins, scones), cereals, crackers, enriched grains, whole grains, noodles, pasta, pancakes, rolls, waffles	The following prepared with egg or egg ingredients: breads, crusts, baked goods (brownies, cakes, cookies, muffins, scones), cereals, crackers, enriched grains, whole grains, noodles, pasta, pancakes, rice, rolls, waffles
Fruits	Pure fruits (fresh, frozen, canned, pureed, juiced, and dried)	Fruits prepared with egg or egg ingredients such as cakes, cookies, sauces, breads.
Vegetables	Pure vegetables (fresh, frozen, canned, pureed, juiced, and dried)	Vegetables prepared with egg or egg ingredients (batters, sauces, toppings, breading) or vegetables prepared in a fryer which is used for egg containing products
Fats/oils	The following prepared without egg or egg ingredients: Butter, cream, margarine, oils; gravies, sauces and salad dressings, plant based mayonnaise substitutes	The following prepared with egg or egg ingredients: gravies, sauces (ie, bearnaise, hollandaise), salad dressings, mayonnaise
Desserts/other	The following prepared without egg or egg ingredients: cakes, cookies, ice cream, popsicles, pudding, frosting, buttercream	The following prepared with egg or egg ingredients: custard, frosting, ice cream, meringue, mousse, nougat, marshmallow, marshmallow spreads, sherbet, sorbet, souffle, marzipan or cake decorations

(continued on next page)

Table 8 (continued)		
Food Group	Foods to Choose	Foods/Ingredients to Avoid
Ingredients	Gelatin, herbs, pepper, spices	Albumin, apovitellin, avidin, egg, egg white, egg yolk, globulin, livetin, lysozyme, ovalbumin, ovoglobulin, ovomucin, ovomucoid, ovovitellin, vitellin

anaphylaxis.[58–60] Reactions can occur in the absence of cofactors, if sufficient wheat has been consumed.[61] Some reactions to wheat products are not owing to wheat allergy; anaphylaxis to pancakes has reported to have been triggered by allergy to cereal mites (insects).[62] This important differential diagnosis emphasizes the need to take a detailed food allergy history.[3] Owing to cross-reactivity, a positive test to wheat may not be clinically relevant in grass-sensitized individuals, whereas the wheat allergen omega 5 gliadin has excellent diagnostic specificity and sensitivity.[63–66]

Wheat can trigger occupational asthma owing to workplace exposure to flour and is also a common trigger of eosinophilic esophagitis.[67–69] Celiac disease (CD), the other major condition linked to wheat ingestion, is an autoimmune disease triggered by gluten causing chronic inflammation, villous atrophy, and malabsorption in the small intestine in genetically predisposed individuals.[70,71] The IgA class of anti–tissue transglutaminase and/or endomysial antibodies can indicate CD but an intestinal biopsy is mandatory to confirm diagnosis.[72] Around 8.4% of individuals are affected by wheat allergy or CD, but many adults consider they are wheat intolerant or have nonceliac gluten sensitivity.[73–75] Symptoms related to suspected nonceliac gluten sensitivity are often not caused by gluten, but by wheat carbohydrates, for example, fructans, prompting the suggestion that nonceliac gluten sensitivity be renamed nonceliac wheat sensitivity.[76,77] Wheat avoidance may also be due to the perception that a wheat-free diet is part of a healthier lifestyle.[78,79]

Table 9 Substitutes for egg in baking and cooking	
Use	Substitute
Baked goods: leavening	In place of one egg: 1½ tbsp water, 1½ tbsp oil and 1 tsp baking powder 1 tsp baking powder, 1 tbsp water, and 1 tbsp vinegar
Baked goods: binding	In place of 1 egg: Mix 1 tbsp ground flaxseed and 3 tbsp warm water; let stand 1 minute before use 1/4 cup either fruit puree (applesauce, banana), silken tofu, or plain yogurt 1 packet gelatin and 2 tbsp warm water Prepackaged egg substitutes often made from potato and tapioca starch Liquid leftover from canned or freshly cooked chickpeas, 3 tbsp Xanthan gum: 1 tsp per recipe can help with binding and texture enhancement
Thickening	Add additional flour, starch

Box 1
Baked milk and baked egg recipes

Basic baked egg muffin recipe
    Developed by The Icahn School of Medicine at Mt. Sinai, NY, NY
    Yield: 6 Muffins
    Serving size: 1
    Egg protein per serving: 2 g

Ingredients
    Dry ingredients
        1 cup (125 g) all-purpose flour (wheat)
        ½ cup (100 g) sugar
        ¼ teaspoon (1.5 g) salt
        1 teaspoon (4.6 g) baking powder
    Wet ingredients
        2 Tablespoons (30 mL) canola oil or other tolerated vegetable oil
        ½ teaspoon (2.5 mL) vanilla extract
        2 large eggs, beaten
        ½ cup (120 mL) milk (cow's milk or plant-based substitute)

Directions
1. Preheat oven to 350° F (180° C). Check the oven is fully preheated.
2. Line a muffin pan with 6 muffin liners or grease the muffin tins with allowed butter (if not cow's milk allergic) margarine or oil spray.
3. Stir together wet ingredients until well combined. Set aside
4. In a separate bowl mix together the dry ingredients.
5. Add wet ingredients to dry ingredients all at once and gently stir until wet and dry ingredients combined. Do not over-mix. Some lumps may remain
6. Divide the batter into the 6 muffin tins, evenly.
7. Bake for 30 to 35 minute or until golden brown and firm to touch. Do not use muffins if soggy, gooey, or unbaked inside.
8. Cool completely before serving.

Baked Egg Muffins, reduced sugar recipe
    This recipe makes 6 muffins.
    Developed by The Icahn School of Medicine at Mt. Sinai, NY, NY
    Developed by Wendy Elverson, RD, LDN
    Yield: 6 muffins
    Serving size: 1 muffin
    Egg protein per serving: 2 g
        Ingredients
            Dry ingredients
                1 ¼ cups (155 g) all-purpose flour (or ½ cup white whole wheat flour and ¾ cup all-purpose flour)
                ¼ cup sugar (50 g)
                ¼ (1.5 g) teaspoon salt
                2 teaspoons (9 g) baking powder
                1 teaspoon (2.5 g) cinnamon (optional)
            Wet ingredients
                1 cup (240 mL) allowed "milk" beverage (cow's milk or plant-based alternative)
                2 Tablespoons (30 mL) canola oil
                1 teaspoon (5 mL) vanilla extract
                2 large eggs, beaten
        Directions
        1. Preheat oven to 350° F (180° C)
        2. Line a 6-cup muffin pan with paper liners, or grease muffin tins with allowed butter, margarine or oil spray.
        3. In a bowl mix together wet ingredient. Set aside.
        4. In a separate bowl mix dry ingredients.

5. Gradually whisk liquid ingredients into dry ingredients until fully combined. It is ok if there are some lumps in the batter.
6. Bake at 350° for 25 to 30 minutes or longer if needed. A toothpick or knife inserted in the middle should come out clean. Do not use muffins if soggy, gooey or unbaked inside.

Basic baked-milk muffin
  Yield: 6 muffins
  Serving size: 1 muffin
  Milk protein per serving: 1.3 g
    Ingredients
      Dry ingredients
        1 $\frac{1}{4}$ cup (155 g) all-purpose flour
        ½ cup (100 g) sugar
        $\frac{1}{4}$ teaspoon (1.5 g) salt
        2 teaspoons (9 g) baking powder
      Wet ingredients
        1 cup (240 mL) milk (Cow's milk or allowed plant based "milk")
        2 Tablespoons (30 mL) canola oil
        1 teaspoon (5 mL) vanilla extract
        1 egg (or equivalent replacer such as Ener-G® foods egg replacer)
    Directions
    1. Preheat oven to 350° F (180° C). Be sure oven is completely to this temperature.
    2. Line a muffin pan with 6 muffin liners or grease times with allowed butter, margarine, or oil spray.
    3. Stir together wet ingredients until well combined (including egg or egg replacer even though egg replacer is a dry ingredient). Set aside.
    4. In a separate bowl mix together the dry ingredients.
    5. Add wet ingredients to dry ingredients all at once and gently stir until wet and dry ingredients are just combined. Do not over-stir. Some small lumps may remain.
    6. Divide batter evenly into the 6 muffin tins.
    7. Bake 30 to 35 minutes or until golden brown and firm to the touch. Do not use muffins if soggy, gooey, or unbaked inside.
    8. Cool completely before serving.

Baked milk 50% whole wheat bread
  Developed by Wendy Elverson, RD, LDN
  ~ 1 ½ pound loaf
  Serving size: 1/12 of loaf, ~2oz (1.2 g milk protein)
  Servings per loaf: 12
  Milk protein per serving: 1.2 g
    Ingredients
      1 cup plus 2 tablespoons room temperature water
      1 tablespoon canola oil
      1 teaspoon salt
      1 ½ cups white whole wheat flour
      1 ½ cups bread flour
      46g nonfat dry milk powder (14 g protein)
      1 tablespoon honey
      2 teaspoons active dry yeast
    Instructions
      Add ingredients to bread machine in the order recommended by your machine.
      Use basic or whole wheat cycle.
      Once bread is ready, remove from the bread maker and place on a wire rack, let it cool fully before slicing. Once baked and cooled, weigh the full loaf. Divide weight by 12, and this value will be the amount of 1 serving of bread. Alternatively, if you do not have a kitchen scale, cut the bread into 12 equal size pieces.
      Serving size: 1 piece

Baked egg and baked milk tips

- Consider a bread maker (46g dry milk powder and/or 1 egg can be added per 1.5 pound or 680 g loaf of bread).
- Pair bread and muffins with a nutrient dense food or spread.
- Add moistness to muffins using pumpkin, apple, banana, or zucchini.
- Cut the sugar: many recipes can decrease the sugar to 2 to 3 tablespoons per 6 muffins.
- Incorporate whole grain flours (oat, buckwheat, whole wheat, or sorghum).
- Add ground flaxseed, wheat germ and nonprocessed wheat bran for fiber.

Developed by The Icahn School of Medicine at Mt. Sinai, NY, NY, and Wendy Elverson, RD, LDN.

Dietary management of wheat and other grain allergies

Wheat allergy and CD require complete exclusion of wheat, including ancient varieties for example, spelt, einkorn, and emmer (**Table 10**).[80] Those who have CD must also avoid barley, rye, and kamut, whereas children allergic to wheat may tolerate rye, although barley may cause symptoms in some children.[81,82] Excluding grains can result in nutritional deficiencies, owing to their importance as a major provider of energy, iron, and B vitamins. Gluten-free products often cost more than comparable wheat-based products; they also contain less protein and fiber, and often more fat and sugar.[83] Studies suggest that, the diets of those with CD are unbalanced, with often poor knowledge of and adherence to a gluten-free diet.[84,85] Thus, the involvement of a dietitian is essential to ensure appropriate nutritional intake in individuals of all ages, for whom the dietary exclusion of wheat and grains is necessary.

Key points regarding wheat allergy

1. Wheat allergy is most prevalent in young children; new-onset wheat allergy in adults often manifests as a trigger of food-dependent exercise-induced anaphylaxis.
2. Wheat can also trigger non–IgE-mediated food allergies, including eosinophilic esophagitis, CD, and occupational asthma.
3. Optimal diagnosis of wheat allergy can be achieved through a detailed diet and clinical history and testing to the wheat allergen omega 5 gliadin.
4. Symptoms attributed to gluten sensitivity are more likely to be due to wheat carbohydrates such as fructans.
5. Excluding wheat and other grains can adversely affect nutritional status; dietary advice from a qualified professional is recommended for those with a wheat allergy or CD.

Soy and Legume Allergies

Soybean (glycine max) is well-recognized as allergenic and is one of the 8 most commonly allergenic foods worldwide. The prevalence of soy protein allergy among all children is 0.4%[86] with a high rate of resolution (45%) by age 6 or 7.[87,88] IgE-mediated reactions, that is, food-dependent exercise-induced anaphylaxis,[89,90] non–IgE-mediated, that is, food protein–induced enterocolitis syndrome,[91] as well as mixed IgE-mediated reactions, that is, eosinophilic esophagitis,[92] have been implicated with soy. Soybeans are rich in isoflavones that have been shown to provide a number of health benefits. The presence of isoflavones in soybeans have also raised concern specifically in women with estrogen-sensitive breast cancer, but clinical research has consistently shown no adverse effects on breast cancer risk.[93] Soy containing foods have a rich nutrient profile including high quality protein, essential fatty acids, and micronutrients (see **Table 2**).

Table 10
Foods to choose and foods to avoid in wheat free diet

Food Group	Foods to Choose	Foods/Ingredients to Avoid
Meat and other protein-rich foods	The following prepared without wheat or wheat ingredients (fresh, frozen, canned, dried, cured, processed, smoked, or brined): beef, pork, lamb, other meats, poultry, fish, seafood, nut, nut butters, seeds, beans, tofu, cheese, eggs	The following prepared with wheat or wheat ingredients (battered, breaded, bread crumbed, floured, cooked in fryer shared with wheat, or wheat containing): beef, pork, lamb, other meats, poultry, fish, seafood, meatloaf, lasagna, sauces, marinades, seitan, haggis
Dairy	The following (fresh, UHT, dried, condensed, or evaporated): cow, goat, and sheep milks, fresh and soured cream, buttermilk, crème fraiche	Milk with added fiber, artificial cream, yogurt or fromage frais containing muesli or cereals
Grains	Grits, corn, corn flour, corn starch, rice, rice flour, arrowroot, amaranth, buckwheat, millet, teff, quinoa, sorghum, soya flour, potato flour, potato starch, modified starch, gram flour, gluten-free oats, gluten-free bread, gluten-free crackers, gluten-free pasta, gluten-free breakfast cereals, gluten-free stuffing mix	Wheat, wheat bran, wheat germ, wheat starch, bulgur wheat, durum wheat, semolina, couscous, barley, malt, malted barley, rye, triticale, kamut, spelt, farro, Freekeh, einkorn, bread, pastry, spaghetti, macaroni, other pastas, oats not labeled gluten free
Fruits	Pure fruits (fresh, frozen, canned, pureed, juiced, and dried)	Fruits prepared or processed with wheat
Vegetables	Pure vegetables (fresh, frozen, canned, pureed, and dried)	Vegetables prepared in batter, bread, bread crumb, flour, or cooked in fryer shared with wheat; that is, potato croquettes
Fats/oils	Butter, margarine, lard, cooking oils, ghee, low-fat spread	Shared oils with wheat
Desserts/other	Plain potato crisps/chips, homemade popcorn, gluten-free baked goods	Ice cream cones and wafers, thickened liquids, baked goods snacks made from wheat, rye, barley and oats, pretzels
Ingredients	Gelatin, bicarbonate of soda, cream of tartar, yeast, artificial sweeteners, Tomato and garlic puree, individual herbs and spices, vinegars, mixed herbs and spices, ground pepper	Wheat starch, wheat protein isolate, hydrolyzed wheat protein, wheat germ oil, cereal extract, vital wheat gluten

Dietary management of soy and other legume allergies

Many foods contain similar nutrients as those found in soy, so the avoidance of soy alone rarely compromises the nutritional quality of the diet, but because soy is often an ingredient in many processed foods, this may limit food choices for individuals with food allergies (**Table 11**). Asian countries have included fermented and

Table 11
Foods to choose and foods to avoid in soy free diet

Food Group	Foods to Choose	Foods/Ingredients to Avoid
Meat and other protein rich foods	The following prepared without soy or soy ingredients (fresh, frozen, canned, dried, cured, processed, smoked, or brined): beef, pork, lamb, other meats, poultry, fish, seafood, nut, nut butters, seeds, no soy beans, cheese, eggs	Tofu, tempeh, texturized vegetable protein, Koyadofu
Dairy alternatives	The following prepared without soy or soy products: seed, tree nut and nonsoy legume-based cheeses, yogurts, ice creams and beverages	The following prepared with soy or soy ingredients: cheese, yogurt, ice cream, beverages
Grains	The following prepared without soy or soy ingredients: breads, baked goods (brownies, cakes, cookies, muffins, scones), cereals, crackers, enriched grains, whole grains, noodles, pasta, pancakes, rolls, waffles	The following prepared with soy or soy ingredients: breads baked goods (brownies, cakes, cookies, muffins, scones), cereals, crackers, enriched grains, whole grains, noodles, pasta, pancakes, rice, rolls, waffles, soy grits.
Fats/oils	The following prepared without soy or soy ingredients: Butter, cream, margarine, oils, gravies, sauces and salad dressings, vegan mayonnaise substitutes	Cold pressed or expeller pressed or extruded or unrefined soy oil.
Desserts/other	The following prepared without soy or soy ingredients: cakes, cookies, ice cream, popsicles, pudding, frosting, buttercream	The following prepared with soy or soy ingredients: cakes, cookies, ice cream, popsicles, pudding, frosting, buttercream
Ingredients	Gelatin, herbs, pepper, spices	Natto, miso, hydrolyzed plant protein, soy sauce, soybean (curds or granules), soy protein (concentrate or isolate), Worcestershire sauce, soy sprouts, tamari, okara, soy albumin

unfermented soy foods into their cuisine for centuries, but the consumption of soy foods has increased in the United States and many Western countries over the past 25 years.[94] Unfermented soy foods include tofu, soy oil, soy flour, and soy milk; fermented soybean products are available as miso, okara, soy sauce, tempeh, or natto. Refined soybean oil is exempt from labeling in the United States because any residual trace amounts of protein that might be in soybean oil have been shown not to cause reactions in soy protein-sensitive individuals.[95] Lecithin derived from soybeans is present in a wide variety of foods in the form of an emulsifier, stabilizer, or releasing agent and does require labeling under the Food Allergen Labeling And Consumer Protection Act (https://www.fda.gov/food/food-allergensgluten-free-guidance-documents-regulatory-information/food-allergen-labeling-and-consumer-protection-act-2004-questions-and-answers). Many health care providers have allowed selected patients to safely consume soy lecithin. Studies have identified the presence of IgE binding proteins in soy lecithin.[96,97] However, the proteins present have little antigenicity and food products would generally not contain sufficient soy protein residues to provoke allergic reactions in the majority of consumers allergic to soy (https://farrp.unl.edu/soy-lecithin). Gholmie and colleagues[98] performed a double-blind cross-over study and found the vast majority of those with non–IgE-mediated soy allergy could safely include soy lecithin in the diet.

Most vegetarian and vegan foods use soy as the main source of protein and warrant careful consideration for macronutrient and micronutrient intake. Infants and children following a vegan diet with food allergy need to be carefully monitored specifically for protein intake, as well as for micronutrient deficiencies[99] As with all foods, soy foods should be considered part of a varied diet.

Legumes may elicit mild to life-threatening allergenic symptoms. Allergens of peanut and soybean are the most well-known and characterized but other leguminous crops such as lentil, chickpea, beans, peas, mung bean, red gram (pigeon pea), and black gram have been implicated in allergenic reactions.[100] In various countries, the comparative prevalence of allergies to various legumes is variable with allergies to lentils common in Spain and to chickpeas, lentils, and black gram in India.[101] Although good comparative studies have not been done in the United States, peanut is surely the most common allergenic legume in the United States, followed by soybean.

Individuals allergic to a single legume often display positive skin prick tests or IgE binding to other legumes that they can safely ingest.[102,103] Serologic cross-sensitization between members of the legume family (Leguminosae) is observed frequently; however, the clinical symptomology is documented to be rare. A major soybean allergen, Gly m 4, is cross-reactive with birch pollen allergen, Bet v 1. Cross-reactivity occurs owing to proteins in 1 substance being similar to proteins in another substance and can occur between one food and another or between pollens and food. It is estimated that 10% of patients allergic to birch pollen allergic also have a soy allergy, typically in the form of an oral allergy syndrome. Individuals with birch pollen and soy allergies may have more severe reactions with the intake of large amounts of soy foods, even if processed soy-containing foods are usually well-tolerated.[104,105]

Key points regarding soy allergy

- Many processed foods contain soy, making a soy elimination diet difficult.
- Soy protein ingredients can be found in some cereals, crackers, canned tuna fish, or even peanut butter.
- Soy lecithin is tolerated by most individuals who are allergic to soy and is not typically avoided on a soy elimination diet.
- Refined soybean oil is exempt from labeling in the United States. Most soybean oil manufactured in the United States and added to food products is highly refined. Avoidance of soy lecithin and soy oil in those with soy allergies are not advised.

Seafood Allergies

Allergy to seafood includes both fish and shellfish. Cartilaginous fish such as shark, ray, skate, and swordfish rarely provoke fish allergy, which is most often triggered by bony finned fish.[106,107] Fish allergy most often involves sensitization to the muscle protein β parvalbumin, although other allergens may be relevant in tropical fish species or in raw fish.[108–114] The prevalence of challenge-confirmed allergy ranges from 0% to 0.3%, with high levels reported in the Philippines and Norway.[106,115,116] Sensitization usually occurs in childhood, with anaphylaxis more likely to be reported in children.[117–119] Resolution of fish allergy was considered to be rare, although 1 study reported that 74% of patients with a fish allergy developed tolerance to at least 1 fish species.[120] Fish and other seafood is also a trigger of non–IgE-mediated food allergies such as food protein–induced enterocolitis syndrome.[121,122] Differential diagnoses for fish allergy include reactions owing to the consumption of raw or lightly cooked fish contaminated with L3 Anisakis spp. larvae,[123] and reactions to fish can also be caused by the breakdown of fish histidine into histamine by marine bacteria in the flesh of caught fish, known as scombroid poisoning.[124]

Edible shellfish include crustaceans (crayfish, lobster, crab, and prawns) and mollusks (oyster, mussel, clam, scallop, octopus, squid, and edible snails).[107] Around 2% of the world's population is affected by a shellfish allergy, with challenge-confirmed allergy reported in up to 0.9% of individuals.[117,125] Shellfish allergy often presents in adult life, with crustaceans rather than mollusks being the most common shellfish involved.[126,127] The primary shellfish allergen is tropomyosin, which is both water soluble and heat stable, but other allergens may be relevant in different species.[107] The lack of similarity between fish and shellfish allergens usually means cross-reactivity is unlikely, although co-sensitization and can also be a potential cause of scombroid poisoning.[128,129]

Dietary management of fish and seafood allergy

The avoidance of fish and/or shellfish may seem to be easy; however, both fish and shellfish allergens are heat stable and fish allergens can also be aerosolized. Thus, cooking vapors or foods cooked in oil or stock contaminated with fish or shellfish may provoke symptoms.[130,131] Seafood can also cause reactions owing to its presence as a minor ingredient, such as in prawn crackers, fish-derived gelatin, and Worcestershire sauce as examples. Health products such as fish oil supplements also need to be avoided because they have been known to provoke reactions.[132] Proper avoidance of seafood and substitutions are noted in **Table 12**. Seafood plays a valuable role in diet diversity and contributes to optimal nutrition owing to its rich nutrient composition, which includes omega-3 fatty acids, vitamins D, riboflavin (B_2), calcium, phosphorous, iron, zinc, magnesium, and potassium. However, those with seafood allergies can optimize nutrition with alternative sources of alpha linolenic acid and docosahexaenoic acid , as noted in **Table 13**.

Key points regarding fish and seafood allergy

1. Fish allergy usually starts in childhood, whereas allergy to shellfish is often an adult-onset condition.
2. The allergens in fish and shellfish are different; allergy to one does not automatically require the avoidance of all seafood.
3. Crustaceans are more frequent triggers of shellfish allergy than mollusks.
4. Seafood allergens are heat stable and can provoke reactions owing to aerosolization.
6. Seafood is an important part of a diverse diet and provides important nutrients, especially omega-3 fatty acids and iodine.

Peanuts, Tree Nuts, and Seeds

Nut and seed allergies are typically severe and lifelong.[133–135] Nut is a culinary term that describes any large, oily kernel within a shell used for food.[136] Tree nut definitions vary worldwide, but commonly include almond, Brazil nut, cashew, hazelnut, macadamia, pecan, pistachio, and walnut. In the United States, beechnut, butternut,

Table 12
Foods to choose and foods to avoid in seafood free diet

Food Group	Foods to Choose	Foods/Ingredients to Avoid
Meat and other protein-rich foods	The following (fresh, frozen, canned, dried, cured, processed, smoked, or brined): beef, pork, lamb, other meats, poultry, nut, nut butters, seeds, beans, tofu, cheese, eggs	Tuna, anchovies, bass, catfish, cod, flounder, grouper, haddock, hake, halibut, herring, mahi mahi, perch, pike, pollock, salmon, scrod, sole, snapper, swordfish, tilapia, trout, barnacle, crab, crawfish, krill, lobster, prawns, shrimp, abalone, clams, cockle, cuttlefish, limpet, mussels, octopus, oysters, periwinkle, sea cucumber, sea urchin, scallops, snails, squid, whelk, fish sticks, and items cooked in a shared fryer with seafood
Dairy	The following (fresh, UHT, dried, condensed, or evaporated): cow, goat, sheep, and other animal milks (camel, buffalo), butter, buttermilk, cheese, cream, creme fraiche curds, custard, ghee, half and half, ice cream, milk fat, milk protein, pudding, sour cream, yogurt, cottage cheese	
Grains	Wheat, bread, pastry, bulgar wheat, spaghetti, macaroni, other pasta, durum wheat, wheat bran, wheat germ, wheat starch, semolina, couscous, barley, malt, malted barley, rye, triticale, kamut, spelt, oats, farro, Freekeh, einkorn	
Fruits	All fruits (fresh, frozen, canned, pureed, juiced, and dried)	
Vegetables	All vegetables (fresh, frozen, canned, pureed, juiced, and dried)	Vegetables prepared in shared fryers with seafood.
Fats/oils	Butter, margarine, lard, cooking oils, ghee, low fat spread	Fish oil
Desserts/other	All baked goods	Any products prepared in a shared fryer with seafood
Ingredients	Bicarbonate of soda, cream of tartar, yeast, artificial sweeteners, individual herbs and spices, vinegars, mixed herbs and spices, ground pepper	Worcestershire sauce, imitation or artificial fish or shellfish, caponata, Caesar salad or Caesar dressing, bouillabaisse, barbecue sauce, surimi, seafood flavoring, glucosamine, cuttlefish ink, fish gelatin

Table 13
Alternative food sources of alpha linolenic acid and docosahexaenoic acid

Category (Serving Size)	Food	Alpha Linolenic Acid (g)	Docosahexaenoic Acid (g)
Seeds (1 tbsp)	Flaxseed	2.35	
	Chia	2.53	
Nuts (1 ounce)	Black walnuts	0.76	
	English walnuts	2.57	
Oils (1 tbsp)	Flaxseed	7.26	
	Soybean	0.92	
	Canola	1.28	
Legumes (1/2 c prepared)	Edamame	0.28	
	Refried beans, canned, vegetarian	0.21	
	Kidney beans	0.1	
Other	1 whole omega-3 enriched egg	.34	.75–2.5

chestnut, chinquapin, coconut, ginkgo, hickory nut, lychees, and shea nut are also included; however, these nuts do not commonly elicit reactions.[136]

Seed allergies are an emerging issue in many countries, with sesame most common. Reactions to linseed (flaxseed), pumpkin, poppy, mustard, and sunflower seeds have also occurred.[137,138] Sesame seed is considered a major allergen in Canada, Australia, and Europe, and the US Food and Drug Administration is considering adding it to its list of major allergens.[139] For food labeling purposes, pine nuts are considered a seed in Europe, but a nut in North America.

The prevalence rates of nut and seed allergies vary between countries, with peanut allergy affecting up to 3.0%,[140–142] tree nut allergy up to 3.0%[143,144] and sesame allergy 0.1% to 0.2%. Other seed allergies seem to be rarer.[142,145–147] Identifying seeds on labels can be difficult because they are often included as seasonings or spices. Nuts and seeds are important sources of nutrients, particularly for the emerging vegetarian/vegan diets in patients with food allergies.[99]

Dietary management and treatment of nut and seed allergies

Affected children usually have an allergy to the peanut or a single tree nut early in life and may develop multiple nut and seed allergies over time.[44,148] **Table 14** provides a list of safe foods to choose and avoid if peanut or tree nuts are eliminated. In the United States, refined peanut oil is considered safe for those with peanut allergy, but unrefined peanut oil should be avoided. The EU recommends the avoidance of all peanut oils. Sesame oil is largely available unrefined and is not safe for individuals allergic to sesame.

The Pronuts study recently reported that 60% of children with nut or seed allergy had more than 1 other nut or seed allergy.[149] Up to 40% of those with peanut allergy have 1 or more tree nut allergy[144,150] and 25% have a sesame allergy.[151] For those with a tree nut allergy, up to 30% have 1 or more additional tree nut allergy.[144,150] Tree nut co-allergy is most commonly reported between the walnut and the pecan (Juglandaceae family) and the cashew and the pistachio (Anacardiaceae family).[144,149,152–154] It is becoming more common to identify tolerated nuts and include

Table 14
Foods to choose and foods to avoid in peanut and tree nut free diet

Food Group	Foods to Choose	Foods/Ingredients to Avoid
Meat and other protein-rich foods	The following (fresh, frozen, canned, dried, cured, processed, smoked, or brined): beef, pork, lamb, other meats, poultry, fish, seafood, seeds, beans, tofu, cheese, eggs	Nuts and nut butters
Dairy	The following (fresh, UHT, dried, condensed, or evaporated): cow, goat, sheep, and other animal milks (camel, buffalo), butter, buttermilk, cheese, cream, creme fraiche curds, custard, ghee, half and half, ice cream, milk fat, milk protein, pudding, sour cream, yogurt, cottage cheese	Flavored cheese, yogurts with toppings
Grains	Wheat, bread, pastry, bulgar wheat, spaghetti, macaroni, other pasta, durum wheat, wheat bran, wheat germ, wheat starch, semolina, couscous, barley, malt, malted barley, rye, triticale, kamut, spelt, oats not labeled gluten-free, farro, Freekeh, einkorn,	Muesli, granola, breakfast cereals, cereal bars
Fruits	All fruits (fresh, frozen, canned, pureed, juiced, and dried)	Fruits prepared or processed with nuts
Vegetables	All vegetables (fresh, frozen, canned, pureed, juiced, and dried)	Vegetables prepared or processed with nuts
Fats/oils	Butter, margarine, lard, cooking oils, ghee, low fat spread	Cold-pressed, expelled or extruded peanut oil, arachis oil
Desserts/other	Baked goods without peanut or tree nut ingredients	Nougat, fudge, Christmas cakes and puddings, fruit cake icing, baklava (Greek pastry), nut-filled chocolates, praline, marzipan, satay sauce, pesto, Asian and Indian foods

(continued on next page)

Table 14 (continued)		
Food Group	**Foods to Choose**	**Foods/Ingredients to Avoid**
Ingredients	Bicarbonate of soda, cream of tartar, yeast, artificial sweeteners, individual herbs and spices, vinegars, mixed herbs and spices, ground pepper,	Lupin, peanut flour, artificial nuts, beer nuts, almond, beechnut, black walnut hull extract, brazil nut, butternut, cashew, chestnut, chinquapin nut, coconut, filbert/hazelnut, gianduja, ginkgo nut, hickory nut, litchi/lichee/lychee nut, macadamia nut, marzipan/almond paste, nangai nut, natural nut extract, nut butters, nut distillates/alcoholic extracts, nut meal, nut meat, nut milk, nut oils, nut paste, nut pieces, pecan, pesto, pili nut, pine nut, pistachio, praline, shea nut, walnut, walnut hull extract.

them in the diet. The proposed benefits and negative considerations of a more liberal approach are summarized in **Table 15**.

Oral immunotherapy for peanut allergy (Palforzia) has been approved by the US Food and Drug Administration[155] to be used with avoidance for those with peanut allergies. Oral immunotherapy is not a cure and has risks (adverse reactions, increased risk for eosinophilic esophagitis, and cost of treatment) that must be weighed against the benefits (increased threshold for reactions, improved quality of life, and reduced anxiety).[156,157] Evidence and expert consensus support introducing peanut in infancy to prevent peanut allergy.[158,159] Caregivers may need assistance to safely introduce peanuts to nonallergic children in households with nut allergic children.

Table 15 Proposed benefits and negative considerations of blanket nut avoidance	
Proposed Benefits	**Negative Considerations**
Improved quality of life owing to less restrictive eating and inclusion of nuts that may have important social or cultural significance.	Diagnostic burden of potentially multiple oral food challenges to determine allergy/tolerance to each nut.
Inclusion of tolerated nuts may halt the progression of multiple nut allergies or facilitate development of cross-tolerance to the index allergic nut	Including multiple nuts in the diet of young children can be challenging owing to choking concerns, taste and texture aversions.
Nuts are a good source of protein and iron, particularly if meat and eggs are excluded from the diet such as those on a vegan diet or with multiple food allergies.	There are no clear guidelines regarding how much and how often nuts should be included.
	Increased burden of managing cross-contamination and labeling issues to identify individual tree nuts on food labels in many countries
	Lack of data regarding potential reactions owing to more liberal approach to nut restriction/eating.

Key points regarding peanut, tree nut and seed allergy

- Blanket avoidance of all nuts or seeds is no longer recommended. Rather, the inclusion of tolerated nuts and seeds should be guided by the allergy-focused history and appropriate allergy testing within an allergy team and ideally supervised by a dietitian.
- Oral immunotherapy for peanut allergy is not a cure, but can decrease the risk of severe reactions.
- In the United States, refined peanut oil is considered to be safe for those with peanut allergy, but unrefined peanut oil should be avoided. The EU recommends the avoidance of refined and unrefined peanut oil stating "However, the risk of severe adverse reactions to highly refined peanut oils seems to be low, although it cannot be ruled out in every highly sensitive peanut allergic individual."[160] Sesame oil is largely available unrefined and is not safe for sesame allergic individuals.

LIFESTYLE ISSUES
Cross-Contact

Cross-contact happens when one food meets another food. This contact results in a food containing small amounts of another food. Although this amount can be miniscule, it may cause an allergic reaction in children with food allergies.

Ways patients can avoid cross-contact include
- Use kitchen equipment that has been washed well with soap and water.
- Always wash hands with soap and water and dry with a hand towel (paper or fabric) before touching other foods or switching between kitchen utensils. Antibacterial gels will not remove food allergens.
- Store allergy-safe foods covered and away from other foods that may splatter or spill.
- Thoroughly wash counters and tables with soap or household cleaner and water after preparing meals.
- Limit the sharing of food, drinks, and utensils. Teach children not to share these items when at school or with friends.
- Encourage hand and face washing for all family members after meals, especially when allergens are present in the meal, to avoid topical exposure with hugs and kisses.
- When shopping, avoid bulk bins, salad or soup or buffet bars, and the deli counter.

Eating away from Home

Banning allergens from public places is controversial; it is supported by limited evidence and may provide a false sense of security. Allergens can be removed using common cleaning methods.[161] The most common lifestyle issues to address in those with food allergies include eating in restaurants and traveling and have been discussed in detail by Venter and colleagues.[162]

Restaurants

The management of food allergy in restaurants can be challenging. Tips for food allergic patients eating out in restaurants include the following.

- Check the restaurant's website for allergen information before visiting. Consider calling ahead to inform staff of food allergies.

- Once at the restaurant, always tell restaurant staff very clearly about which food allergens require avoidance. Ask about ingredients and food preparation methods.
- Recommend using a "chef card" or "translation card" to help to assist with communication. These can be found at www.foodallergy.org
- Avoid peak times, such as lunch and dinner rushes, when staff are more distracted.
- Be aware of cross-contact. Avoid restaurants that are high risk for cross-contact, such as buffets or all-you-can-eat restaurants. Avoid fried foods if fryers are used for multiple menu items (chicken nuggets, cheese sticks, popcorn shrimp). Ask for meat and vegetables to be wrapped in foil before being placed on the grill. Ask line servers to change their gloves.
- In case of any doubt, ask the waiter or ideally the chef to double check. Do not hesitate to send food back.
- Have a backup plan by having and allergy friendly snack available.

Travel

Travel raises issues regarding food avoidance and choosing suitable foods. Airline, railway, and nautical policies around the world differ and the safest option may be to take allergen-safe foods along and avoid all foods provided by the airline. For example, food allergen labeling of nonpackaged foods served on airplanes is not currently enforced for flights departing from the United States.[163] EU food labeling laws,[164] however, dictate that allergens must either be listed on the packaging, menu, recipe, or ticket or be available from a crew member for flights leaving from the EU or UK. In case the family opts to consume foods provided by their traveling option, it is advisable to be aware of the national allergen policies and travel method specific policies. It is important to contact the carrier beforehand about any food allergen–related restrictions. Verify information upon check-in; boarding the train, aircraft, or boat; and once again when the food is served. Ask to be provided with an ingredient list if possible. Always travel with the required emergency medication at hand. It may be worth checking with the airline or carrier about the availability of emergency medication on board the aircraft, train, or boat as well.

SUMMARY

Food allergy is increasing worldwide. There are several major food allergens; however, any food can potentially become an allergen and we should still be wary of novel allergens. Recently, the move toward individualized management of food allergy has led to subtlety in management strategies such as encouraging intake of baked egg and baked milk when tolerated and inclusion of tolerated tree nuts and fish, rather than elimination of complete food groups. This has the advantage of less limited diets and improved quality of life.

Important factors to address during a nutritional consultation include allergen avoidance and ensuring the diet is nutritionally balanced. Allergen avoidance requires label reading skills and an understanding of food allergy labeling laws, which differ among countries or regions. Other avoidance education needs are understanding cross-contact, how to eat away from home, and how to travel. The risk of accidental exposure to allergens can be mitigated through adequate knowledge and suitable precautions taken by both patients and caregivers.

It is important to recognize and support the patients' nutritional requirements and quality of life, and this is particularly important for infants and young children where appropriate growth and development of normal feeding skills should be assessed as part of ongoing nutritional management. Given the risks of inadequate allergen elimination diets, dietary guidance is vital as the prevalence of allergies to the most common foods, and allergies to multiple foods is increasing. Moving forward, the value of a dietitian on the food allergy clinic team is immeasurable as the intricacy of management is ever evolving and stretches beyond simply avoiding the allergen.[33]

CLINICS CARE POINTS

- Comprehensive and individualized avoidance education is a safety necessity.
- Appropriate substitutions aid in the management of food allergy.
- Nutritional complete diets ensure adequate nutrition for optional growth.
- Reading food allergen labels is a necessary and fundamental skill of allergy management.
- Recently, the move toward individualized management of food allergy has led to subtlety in management strategies such as encouraging intake of baked egg and baked milk when tolerated and inclusion of tolerated tree nuts and fish, rather than the elimination of complete food groups.
- Lifestyle factors vary among individuals and play an integral part in allergy management.
- Dietary input from a registered dietitian as part of a multidisciplinary team improves both growth parameters and nutritional biomarkers and supports patient self-efficacy.

ACKNOWLEDGMENTS

The authors would like to acknowledge Ilina Goyal for searching the food label information and preparing the table on food labeling with information from the United States, Europe, and Canada.

DISCLOSURE

Conflicts of interest: R. Durban has received consultancy fees from AstraZeneca and Mead Johnson Nutrition, and lecture fees from Abbott, Nutricia North America, and Mead Johnson Nutrition. M. Groetch has no commercial interests to disclose. S. Coleman is a consultant to the National Peanut Board. W. Elverson has received an educational grant and consulting fees from Nutricia Danone. V. McWilliam has received lecture fees for Aspen Global, Abbott Australasia, and Nestle Health Sciences, and consultancy fees from Nestle and Nutricia outside the submitted work. R. Meyer has completed academic lectures for Danone/Nutricia, Abbott, Mead Johnson, and Nestle, and received an academic grant from Danone. M. Netting's research team receives research funding from Nestlé Nutrition Institute. B. Vlieg–Boerstra received research funding from Nutricia, and consulting or speaker's fees from Marfo Food groups, Nutricia, and Abbott. C. Venter has provided and reviewed educational material for Danone, Recktrt Benckiser, Abbott Nutrition, DBV technologies, and the Nestle Nutrition Institute.

REFERENCES

1. World Allergy Organization. World Allergy Organization White Book on Allergy. 2011. Available at: http://www.worldallergy.org/UserFiles/file/WAO-White-Book-on-Allergy_web.pdf. Accessed March, 2021.

2. Institute of Medicine. Food allergies: global burden, causes, treatment, prevention and public policy. 2017. Available at: http://www.nationalacademies.org/hmd/Activities/Nutrition/FoodAllergies.aspx. Accessed March, 2021.
3. Skypala IJ, Venter C, Meyer R, et al. The development of a standardised diet history tool to support the diagnosis of food allergy. Clin Transl Allergy 2015;5:7.
4. Zurzolo GA, Koplin JJ, Ponsonby AL, et al. Consensus of stakeholders on precautionary allergen labelling: a report from the Centre for Food and Allergy Research. J Paediatr Child Health 2016;52(8):797–801.
5. Carruth BR, Skinner JD. Feeding behaviors and other motor development in healthy children (2-24 months). JAmCollNutr 2002;21(2):88–96.
6. Maslin K, Dean T, Arshad SH, et al. Fussy eating and feeding difficulties in infants and toddlers consuming a cows' milk exclusion diet. Pediatr Allergy Immunol 2015;26(6):503–8.
7. Mehta H, Groetch M, Wang J. Growth and nutritional concerns in children with food allergy. Curr Opinallergy Clinimmunol 2013;13(3):275–9.
8. Meyer R, De Koker C, Dzubiak R, et al. The impact of the elimination diet on growth and nutrient intake in children with food protein induced gastrointestinal allergies. Clin Transl Allergy 2016;6:25.
9. Flammarion S, Santos C, Guimber D, et al. Diet and nutritional status of children with food allergies. Pediatr Allergy Immunol 2011;22(2):161–5.
10. Meyer R, De KC, Dziubak R, et al. Malnutrition in children with food allergies in the UK. J Humnutrdiet 2014;27(3):227–2235.
11. Liu T, Howard RM, Mancini AJ, et al. Kwashiorkor in the United States: fad diets, perceived and true milk allergy, and nutritional ignorance 1. Arch Dermatol 2001;137(5):630–6.
12. Keller MD, Shuker M, Heimall J, et al. Severe malnutrition resulting from use of rice milk in food elimination diets for atopic dermatitis. Isr Med Assoc J 2012;14(1):40–2.
13. Vassilopoulou E, Christoforou C, Andreou E, et al. Effects of food allergy on the dietary habits and intake of primary schools' Cypriot children. Eur Ann Allergy Clin Immunol 2017;49(4):181–5.
14. Christie L, Hine RJ, Parker JG, et al. Food allergies in children affect nutrient intake and growth. J Am Diet Assoc 2002;102(11):1648–51.
15. Meyer R, De KC, Dziubak R, et al. A practical approach to vitamin and mineral supplementation in food allergic children. Clin Transl Allergy 2015;5:11.
16. Ojuawo A, Lindley KJ, Milla PJ. Serum zinc, selenium and copper concentration in children with allergic colitis. East Afr Med J 1996;73(4):236–8.
17. Beck C, Koplin J, Dharmage S, et al. Persistent food allergy and food allergy coexistent with eczema is associated with reduced growth in the first 4 years of life. J Allergy Clinimmunol Pract 2016;4(2):248–56.
18. Isolauri E, Sutas Y, Salo MK, et al. Elimination diet in cow's milk allergy: risk for impaired growth in young children. J Pediatr 1998;132(6):1004–9.
19. Meyer R, Rommel N, Van OL, et al. Feeding difficulties in children with food protein-induced gastrointestinal allergies. J Gastroenterolhepatol 2014;29(10):1764–9.
20. Mukkada VA, Haas A, Greskoff Maune N, et al. Feeding dysfunction in children with eosinophilic gastrointestinal diseases. Pediatrics 2011;126:e672–7.
21. Chehade M, Meyer R, Beauregard A. Feeding difficulties in children with non-IgE mediated food allergic gastrointestinal disorders. Ann Allergy asthma Immunol 2019;122(6):603–9.

22. Harris G. Development of taste and food preferences in children. Curr Opin Clin Nutr Metab Care 2008;11(3):315–9.
23. Taylor CM, Emmett PM. Picky eating in children: causes and consequences. Proc Nutr Soc 2019;78(2):161–9.
24. Rouf K, White L, Evans K. A qualitative investigation into the maternal experience of having a young child with severe food allergy. Clin Child Psychol Psychiatry 2012;17(1):49–64.
25. Somers LS. Peanut allergy: case of an 11-year-old boy with a selective diet. J Am Diet Assoc 2011;111(2):301–6.
26. Canani RB, Leone L, D'Auria E, et al. The effects of dietary counseling on children with food allergy: a prospective, multicenter intervention study. J Acad Nutr Diet 2014;114(9):1432–9.
27. WHO/FAO/UNU. Protein and amino acid requirements in human nutrition. Geneva: WHO; 2001.
28. Gerasimidis K, Bronsky J, Catchpole A, et al. Assessment and interpretation of vitamin and trace element status in sick children: a position paper from the European Society for Paediatric Gastroenterology Hepatology, and Nutrition Committee on Nutrition. J Pediatr Gastroenterol Nutr 2020;70(6):873–81.
29. Fiocchi A, Brozek J, Schunemann H, et al. World Allergy Organization (WAO) diagnosis and rationale for action against cow's milk allergy (DRACMA) guidelines. Pediatr Allergy Immunol 2010;21(Suppl 21):1–125.
30. Boyce JA, Assa'a A, Burks AW, et al. Guidelines for the diagnosis and management of food allergy in the United States: summary of the NIAID-Sponsored Expert Panel Report. Nutrition 2011;27(2):253–67.
31. Fiocchi A, Schunemann HJ, Brozek J, et al. Diagnosis and Rationale for Action Against Cow's Milk Allergy (DRACMA): a summary report. J Allergy Clin Immunol 2010;126(6):1119–28.e2.
32. Skripak JM, Matsui EC, Mudd K, et al. The natural history of IgE-mediated cow's milk allergy. J Allergy Clin Immunol 2007;120(5):1172–7.
33. Venter C, Groetch M, Netting M, et al. A patient-specific approach to develop an exclusion diet to manage food allergy in infants and children. Clin Exp Allergy 2018;48(2):121–37.
34. Rajani PS, Martin H, Groetch M, et al. Presentation and Management of Food Allergy in Breastfed Infants and Risks of Maternal Elimination Diets. J Allergy Clin Immunol Pract 2020;8(1):52–67.
35. Netting MJ, Allen KJ. Reconciling breast-feeding and early food introduction guidelines in the prevention and management of food allergy. J Allergy Clin Immunol 2019;144(2):397–400.e1.
36. Meyer R, Chebar Lozinsky A, Fleischer DM, et al. Diagnosis and management of non-IgE gastrointestinal allergies in breastfed infants-An EAACI Position Paper. Allergy 2020;75(1):14–32.
37. Fiocchi A, Dahda L, Dupont C, et al. Cow's milk allergy: towards an update of DRACMA guidelines. World Allergy Organ J 2016;9(1):35.
38. American Academy of Pediatrics. Committee on Nutrition. Hypoallergenic infant formulas. Pediatrics 2000;106(2 Pt 1):346–9.
39. Host A, Halken S. Hypoallergenic formulas–when, to whom and how long: after more than 15 years we know the right indication. Allergy 2004;59(Suppl 78):45–52.
40. Egan M, Lee T, Andrade J, et al. Partially hydrolyzed whey formula intolerance in cow's milk allergic patients. Pediatr Allergy Immunol 2017;28(4):401–5.

41. Luyt D, Ball H, Makwana N, et al. BSACI guideline for the diagnosis and management of cow's milk allergy. Clin Exp Allergy 2014;44(5):642–72.

42. Meyer R, Wright K, Vieira MC, et al. International survey on growth indices and impacting factors in children with food allergies. J Hum Nutr Diet 2018;32(2): 175–84.

43. Merritt RJ, Fleet SE, Fifi A, et al. North American Society for Pediatric Gastroenterology, Hepatology, and Nutrition position paper: plant-based milks. J Pediatr Gastroenterol Nutr 2020;71(2):276–81.

44. Savage J, Sicherer S, Wood R. The natural history of food allergy. J Allergy Clin Immunol Pract 2016;4(2):196–203 [quiz: 204].

45. Nowak-Wegrzyn A, Bloom KA, Sicherer SH, et al. Tolerance to extensively heated milk in children with cow's milk allergy. J Allergy Clin Immunol 2008;122(2): 342–7, 347 e341–342.

46. Rona RJ, Keil T, Summers C, et al. The prevalence of food allergy: a meta-analysis. J Allergy Clin Immunol 2007;120(3):638–46.

47. Osborne N, Gurrin L, Koplin J, et al. Prevalence of food challenge: confirmed food allergies in a large pediatric population based study in Melbourne, Australia. Allergy 2010;65:375.

48. Savage JS, Fisher JO, Birch LL. Parental influence on eating behavior: conception to adolescence. J L Med Ethics 2007;35(1):22–34.

49. Clark A, Islam S, King Y, et al. A longitudinal study of resolution of allergy to well-cooked and uncooked egg. Clin Exp Allergy 2011;41(5):706–12.

50. Leonard SA, Caubet JC, Kim JS, et al. Baked milk- and egg-containing diet in the management of milk and egg allergy. J Allergy Clin Immunol Pract 2015; 3(1):13–23 [quiz: 24].

51. Nwaru BI, Panesar SS, Hickstein L, et al. The epidemiology of food allergy in Europe: protocol for a systematic review. Clin Transl Allergy 2013;3(1):13.

52. Cianferoni A. Wheat allergy: diagnosis and management. J Asthma Allergy 2016;9:13–25.

53. Srisuwatchari W, Vichyanond P, Jirapongsananuruk O, et al. Characterization of children with IgE-mediated wheat allergy and risk factors that predict wheat anaphylaxis. Asian Pac J Allergy Immunol 2020. https://doi.org/10.12932/AP-130919-0645.

54. Lee E, Jeong K, Lee J, et al. Clinical and laboratory findings of barley allergy in Korean children: a single hospital based retrospective study. J Korean Med Sci 2020;35(3):e23.

55. Satoh R, Jensen-Jarolim E, Teshima R. Understanding buckwheat allergies for the management of allergic reactions in humans and animals. Breed Sci 2020;70(1):85–92.

56. Hong J, Convers K, Reeves N, et al. Anaphylaxis to quinoa. Ann Allergy Asthma Immunol 2013;110(1):60–1.

57. Ricci G, Andreozzi L, Cipriani F, et al. Wheat allergy in children: a comprehensive update. Medicina (Kaunas) 2019;55(7):400.

58. Bartra J, Araujo G, Muñoz-Cano R. Interaction between foods and nonsteroidal anti-inflammatory drugs and exercise in the induction of anaphylaxis. Curr Opin Allergy Clin Immunol 2018;18(4):310–6.

59. Hompes S, Dolle S, Grunhagen J, et al. Elicitors and co-factors in food-induced anaphylaxis in adults. Clin Transl Allergy 2013;3(1):38.

60. Christensen MJ, Eller E, Mortz CG, et al. Wheat-dependent cofactor-augmented anaphylaxis: a prospective study of exercise, aspirin, and alcohol efficacy as cofactors. J Allergy Clin Immunol Pract 2019;7(1):114–21.

61. Christensen MJ, Eller E, Mortz CG, et al. Exercise lowers threshold and increases severity, but wheat-dependent, exercise-induced anaphylaxis can be elicited at rest. J Allergy Clin Immunol Pract 2018;6(2):514–20.

62. Sánchez-Borges M, Capriles-Hulett A, Fernandez-Caldas E. Oral mite anaphylaxis: who, when, and how? Curr Opin Allergy Clin Immunol 2020;20(3):242–7.

63. Jones SM, Magnolfi CF, Cooke SK, et al. Immunologic cross-reactivity among cereal grains and grasses in children with food hypersensitivity. J Allergy Clin Immunol 1995;96(3):341–51.

64. Venter C, Maslin K, Arshad SH, et al. Very low prevalence of IgE mediated wheat allergy and high levels of cross-sensitisation between grass and wheat in a UK birth cohort. Clin Transl Allergy 2016;6:22.

65. Nilsson N, Sjölander S, Baar A, et al. Wheat allergy in children evaluated with challenge and IgE antibodies to wheat components. Pediatr Allergy Immunol 2015;26(2):119–25.

66. Le TA, Al Kindi M, Tan JA, et al. The clinical spectrum of omega-5-gliadin allergy. Intern Med J 2016;46(6):710–6.

67. Wiszniewska M, Walusiak-Skorupa J. Diagnosis and frequency of work-exacerbated asthma among bakers. Ann Allergy Asthma Immunol 2013; 111(5):370–5.

68. Molina-Infante J, Lucendo AJ. Approaches to diet therapy for eosinophilic esophagitis. Curr Opin Gastroenterol 2020;36(4):359–63.

69. Lucendo AJ, Molina-Infante J. Treatment of eosinophilic esophagitis with diets. Minerva Gastroenterol Dietol 2020;66(2):124–35.

70. Al-Toma A, Volta U, Auricchio R, et al. European Society for the Study of Coeliac Disease (ESsCD) guideline for coeliac disease and other gluten-related disorders. United Eur Gastroenterol J 2019;7(5):583–613.

71. Lebwohl B, Sanders DS, Green PHR. Coeliac disease. Lancet 2018;391(10115): 70–81.

72. Fasano A, Catassi C. Current approaches to diagnosis and treatment of celiac disease: an evolving spectrum. Gastroenterology 2001;120(3):636–51.

73. van Gils T, Nijeboer P, IJssennagger CE, et al. Prevalence and Characterization of Self-Reported Gluten Sensitivity in The Netherlands. Nutrients 2016; 8(11):714.

74. Golley S, Corsini N, Topping D, et al. Motivations for avoiding wheat consumption in Australia: results from a population survey. Public Health Nutr 2015;18(3): 490–9.

75. Potter M, Jones MP, Walker MM, et al. Incidence and prevalence of self-reported non-coeliac wheat sensitivity and gluten avoidance in Australia. Med J Aust 2020;212(3):126–31.

76. Barmeyer C, Schumann M, Meyer T, et al. Long-term response to gluten-free diet as evidence for non-celiac wheat sensitivity in one third of patients with diarrhea-dominant and mixed-type irritable bowel syndrome. Int J Colorectal Dis 2017;32(1):29–39.

77. Biesiekierski JR, Peters SL, Newnham ED, et al. No effects of gluten in patients with self-reported non-celiac gluten sensitivity after dietary reduction of fermentable, poorly absorbed, short-chain carbohydrates. Gastroenterology 2013; 145(2):320–8.e1-3.

78. Sharma N, Bhatia S, Chunduri V, et al. Pathogenesis of celiac disease and other gluten related disorders in wheat and strategies for mitigating them. Front Nutr 2020;7:6.

79. Araya M, Bascuñán KA, Alarcón-Sajarópulos D, et al. Living with gluten and other food intolerances: self-reported diagnoses and management. Nutrients 2020;12(6):1892.

80. Sievers S, Rohrbach A, Beyer K. Wheat-induced food allergy in childhood: ancient grains seem no way out. Eur J Nutr 2020;59(6):2693–707.

81. Srisuwatchari W, Piboonpocanun S, Wangthan U, et al. Clinical and in vitro cross-reactivity of cereal grains in children with IgE-mediated wheat allergy. Allergol Immunopathol (Madr) 2020;48(6):589–96.

82. Burman J, Palosuo K, Kukkonen K, et al. Children with wheat allergy usually tolerate oats. Pediatr Allergy Immunol 2019;30(8):855–7.

83. Babio N, Lladó Bellette N, Besora-Moreno M, et al. A comparison of the nutritional profile and price of gluten-free products and their gluten-containing counterparts available in the Spanish market. Nutr Hosp 2020;37(4):814–22.

84. Suárez-González M, Bousoño García C, Jiménez Treviño S, et al. Influence of nutrition education in paediatric coeliac disease: impact of the role of the registered dietitian: a prospective, single-arm intervention study. J Hum Nutr Diet 2020;33(6):775–85.

85. Gładyś K, Dardzińska J, Guzek M, et al. Celiac dietary adherence test and standardized dietician evaluation in assessment of adherence to a gluten-free diet in patients with celiac disease. Nutrients 2020;12(8):2300.

86. Gupta RS, Springston EE, Warrier MR, et al. The prevalence, severity, and distribution of childhood food allergy in the United States. Pediatrics 2011;128: e9–16.

87. Sicherer SH, Sampson HA. Food allergy: a review and update on epidemiology, pathogenesis, diagnosis, prevention, and management. J Allergy Clin Immunol 2018;141(1):41–58.

88. Savage JH, Kaeding AJ, Matsui EC, et al. The natural history of soy allergy. J Allergy Clin Immunol 2010;125:683–6.

89. Izadi N, Rabinovitch N. Food-dependent exercise-induced anaphylaxis to soybean. J Allergy Clin Immunol Pract 2019;7(1):303–4.

90. Hayashi M, Pawankar R, Yamanishi S, et al. Food-dependent exercise-induced anaphylaxis to soybean: Gly m 5 and Gly m 6 as causative allergen components. World Allergy Organ J 2020;13(7):100439.

91. Nowak-Wegrzyn A, Berin MC, Mehr S. Food Protein-Induced Enterocolitis Syndrome. J Allergy Clin Immunol Pract 2020;8(1):24–35.

92. Groetch M, Venter C, Skypala I, et al. Dietary therapy and nutrition management of eosinophilic esophagitis: a work group report of the American Academy of Allergy, Asthma, and Immunology. J Allergy Clin Immunol Pract 2017;5(2): 312–24.e9.

93. Messina M, Rogero MM, Fisberg M, et al. Health impact of childhood and adolescent soy consumption. Nutr Rev 2017;75(7):500–15.

94. Ballmer-Weber BK, Vieths S. Soy allergy in perspective. Curr Opin Allergy Clin Immunol 2008;8:270–5.

95. Bush RK, Taylor SL, Nordlee JA, et al. Soybean oil is not allergenic to soybean-sensitive individuals. J Allergy Clin Immunol 1985;76:242–5.

96. Awazuhara H, Kawai H, Baba M, et al. Antigenicity of the proteins in soy lecithin and soy oil in soybean allergy. Clin Exp Allergy 1998;28(12):1559–64.

97. Gu X, Beardslee T, Zeece M, et al. Identification of IgE-binding proteins in soy lecithin. Int Arch Allergy Immunol 2001;126:218–25.

98. Gholmie Y, Lozinsky AC, Godwin H, et al. Tolerance of soya lecithin in children with non-immunoglobulin E-mediated soya allergy: a randomised, double-blind, cross-over trial. J Hum Nutr Diet 2020;33(2):232–40.

99. Protudjer JLP, Mikkelsen A. Veganism and paediatric food allergy: two increasingly prevalent dietary issues that are challenging when co-occurring. BMC Pediatr 2020;20(1):341.

100. Verma AK, Kumar S, Das M, et al. A comprehensive review of legume allergy. Clin Rev Allergy Immunol 2013;45(1):30–46.

101. Martínez San Ireneo M, Ibáñez Sandín MD, Fernández-Caldas E. Hypersensitivity to members of the botanical order Fabales (legumes). J Investig Allergol Clin Immunol 2000;10:187–99.

102. Bernhisel-Broadbent J, Sampson HA. Cross-allergenicity in the legume botanical family in children with food hypersensitivity. J Allergy Clin Immunol 1989; 83(2):435–40.

103. Kazatsky AM, Wood RA. Classification of Food Allergens and Cross-Reactivity. Curr Allergy Asthma Rep 2016;16(3):1–7.

104. Oesterlin C, Kugler C, Darsow U, et al. Soy in vegan nutrition - lifestyle products with risk potential for people with birch pollen allergy. Aktuelle Dermatol 2019; 45(6):273–6.

105. Skypala IJ. Can patients with oral allergy syndrome be at risk of anaphylaxis? Curr Opin Allergy Clin Immunol 2020;20(5):459–64.

106. Stephen JN, Sharp MF, Ruethers T, et al. Allergenicity of bony and cartilaginous fish - molecular and immunological properties. Clin Exp Allergy 2017;47(3): 300–12.

107. Ruethers T, Taki AC, Johnston EB, et al. Seafood allergy: a comprehensive review of fish and shellfish allergens. Mol Immunol 2018;100:28–57.

108. Kalic T, Morel-Codreanu F, Radauer C, et al. Patients allergic to fish tolerate ray based on the low allergenicity of its parvalbumin. J Allergy Clin Immunol Pract 2019;7(2):500–8.e1.

109. Hansen TK, Bindslev-Jensen C, Skov PS, et al. Codfish allergy in adults: IgE cross-reactivity among fish species. Ann Allergy Asthma Immunol 1997;78(2): 187–94.

110. Griesmeier U, Vázquez-Cortés S, Bublin M, et al. Expression levels of parvalbumins determine allergenicity of fish species. Allergy 2010;65(2):191–8.

111. Schulkes KJ, Klemans RJ, Knigge L, et al. Specific IgE to fish extracts does not predict allergy to specific species within an adult fish allergic population. Clin Transl Allergy 2014;4:27.

112. Kobayashi A, Kobayashi Y, Shiomi K. Fish allergy in patients with parvalbumin-specific immunoglobulin E depends on parvalbumin content rather than molecular differences in the protein among fish species. Biosci Biotechnol Biochem 2016;80(10):2018–21.

113. Kobayashi Y, Akiyama H, Huge J, et al. Fish collagen is an important panallergen in the Japanese population. Allergy 2016;71(5):720–3.

114. Kuehn A, Hilger C, Lehners-Weber C, et al. Identification of enolases and aldolases as important fish allergens in cod, salmon and tuna: component resolved diagnosis using parvalbumin and the new allergens. Clin Exp Allergy 2013; 43(7):811–22.

115. Connett GJ, Gerez I, Cabrera-Morales EA, et al. A population-based study of fish allergy in the Philippines, Singapore and Thailand. Int Arch Allergy Immunol 2012;159(4):384–90.

116. Eggesbø M, Halvorsen R, Tambs K, et al. Prevalence of parentally perceived adverse reactions to food in young children. Pediatr Allergy Immunol 1999; 10(2):122–32.

117. Moonesinghe H, Mackenzie H, Venter C, et al. Prevalence of fish and shellfish allergy: a systematic review. Ann Allergy Asthma Immunol 2016;117(3): 264–72.e4.

118. Kourani E, Corazza F, Michel O, et al. What do we know about fish allergy at the end of the decade? J Investig Allergol Clin Immunol 2019;29(6):414–21.

119. Worm M, Eckermann O, Dölle S, et al. Triggers and treatment of anaphylaxis: an analysis of 4,000 cases from Germany, Austria and Switzerland. Dtsch Arztebl Int 2014;111(21):367–75.

120. Carvalho S, Marcelino J, Cabral Duarte M, et al. Contribution of recombinant Parvalbumin Gad c 1 in the diagnosis and prognosis of fish allergy. J Investig Allergol Clin Immunol 2019;0.

121. Miceli Sopo S, Monaco S, Badina L, et al. Food protein-induced enterocolitis syndrome caused by fish and/or shellfish in Italy. Pediatr Allergy Immunol 2015;26(8):731–6.

122. Infante S, Marco-Martín G, Sánchez-Domínguez M, et al. Food protein-induced enterocolitis syndrome by fish: not necessarily a restricted diet. Allergy 2018; 73(3):728–32.

123. Seneviratne R, Gunawardena NS. Prevalence and associated factors of wheezing illnesses of children aged three to five years living in under-served settlements of the Colombo Municipal Council in Sri Lanka: a cross-sectional study. BMC Public Health 2018;18(1):127.

124. Colombo FM, Cattaneo P, Confalonieri E, et al. Histamine food poisonings: a systematic review and meta-analysis. Crit Rev Food Sci Nutr 2018;58(7): 1131–51.

125. Lopata AL, Kleine-Tebbe J, Kamath SD. Allergens and molecular diagnostics of shellfish allergy: part 22 of the Series Molecular Allergology. Allergo J Int 2016; 25(7):210–8.

126. Kamdar TA, Peterson S, Lau CH, et al. Prevalence and characteristics of adult-onset food allergy. J Allergy Clin Immunol Pract 2015;3(1):114–5.e1.

127. Khan F, Orson F, Ogawa Y, et al. Adult seafood allergy in the Texas Medical Center: a 13-year experience. Allergy Rhinol (Providence) 2011;2(2):e71–7.

128. González-Fernández J, Alguacil-Guillén M, Cuéllar C, et al. Possible Allergenic Role of Tropomyosin in Patients with Adverse Reactions after Fish Intake. Immunol Invest 2018;47(4):416–29.

129. Tan JA, Smith WB. Non-IgE-mediated gastrointestinal food hypersensitivity syndrome in adults. J Allergy Clin Immunol Pract 2014;2(3):355–7.e1.

130. James JM, Crespo JF. Allergic reactions to foods by inhalation. Curr Allergy Asthma Rep 2007;7(3):167–74.

131. Lopata AL, O'Hehir RE, Lehrer SB. Shellfish allergy. Clin Exp Allergy 2010;40(6): 850–8.

132. Howard-Thompson A, Dutton A, Hoover R, et al. Flushing and pruritus secondary to prescription fish oil ingestion in a patient with allergy to fish. Int J Clin Pharm 2014;36(6):1126–9.

133. Turner PJ, Gowland MH, Sharma V, et al. Increase in anaphylaxis-related hospitalizations but no increase in fatalities: an analysis of United Kingdom national anaphylaxis data, 1992-2012. J Allergy Clin Immunol 2015;135(4):956–63.e1.

134. Bock SA, Munoz-Furlong A, Sampson HA. Fatalities due to anaphylactic reactions to foods. J Allergy Clin Immunol 2001;107(1):191–3.

135. Liew WK, Williamson E, Tang ML. Anaphylaxis fatalities and admissions in Australia. J Allergy Clin Immunol 2009;123(2):434–42.
136. Weinberger T, Sicherer S. Current perspectives on tree nut allergy: a review. J Asthma Allergy 2018;11:41–51.
137. Patel A, Bahna SL. Hypersensitivities to sesame and other common edible seeds. Allergy 2016;71(10):1405–13.
138. Lyons SA, Clausen M, Knulst AC, et al. Prevalence of Food Sensitization and Food Allergy in Children across Europe. J Allergy Clin Immunol Pract 2020; 8(8):2736–46.e9.
139. Messina M, Venter C. Recent surveys on food allergy prevalence. Nutr Today 2020;55(1):22–9.
140. Gupta RS, Warren CM, Smith BM, et al. Prevalence and severity of food allergies among US Adults. JAMA Netw Open 2019;2(1):e185630.
141. Gupta RS, Warren CM, Smith BM, et al. The Public Health Impact of Parent-Reported Childhood Food Allergies in the United States. Pediatrics 2018; 142(6):e20181235.
142. Osborne NJ, Koplin JJ, Martin PE, et al. Prevalence of challenge-proven IgE-mediated food allergy using population-based sampling and predetermined challenge criteria in infants. J Allergy Clin Immunol 2011;127(3):668–76.e1–2.
143. McWilliam V, Koplin J, Lodge C, et al. The prevalence of tree nut allergy: a systematic review. Curr Allergy asthma Rep 2015;15(9):54.
144. McWilliam V, Peters R, Tang MLK, et al. Patterns of tree nut sensitization and allergy in the first 6 years of life in a population-based cohort. J Allergy Clin Immunol 2018;143(2):644–50.e5.
145. Ben-Shoshan M, Harrington DW, Soller L, et al. A population-based study on peanut, tree nut, fish, shellfish, and sesame allergy prevalence in Canada. J Allergy Clin Immunol 2010;125(6):1327–35.
146. Sicherer SH, Munoz-Furlong A, Godbold JH, et al. US prevalence of self-reported peanut, tree nut, and sesame allergy: 11-year follow-up. J Allergy Clin Immunol 2010;125(6):1322–6.
147. Warren CM, Chadha AS, Sicherer SH, et al. Prevalence and Severity of Sesame Allergy in the United States. JAMA Netw Open 2019;2(8):e199144.
148. Clark AT, Ewan PW. The development and progression of allergy to multiple nuts at different ages. Pediatr Allergy Immunol 2005;16(6):507–11.
149. Brough HA, Caubet JC, Mazon A, et al. Defining challenge-proven coexistent nut and sesame seed allergy: a prospective multicenter European study. J Allergy Clin Immunol 2020;145(4):1231–9.
150. Sasaki M, Koplin JJ, Dharmage SC, et al. Prevalence of clinic-defined food allergy in early adolescence: the SchoolNuts study. J Allergy Clin Immunol 2017;141(1):391–8.e4.
151. Du Toit G, Katz Y, Sasieni P, et al. Early consumption of peanuts in infancy is associated with a low prevalence of peanut allergy. J Allergy Clin Immunol 2008;122(5):984–91.
152. Maloney JM, Rudengren M, Ahlstedt S, et al. The use of serum-specific IgE measurements for the diagnosis of peanut, tree nut, and seed allergy. J Allergy Clin Immunol 2008;122(1):145–51.
153. Geiselhart S, Hoffmann-Sommergruber K, Bublin M. Tree nut allergens. Mol Immunol 2018;100:71–81.
154. Elizur A, Appel MY, Nachshon L, et al. NUT Co Reactivity - Acquiring Knowledge for Elimination Recommendations (NUT CRACKER) Study. Allergy 2017;73(3): 593–601.

155. FDA. Palforzia. US Food & Drug Administration website. 2020. Available at: https://www.fda.gov/vaccines-blood-biologics/allergenics/palforzia. Accessed August 24, 2020.
156. Blackman AC, Staggers KA, Kronisch L, et al. Quality of life improves significantly after real-world oral immunotherapy for children with peanut allergy. Ann Allergy asthma Immunol 2020;125(2):196–201.e1.
157. Patrawala M, Shih J, Lee G, et al. Peanut oral immunotherapy: a current perspective. Curr Allergy asthma Rep 2020;20(5):14.
158. Fleischer DM, Sicherer S, Greenhawt M, et al. Consensus communication on early peanut introduction and the prevention of peanut allergy in high-risk infants. World Allergy Organ J 2015;8(1):27.
159. de Silva D, Halken S, Singh C, et al. Preventing food allergy in infancy and childhood: systematic review of randomised controlled trials. Pediatr Allergy Immunol 2020;31(7):813–26.
160. Panel on Dietetic Products NaA. Scientific Opinion on the evaluation of allergenic foods and food ingredients for labelling purposes. EFSA J 2014; 12(11):286.
161. Perry TT, Conover-Walker MK, Pomes A, et al. Distribution of peanut allergen in the environment. J Allergy Clin Immunol 2004;113(5):973–6.
162. Venter C, Sicherer SH, Greenhawt M. Management of peanut allergy. J Allergy Clin Immunol Pract 2019;7(2):345–55.e2.
163. Available at: http://allergicliving.com/index.php/2010/08/30/comparing-airlines/. Accessed June 13, 2012.
164. Agency FS. Food allergen labelling and information requirements under the EU Food Information for Consumers Regulation No. 1169/2011: technical guidance. 2015. Available at: https://www.food.gov.uk/sites/default/files/media/document/food-allergen-labelling-technical-guidance.pdf. Accessed March, 2018.

Biologics and Novel Therapies for Food Allergy

Sultan Albuhairi, MD[a], Rima Rachid, MD[b,c,*]

KEYWORDS

- Food allergy • Biologics • Microbiome • Fecal microbiota transplantation
- Omalizumab • Dupilumab

KEY POINTS

- New therapeutic modalities in food allergy are needed to minimize the risk of anaphylaxis and improve associated anxiety, nutritional deficiencies, and patient's quality of life.
- Biologics are promising modalities, as they may potentially target multiple food allergies instead of one, in addition to possibly treating other concomitant atopic diseases.
- Although omalizumab has been evaluated extensively in allergic diseases, most biologics are more novel and have broader immunologic impact. Hence, careful evaluation of their safety and their modulation of the immune system should be conducted.

INTRODUCTION

Food allergy is a significant public health burden with a significant increase in its prevalence over the last decades globally. In the United States, food allergy affects around 10% of adults and 8% of children.[1–3] The potential risk of severe or fatal anaphylaxis, the associated anxiety and nutritional issues of the affected patients, and the significantly negative impact on quality of life all underscore the need for developing effective therapeutic options for food allergy.[4,5]

Although the current standard of care for most food allergy consists of avoiding the culprit allergens and keeping rescue medicine available for emergency use, AR101, the first treatment of peanut oral immunotherapy (OIT), received Food and Drug

Conflict of Interest: S. Albuhairi reports no financial disclosure. R. Rachid is an inventor on published US patent application, 15/801,811, that covers methods and compositions for the prevention and treatment of food allergy using microbial treatments. R. Rachid has pending patent applications related to the use of probiotics in enforcing oral tolerance in food allergy (62/758,161, and 62/823,866). R. Rachid has equity in Pareto Bio. R. Rachid received research support from Aimmune Therapeutics and End-Allergies-Together.
Source of funding: None.
[a] Department of Pediatrics, Allergy and Immunology Section, King Faisal Specialist Hospital and Research Centre, Riyadh 11211, Saudi Arabia; [b] Division of Immunology, Boston Children's Hospital, 300 Longwood Avenue, Boston, MA 02115, USA; [c] Department of Pediatrics, Harvard Medical School, Boston, MA, USA
* Corresponding author.
E-mail address: Rima.Rachid@childrens.harvard.edu

Administration (FDA) approval in January 2020.[6,7] OIT is the most evaluated therapeutic approach in food allergy. Desensitization is achieved in most of the patients.[7–10] However, OIT has many limitations, including the risk of allergic reactions from the food itself, taste aversion to the food as well as variable rates of sustained unresponsiveness (SU) after stopping it.[11–13] Compliance with therapy over time can be a significant barrier, as the food needs to be taken regularly in order to maintain desensitization. SU was demonstrated in 50% of patients who stopped OIT for 4 weeks after up to 5 years of therapy,[12] whereas it was achieved in only 15% of subjects 6 months after discontinuation.[12,13] Other immunotherapy approaches using the sublingual, epicutaneous, and subcutaneous routes are under evaluation.[14–16] None of these are known to lead to a cure.

There is therefore an unmet need for evaluating other therapeutic approaches in food allergy. Biologics are particularly attractive, as by modifying the allergic response, they can potentially target multiple food allergies instead of one, in addition to possibly treating other concomitant atopic diseases. In addition, as they are administered often intermittently as opposed to the daily or regular dosing of food immunotherapies, they are likely to be associated with better compliance and possibly patient satisfaction with the therapy.

In this article, the authors review the biological therapies that are currently under evaluation for food allergy treatment, as well as some of the potential candidates that could be used for further investigation (**Table 1**).

ANTI-IMMUNOGLOBULIN E ANTIBODY

The hallmark of the allergic reaction is the release of inflammatory mediators including histamine, leukotriene, cytokines, and prostaglandins that are activated after cross-linking of antigen-specific immunoglobulin E (IgE) complex on the surface of the mast cells and basophils on exposure to the antigen.[17,18] Omalizumab is antihuman IgE monoclonal antibody that binds to the 2 constant domains of free IgE, thus forming an IgE/anti-IgE immune complex that impedes the IgE linkage to its receptors on mast cells and basophils, hence inhibiting antigen-triggered degranulation.[19]

Omalizumab has been evaluated as monotherapy in small trials that demonstrated significant increase in threshold of reactivity to peanut after 3 to 24 weeks of therapy.[20,21] Asthmatic children given omalizumab for asthma therapy for 4 months showed an increased threshold of reactivity for multiple food allergens including cow's milk, egg, wheat, and hazelnut.[22]

As an adjunct therapy to OIT, omalizumab had been successfully used to facilitate rapid updosing.[23–29] The authors have shown that omalizumab can rapidly desensitize patients who were reactive to less than 50 mg peanut protein at study entry to 2000 mg 20 weeks later. In that study, participants received omalizumab first for 12 weeks, followed by an additional 8 weeks of therapy combined with peanut OIT.[27] In a double-blinded placebo-controlled milk OIT trial, participants received omalizumab or placebo for 4 months before initiation of milk OIT and continued on the assigned therapy for 24 months. Although there was no differences in efficacy, the omalizumab-treated group had significantly less allergic reactions to OIT.[26] Omalizumab also has been used successfully to facilitate rapid desensitization in multiallergen food OIT.[28,29] Androf and colleagues[28] found that 83% of patients who received omalizumab combined with multifood OIT passed a food challenge to 2 or more food up to 2000 mg of protein compared with 33% patients who received placebo with OIT.

A multicenter double-blinded placebo-controlled phase III trial is currently evaluating the use of omalizumab as monotherapy and as adjunct to multiallergen food

Table 1
List of biologics that are either currently evaluated or are potential investigational therapies in food allergy

Therapeutic Agents	Clinical Use in Food Allergy or Other Atopic Diseases
Anti-IgE	
Omaliuzumab (anti-IgE mAb)	Currently investigated in phase III trials as monotherapy or as adjunct therapy to food OIT.
Ligelizumab (anti-IgE mAb)	Evaluated in chronic spontaneous urticaria and asthma. Not evaluated yet in food allergy.
Anti-TH2 cytokines antibodies	
Anti-IL-4R	Dupilumab is currently investigated as monotherapy or as adjunct therapy to food OIT in phase II trials.
Anti-IL-5 and anti-IL-5R	Mepolizumab (anti-IL-5 mAb), reslizumab (anti-IL-5 mAb), and benralizumab (Anti IL-5-R mAb) are FDA approved for treatment of eosinophilic asthma. They have not been evaluated yet in food allergy.
Anti-IL-13	Lebrikizumab and tralokinumab are currently being evaluated in phase III for asthma and atopic dermatitis. They have not been evaluated yet in for food allergy.
Acalabrutinib (Bruton's tyrosine kinase inhibitor) Ruxolitinib (JAK 1/2 inhibitor) Syk inhibitor	All effective in preventing anaphylaxis reaction in food-allergic mouse model.
Epithelial cytokines	
Anti-IL-33	Etokimab (anti-IL-33 Ab) was evaluated in a phase IIa trial for peanut allergy.
Anti-TSLP	Tezepelumab (anti-TSLP mAb) currently investigated for asthma and atopic dermatitis. It has not been evaluated yet in food allergy.
TH1 adjuvants	
Glucopyranosyl lipid A (GLA)	GLA is being investigated as an adjunct therapy to peanut sublingual immunotherapy in a phase I trial.
Monophosphoryl lipid A (MPL) and CpG oligodeoxynucleotides	Both were investigated in treatment of allergic rhinitis but not in food allergy yet.
DNA vaccines	ASP0892 (ARA-LAMP-vax) is being investigated in phase I peanut allergy trial.
Modified food allergen proteins	Encapsulated, Recombinant Modified Peanut Proteins Ara h 1, Ara h 2, and Ara h 3 (EMP-123) was investigated in peanut allergy. HAL-MPE1 is currently being evaluated for peanut allergy in a phase I trial.

(*continued on next page*)

Table 1 (continued)	
Therapeutic Agents	**Clinical Use in Food Allergy or Other Atopic Diseases**
Anti-sialic acid–binding immunoglobulin-like lectin 8 (Siglec-8) antibody (AK002)	Currently evaluated in eosinophilic esophagitis, eosinophilic gastritis, and eosinophilic duodenitis. Not evaluated yet in IgE-mediated food allergy.
Microbiome interventions	
Probiotics	Lactobacillus GG (LGG), bifidobacterium, and lactobacillus lactis supplemented with extensively hydrolyzed milk formula were evaluated in cow's milk allergy. Lactobacillus rhamnosus was evaluated in combination with peanut OIT. VE416 is currently being evaluated with and without peanut OIT in phase I/II trial.
Fecal microbiota transplantation (FMT)	FMT is being currently investigated in a phase I clinical trial in peanut allergy.

OIT (including milk, egg, wheat, cashew, hazelnut, or walnut (https://clinicaltrials.gov/show/NCT03881696)).

Ligelizumab (QGE031) is an anti-IgE antibody that binds with higher affinity to serum IgE than omalizumab.[30] QGE031 was found to have greater efficacy than omalizumab on inhaled and skin allergen responses in patients with mild allergic asthma.[31] A phase II study comparing QGE031 with omalizumab and placebo in severe asthma has been conducted but the results have not been published yet (https://clinicaltrials.gov/show/NCT01716754). Ligelizumab was found to be more effective in complete control of chronic urticaria symptoms compared with omalizumab and placebo.[32] Another phase II trial assessed QGE031 for the treatment of atopic dermatitis but the results have not published yet (https://clinicaltrials.gov/show/NCT01552629). Ligelizumab has not been evaluated yet in food allergy. Given its higher affinity to IgE, it potentially may have better efficacy allowing for higher levels of desensitization or quicker updosing and/or a higher safety profile as a monotherapy or as an adjunct therapy to OIT compared with omalizumab.

ANTI-T HELPER CELLS TYPE 2 CYTOKINES ANTIBODIES

The interleukin-4 (IL-4) receptor and its ligands IL-4 and IL-13 play a central role in allergic inflammation and the promotion of T helper cells type 2 (TH2) differentiation. Dupilumab is a humanized IgG4 monoclonal antibody that targets the IL-4 receptor alpha chain (IL-4Rα), which is common to both IL-4R complexes: type 1 (IL-4Rα/γc; IL-4 specific) and type 2 (IL-4Rα/IL-13Rα1; IL-4 and IL-13 specific). There is little published in vitro or in vivo data on the precise mechanism of action of Dupilumab. However, proposed mechanisms of action of Dupilumab have been described by Harb and Chatila.[33] Dupilumab is FDA approved for the treatment of moderate-to-severe asthma, chronic rhinosinusitis with nasal polyposis, and atopic dermatitis.[34–37]

The authors have shown in patients who received omalizumab as an adjunct therapy to OIT that peanut-specific regulatory T cells (Treg cells), which at baseline exhibited a TH2 cell-like phenotype, characterized by increased IL-4 expression, progressively reversed on OIT administration. Peanut-specific Treg cell suppressor activity was initially absent at the start of omalizumab/OIT therapy; however, it became robust with OIT. Furthermore, the absent peanut-specific Treg cell function was recovered by the acute blockade of IL-4/IL-4R receptor signaling in Treg cells, which inhibited their IL-4 production.[38] These findings highlight the potential therapeutic effect of IL-4 signalizing inhibition in food allergy. Interestingly, a 30-year-old patient with a history of pistachio allergy and corn anaphylaxis was treated with dupilumab for severe atopic dermatitis. Three months after treatment with Dupilumab, pistachio and corn were tolerated during an open food challenge.[39] Currently, there are 3 ongoing phase II clinical trials evaluating dupilumab in peanut allergy, one as a monotherapy (https://clinicaltrials.gov/show/NCT03793608) and another one an adjunct therapy to peanut OIT (https://clinicaltrials.gov/show/NCT03682770). The third trial evaluates omalizumab alone, dupilumab alone, or omalizumab followed by dupilumab therapy, in patients on multifood OIT (https://clinicaltrials.gov/show/NCT03679676).

Lebrikizumab and QAX576 are both anti-IL-13 monoclonal antibodies that have been evaluated in asthma and eosinophilic esophagitis, respectively.[40–42] In a meta-analysis of 5 trials, lebrikizumab was shown to be effective in decreasing the asthma exacerbations and improving the lung function and had a greater efficacy in asthmatics with high periostin level.[41] In adults with eosinophilic esophagitis, esophageal eosinophil counts were decreased by 60% in patients who received QAX576 compared with an increase of 23% in patients who received placebo.[42] Monoclonal antibodies mepolizumab and reslizumab that bind to IL-5 and benralizumab that binds to IL-5Ra are FDA approved for treatment of eosinophilic asthma.[43,44] These antibodies have not been evaluated yet in food allergy.

SPLEEN TYROSINE KINASE

Spleen tyrosine kinase (Syk) plays a key role in the allergic response early in the signaling cascade following binding of allergen to receptor-bound IgE on the mast cell.

In an adjuvant-free mouse model of peanut allergy, mast cell–targeted genetic deletion of *Syk* or Syk blockade prevented peanut sensitization. In mice with established peanut allergy, Syk blockade facilitated desensitization and induction of Treg cells. In addition, when Syk inhibitor was administered with peanut immunotherapy, it completely protected from anaphylaxis to peanut after interruption of therapy.[45]

BRUTON'S TYROSINE KINASE

Bruton's tyrosine kinase (BTK) has been identified as a key downstream component of FcεRI signaling in human mast cells and basophils.[46] IgE-receptor crosslinking in basophils is followed by phosphorylation of Syk, which, once activated, phosphorylates BTK.[47] Ibrutinib and acalabrutinib are both oral FDA-approved irreversible BTK inhibitors for the treatment of B cell malignancies.[48] In a small pilot study, 2 standard doses of ibrutinib reduced or eliminated skin prick test reactivity to peanut and tree nuts in food-allergic adults. In a humanized mouse model, pretreatment with 2 oral doses of acalabrutinib completely prevented moderate IgE-mediated anaphylaxis and also significantly protected against death during severe anaphylaxis.[49]

JANUS KINASE INHIBITORS

The Janus kinase–signal transducer and activator of transcription pathway is used by different cytokines such as interleukins and interferons to transmit signals intracellularly from the cell membrane to the nucleus.[50] They are FDA approved for conditions such as rheumatoid arthritis, polycythemia vera, and myelofibrosis.[50] Several JAK inhibitors are in phase II and III clinical trials as oral therapies for moderate-to-severe atopic dermatitis or as topical treatments for mild-to-moderate atopic dermatitis.[51] Recently, in large international phase III trial, a once daily dose of abrocitinib, a selective JAK 1 inhibitor, for 12 weeks demonstrated significant efficacy and tolerability in adolescent and adults with moderate-to-severe atopic dermatitis.[52] JAK inhibitors have not been investigated in food allergy clinical trials. However, in murine studies, administration of ruxolitinib, a JAK 1/2 inhibitor, reduced anaphylaxis to ovalbumin and inhibited proliferation and degranulation of mast cells.[53]

ANTI-SIALIC ACID–BINDING IMMUNOGLOBULIN-LIKE LECTIN 8 ANTIBODY

Sialic acid–binding immunoglobulin-like lectin (Siglec)-8 is an inhibitory receptor of the CD33-related subfamily of Siglecs expressed on mature mast cells, eosinophils, and to a lesser extent basophils. When bound to anti-Siglec-8 antibody, it induces apoptosis in eosinophils and inhibits mast cell activity.[54] Lirentelimab or AK002, a humanized anti-Siglec-8 antibody, induced apoptosis of IL-5 ex vivo. Its murine precursor mAK002 prevented passive systemic anaphylaxis through mast cell inhibition in humanized mice.[55] Lirentelimab is currently being investigated as a therapy in eosinophilic esophagitis (NCT04322708) and eosinophilic duodenitis and gastritis (NCT04322604).

EPITHELIAL CYTOKINES: INTERLEUKIN-33 AND THYMIC STROMAL LYMPHOPOIETIN

On allergen exposure, the gut epithelium actively produces cytokines and chemokines, including thymic stromal lymphopoietin (TSLP) and IL-33, which promote dendritic cell activation and TH2 upregulation.[17] IL-33 was shown to be necessary for sensitization to peanut allergens and allergic responses in murine studies.[56] Etokimab (ANB020), an anti-IL-33 monoclonal antibody, was evaluated in a small phase IIa multisite double-blind placebo-controlled trial. Fifteen days after a single dose of etokimab administered to peanut-allergic adults, 73% of those on active therapy tolerated a cumulative dose of 275 mg peanut protein compared with 0% of placebo group.[57]

In a phase II clinical trial, patients receiving Tezepelumab, an anti-TLSP antibody, experienced lower rates of asthma exacerbation compared with those on placebo.[58] A large multicenter double-blind placebo-controlled phase III clinical trial evaluating tezepelumab in adults and adolescents with severe uncontrolled asthma is ongoing (NCT03347279). Adult patients with moderate-to-severe atopic dermatitis actively treated with tezepelumab had improvement in the eczema area and severity index compared with those who received placebo, although the difference between the 2 treatment groups did not reach statistical significance.[59] Tezepelumab has not been investigated yet in treatment of food allergy.

TH1 ADJUVANTS

TH1 adjuvants combined with an allergen may be used to skew the immunologic response toward Th1 polarization. Toll-like receptor (TLR) agonists combined with an allergen such as CpG oligodeoxynucleotides may be another potential therapeutic approach for allergic diseases.[60] Anaphylaxis was reduced when CpG oligodeoxynucleotides were coadministered with ovalbumin and peanut allergen in murine studies.[61–64] In humans, the administration of CpG combined with ragweed allergen has shown efficacy in allergic rhinitis.[65,66]

TLR4 agonist monophosphoryl lipid A (MPL) is another Th1 adjuvant that has shown to improve the clinical symptoms of allergic rhinitis.[67–69] A synthetic form of MPL, glucopyranosyl lipid A, is currently being investigated in a phase I double-blind, placebo-controlled study as adjunctive therapy to peanut SLIT (https://clinicaltrials.gov/show/NCT03463135).

DNA VACCINES

DNA vaccines consist of a bacterial plasmid vectors expressing a target protein gene for *in vivo* administration and transfection. Inclusion of a lysosomal associated membrane protein 1 (LAMP-1) to the DNA plasmid directs the antigen from a proteasomal class I pathway toward a lysosomal class II pathway, hence enhancing their immunogenicity.[70,71] Phase I trials in peanut-allergic adults and teenagers are evaluating the safety, tolerability, and immune response of intradermal and intramuscular ASP0892 (ARA-LAMP-vax), which is a single multivalent peanut (Ara h1, h2, h3) LAMP-DNA plasmid vaccine (https://clinicaltrials.gov/ct2/show/NCT02851277 and https://clinicaltrials.gov/show/NCT03755713).

MODIFIED FOOD ALLERGEN PROTEINS

Modifying an allergen protein may potentially lead to a decreased risk of allergic reaction during desensitization compared with natural protein. Modified food allergen protein was investigated in a phase I trial as a potential therapy for peanut-allergic patients using rectal administered, Heat/Phenol Killed, E. coli Encapsulated, Recombinant Modified Peanut Proteins Ara h 1, Ara h 2, and Ara h 3 (EMP-123). This study demonstrated frequent adverse events including anaphylaxis in 20% of peanut-allergic patients compared with none in healthy control subjects.[72]

A randomized, double-blind, placebo-controlled phase I trial evaluatesthe safety, tolerability, and immunologic effects of subcutaneous HAL-MPE1, a chemically modified adsorbed aluminum hydroxide to peanut extract, in adult and pediatric subjects with peanut allergy (https://clinicaltrials.gov/show/NCT02991885).

TARGETING THE MICROBIOME FOR THE TREATMENT OF FOOD ALLERGY

There is now substantial evidence that the gut microbiota play is a significant role in the pathogenesis of food allergy.[73] The natural immune tolerance promoted by healthy commensal gut bacteria targets both innate and adaptive immune response and protects the intestinal mucosa barrier. Several environmental factors such as diet, antibiotics, cesarean section, and western lifestyle may affect the gut microbiome compositions that subsequently could alter immune tolerance, hence increasing susceptibility to atopic diseases.[74] Conversely, other factors may protect from atopic diseases, such as increased family size and early childhood exposure to pets due to more commensal microbiota diversity.[74,75] Although several studies have evaluated dysbiosis in food allergy, comparison between studies is difficult however, given the significant variability in study design, methods of microbiome analysis, geographic location, and inclusion/exclusion criteria to name a few.[74] The authors recently showed in a prospective study that there is evolving dysbiosis in food-allergic infants that affects 77 different bacterial taxa.[76] Administration of bacteriotherapy including 6 Clostridiales strains and separately 5 Bacteroidales strains, which were affected by the dysbiosis in infants, to a highly allergic food allergy mouse model ($Il4ra^{F709}$ mice) prevented food allergy and completely suppressed anaphylaxis.[76] The authors' studies have demonstrated that the mechanism by which bacteriotherapy regulates food tolerance is complex and depends on TGFβ-1, as well as upregulation of RoRγ +t Treg cells via a TLR/MyD88-dependent mechanism, as well as downregulation of the allergic phenotype of Treg cells, such as GATA3 transcription factor or IL-4 expression.[76] Hence these studies suggest that targeted bacteriotherapy is a promising approach in food allergy treatment. However, the role of the clinically available probiotics in food allergy remains unclear. Infants with cow's milk allergy who received extensively hydrolyzed milk formula (EHMF) supplemented with Lactobacillus GG demonstrated quicker acquisition of tolerance compared with those who received EHMF without probiotic.[77] Patients with cow's milk anaphylaxis or other food allergies were however excluded from the trial. Conversely, a randomized, double-blind placebo-controlled trial among cow's milk allergic infants showed no difference in acquisition of tolerance between infants who received EHMF supplemented with Lactobacillus casei and Bifidobacterium lactis versus those who received EHMF alone.[78] Moreover, the potential role in reducing the risk of atopic diseases and food hypersensitivity was examined in a systematic review that included 2947 infants from 17 studies. Although the study suggested the probiotics could reduce the risk of atopy and food sensitivity when administered prenatally to pregnant women and postnatally to the child, a similar outcome was not observed when the probiotics were given either only prenatally or postnatally.[79]

Lactobacillus rhamnosus CGMCC combined with peanut OIT was evaluated in a randomized double-blind placebo-controlled trial in 62 children aged from 1 to 10 years. Sustained unresponsiveness, evaluated after discontinuation of therapy for 2 to 5 weeks, was noted in 82% of children who received probiotic and peanut OIT compared with 3.6% in the placebo group.[80] However, no solid conclusion could be drawn, given the lack of a comparative treatment arm (peanut OIT with placebo). VE416 is bacterial consortium currently being evaluated as a monotherapy or in combination with peanut OIT in adults and teenagers in a phase I/II trial (NCT03936998).

Fecal microbiota transplantation (FMT) is the transfer of a healthy donor's feces to the gastrointestine of the diseased recipient with the aim of reestablishing the normal microbiome. FMT can be administered via enema, nasogastric route, orally, or by colonoscopy. It has been evaluated very successfully in the treatment of recurrent Clostridium difficile colitis.[81,82] The authors have shown that administering FMT from healthy human babies into $Il4ra^{F709}$ mice rescued the mice from severe anaphylaxis, unlike when FMT from FA babies was administered into these mice.[76] Similar results were observed in a different mouse model sensitized to milk. FMT from healthy babies into mice that were subsequently sensitized to cow's milk allergen β-lactoglobulin protected from anaphylaxis, unlike FMT taken from milk allergic infants.[83] Given these promising results, the authors are currently evaluating in a phase I open-label trial the safety and efficacy of oral, frozen encapsulated FMT in peanut allergic adults aged 18 to 40 years with and without pretreatment with antibiotics (NCT02960074).

SUMMARY

Earlier this year, the first oral immunotherapy for food allergy was FDA approved. New therapeutic approaches are however urgently needed to improve treatment outcome. Biologics are attractive options either as monotherapy or as adjunct to food immunotherapy, as they may improve compliance, target multiple food allergies, and treat other concomitant atopic diseases. Although omalizumab has been evaluated extensively in allergic diseases, most biologics are more novel and have broader immunologic impact. Hence, although many of these biologics have very promising preliminary data on suppressing the allergic response, careful evaluation of their safety and their modulation of the immune system should be conducted.

CLINICS CARE POINTS

- AR101 (Palforzia) is the first FDA-approved oral immunotherapy for peanut allergy. There is an unmet need for investigating other therapies.
- There are currently no biologics approved for food allergy treatment, but studies are on the way for some.
- Careful evaluation of the safety of these biologics and their effect on immunomodulation in vivo should be conducted.

REFERENCES

1. Gupta RS, Springston EE, Warrier MR, et al. The prevalence, severity, and distribution of childhood food allergy in the United States. Pediatrics 2011;128(1): e9–17.
2. Gupta RS, Warren CM, Smith BM, et al. Prevalence and Severity of Food Allergies Among US Adults. JAMA Netw Open 2019;2(1):e185630.
3. Jackson KD, Howie LD, Akinbami LJ. Trends in allergic conditions among children: United States, 1997-2011. NCHS Data Brief 2013;(121):1–8.
4. Patel N, Herbert L, Green TD. The emotional, social, and financial burden of food allergies on children and their families. Allergy Asthma Proc 2017;38(2):88–91.
5. Sicherer SH, Sampson HA. Food allergy: Epidemiology, pathogenesis, diagnosis, and treatment. J Allergy Clin Immunol 2014;133(2):291–307 [quiz: 308].
6. Patrawala M, Shih J, Lee G, et al. Peanut oral immunotherapy: a current perspective. Curr Allergy Asthma Rep 2020;20(5):14.
7. Vickery BP, Vereda A, Casale TB, et al. AR101 oral immunotherapy for peanut allergy. N Engl J Med 2018;379(21):1991–2001.
8. Yee CS, Rachid R. The Heterogeneity of Oral Immunotherapy Clinical Trials: Implications and Future Directions. Curr Allergy Asthma Rep 2016;16(4):25.
9. Varshney P, Jones SM, Scurlock AM, et al. A randomized controlled study of peanut oral immunotherapy: clinical desensitization and modulation of the allergic response. J Allergy Clin Immunol 2011;127(3):654–60.
10. Akashi M, Yasudo H, Narita M, et al. Randomized controlled trial of oral immunotherapy for egg allergy in Japanese patients. Pediatr Int 2017;59(5):534–9.
11. Chu DK, Wood RA, French S, et al. Oral immunotherapy for peanut allergy (PACE): a systematic review and meta-analysis of efficacy and safety. Lancet 2019;393(10187):2222–32.
12. Vickery BP, Scurlock AM, Kulis M, et al. Sustained unresponsiveness to peanut in subjects who have completed peanut oral immunotherapy. J Allergy Clin Immunol 2014;133(2):468–75.
13. Syed A, Garcia MA, Lyu SC, et al. Peanut oral immunotherapy results in increased antigen-induced regulatory T-cell function and hypomethylation of forkhead box protein 3 (FOXP3). J Allergy Clin Immunol 2014;133(2):500–10.
14. Fleischer DM, Greenhawt M, Sussman G, et al. Effect of epicutaneous immunotherapy vs placebo on reaction to peanut protein ingestion among children with peanut allergy: the PEPITES randomized clinical trial. JAMA 2019;321(10): 946–55.
15. Kim EH, Yang L, Ye P, et al. Long-term sublingual immunotherapy for peanut allergy in children: Clinical and immunologic evidence of desensitization. J Allergy Clin Immunol 2019;144(5):1320–6.e1.

16. Waldron J, Kim EH. Sublingual and patch immunotherapy for food allergy. Immunol Allergy Clin North Am 2020;40(1):135–48.
17. Bauer RN, Manohar M, Singh AM, et al. The future of biologics: applications for food allergy. J Allergy Clin Immunol 2015;135(2):312–23.
18. Sampath V, Sindher SB, Zhang W, et al. New treatment directions in food allergy. Ann Allergy Asthma Immunol 2018;120(3):254–62.
19. Liu J, Lester P, Builder S, et al. Characterization of complex formation by humanized anti-IgE monoclonal antibody and monoclonal human IgE. Biochemistry 1995;34(33):10474–82.
20. Sampson HA, Leung DY, Burks AW, et al. A phase II, randomized, double-blind, parallel-group, placebo-controlled oral food challenge trial of Xolair (omalizumab) in peanut allergy. J Allergy Clin Immunol 2011;127(5):1309–10.e1.
21. Savage JH, Courneya JP, Sterba PM, et al. Kinetics of mast cell, basophil, and oral food challenge responses in omalizumab-treated adults with peanut allergy. J Allergy Clin Immunol 2012;130(5):1123–9.e2.
22. Fiocchi A, Artesani MC, Riccardi C, et al. Impact of omalizumab on food allergy in patients treated for asthma: a real-life study. J Allergy Clin Immunol Pract 2019; 7(6):1901–9.e5.
23. Nadeau KC, Schneider LC, Hoyte L, et al. Rapid oral desensitization in combination with omalizumab therapy in patients with cow's milk allergy. J Allergy Clin Immunol 2011;127(6):1622–4.
24. Andorf S, Manohar M, Dominguez T, et al. Observational long-term follow-up study of rapid food oral immunotherapy with omalizumab. Allergy Asthma Clin Immunol 2017;13:51.
25. MacGinnitie AJ, Rachid R, Gragg H, et al. Omalizumab facilitates rapid oral desensitization for peanut allergy. J Allergy Clin Immunol 2017;139(3):873–81.e8.
26. Wood RA, Kim JS, Lindblad R, et al. A randomized, double-blind, placebo-controlled study of omalizumab combined with oral immunotherapy for the treatment of cow's milk allergy. J Allergy Clin Immunol 2016;137(4):1103–10.e1.
27. Schneider LC, Rachid R, LeBovidge J, et al. A pilot study of omalizumab to facilitate rapid oral desensitization in high-risk peanut-allergic patients. J Allergy Clin Immunol 2013;132(6):1368–74.
28. Andorf S, Purington N, Block WM, et al. Anti-IgE treatment with oral immunotherapy in multifood allergic participants: a double-blind, randomised, controlled trial. Lancet Gastroenterol Hepatol 2018;3(2):85–94.
29. Andorf S, Purington N, Kumar D, et al. A phase 2 randomized controlled multisite study using omalizumab-facilitated rapid desensitization to test continued vs discontinued dosing in multifood allergic individuals. EClinicalMedicine 2019;7: 27–38.
30. Kocatürk E, Zuberbier T. New biologics in the treatment of urticaria. Curr Opin Allergy Clin Immunol 2018;18(5):425–31.
31. Gauvreau GM, Arm JP, Boulet LP, et al. Efficacy and safety of multiple doses of QGE031 (ligelizumab) versus omalizumab and placebo in inhibiting allergen-induced early asthmatic responses. J Allergy Clin Immunol 2016;138(4):1051–9.
32. Maurer M, Giménez-Arnau AM, Sussman G, et al. Ligelizumab for chronic spontaneous urticaria. N Engl J Med 2019;381(14):1321–32.
33. Harb H, Chatila TA. Mechanisms of Dupilumab. Clin Exp Allergy 2020;50(1):5–14.
34. Rabe KF, Nair P, Brusselle G, et al. Efficacy and safety of dupilumab in glucocorticoid-dependent severe asthma. N Engl J Med 2018;378(26):2475–85.
35. Bachert C, Han JK, Desrosiers M, et al. Efficacy and safety of dupilumab in patients with severe chronic rhinosinusitis with nasal polyps (LIBERTY NP SINUS-24

and LIBERTY NP SINUS-52): results from two multicentre, randomised, double-blind, placebo-controlled, parallel-group phase 3 trials. Lancet 2019; 394(10209):1638–50.

36. Beck LA, Thaçi D, Hamilton JD, et al. Dupilumab treatment in adults with moderate-to-severe atopic dermatitis. N Engl J Med 2014;371(2):130–9.

37. Paller AS, Siegfried EC, Thaçi D, et al. Efficacy and safety of dupilumab with concomitant topical corticosteroids in children 6 to 11 years old with severe atopic dermatitis: a randomized, double-blinded, placebo-controlled phase 3 trial. J Am Acad Dermatol 2020;83(5):1282–93.

38. Abdel-Gadir A, Schneider L, Casini A, et al. Oral immunotherapy with omalizumab reverses the Th2 cell-like programme of regulatory T cells and restores their function. Clin Exp Allergy 2018;48(7):825–36.

39. Rial MJ, Barroso B, Sastre J. Dupilumab for treatment of food allergy. J Allergy Clin Immunol Pract 2018;7(2):673–4.

40. Hanania NA, Korenblat P, Chapman KR, et al. Efficacy and safety of lebrikizumab in patients with uncontrolled asthma (LAVOLTA I and LAVOLTA II): replicate, phase 3, randomised, double-blind, placebo-controlled trials. Lancet Respir Med 2016;4(10):781–96.

41. Liu Y, Zhang S, Chen R, et al. Meta-analysis of randomized controlled trials for the efficacy and safety of anti-interleukin-13 therapy with lebrikizumab in patients with uncontrolled asthma. Allergy Asthma Proc 2018;39(5):332–7.

42. Rothenberg ME, Wen T, Greenberg A, et al. Intravenous anti-IL-13 mAb QAX576 for the treatment of eosinophilic esophagitis. J Allergy Clin Immunol 2015;135(2):500–7.

43. Farne HA, Wilson A, Powell C, et al. Anti-IL5 therapies for asthma. Cochrane Database Syst Rev 2017;9(9):Cd010834.

44. Matera MG, Calzetta L, Rogliani P, et al. Monoclonal antibodies for severe asthma: Pharmacokinetic profiles. Respir Med 2019;153:3–13.

45. Burton OT, Noval Rivas M, Zhou JS, et al. Immunoglobulin E signal inhibition during allergen ingestion leads to reversal of established food allergy and induction of regulatory T cells. Immunity 2014;41(1):141–51.

46. Kim MS, Rådinger M, Gilfillan AM. The multiple roles of phosphoinositide 3-kinase in mast cell biology. Trends Immunol 2008;29(10):493–501.

47. Smiljkovic D, Blatt K, Stefanzl G, et al. BTK inhibition is a potent approach to block IgE-mediated histamine release in human basophils. Allergy 2017;72(11):1666–76.

48. Isaac K, Mato AR. Acalabrutinib and Its Therapeutic Potential in the Treatment of Chronic Lymphocytic Leukemia: A Short Review on Emerging Data. Cancer Manag Res 2020;12:2079–85.

49. Dispenza MC, Krier-Burris RA, Chhiba KD, et al. Bruton's tyrosine kinase inhibition effectively protects against human IgE-mediated anaphylaxis. J Clin Invest 2020; 130(9):4759–70.

50. Damsky W, King BA. JAK inhibitors in dermatology: The promise of a new drug class. J Am Acad Dermatol 2017;76(4):736–44.

51. Rodrigues MA, Torres T. JAK/STAT inhibitors for the treatment of atopic dermatitis. J Dermatolog Treat 2020;31(1):33–40.

52. Silverberg JI, Simpson EL, Thyssen JP, et al. Efficacy and Safety of Abrocitinib in Patients With Moderate-to-Severe Atopic Dermatitis: A Randomized Clinical Trial. JAMA Dermatol 2020;156(8):863–73.

53. Yamaki K, Yoshino S. Remission of food allergy by the Janus kinase inhibitor ruxolitinib in mice. Int Immunopharmacol 2014;18(2):217–24.

54. Nutku E, Aizawa H, Hudson SA, et al. Ligation of Siglec-8: a selective mechanism for induction of human eosinophil apoptosis. Blood 2003;101(12):5014–20.

55. Youngblood BA, Brock EC, Leung J, et al. AK002, a Humanized Sialic Acid-Binding Immunoglobulin-Like Lectin-8 Antibody that Induces Antibody-Dependent Cell-Mediated Cytotoxicity against Human Eosinophils and Inhibits Mast Cell-Mediated Anaphylaxis in Mice. Int Arch Allergy Immunol 2019;180(2): 91–102.

56. Chu DK, Llop-Guevara A, Walker TD, et al. IL-33, but not thymic stromal lympho-poietin or IL-25, is central to mite and peanut allergic sensitization. J Allergy Clin Immunol 2013;131(1):187–200.e1-8.

57. Chinthrajah S, Cao S, Liu C, et al. Phase 2a randomized, placebo-controlled study of anti-IL-33 in peanut allergy. JCI Insight 2019;4(22):e131347.

58. Corren J, Parnes JR, Wang L, et al. Tezepelumab in adults with uncontrolled asthma. N Engl J Med 2017;377(10):936–46.

59. Simpson EL, Parnes JR, She D, et al. Tezepelumab, an anti-thymic stromal lym-phopoietin monoclonal antibody, in the treatment of moderate to severe atopic dermatitis: A randomized phase 2a clinical trial. J Am Acad Dermatol 2019; 80(4):1013–21.

60. Keet CA, Wood RA. Emerging therapies for food allergy. J Clin Invest 2014; 124(5):1880–6.

61. Adel-Patient K, Ah-Leung S, Bernard H, et al. Oral sensitization to peanut is highly enhanced by application of peanut extracts to intact skin, but is prevented when CpG and cholera toxin are added. Int Arch Allergy Immunol 2007;143(1):10–20.

62. Kulis M, Gorentla B, Burks AW, et al. Type B CpG oligodeoxynucleotides induce Th1 responses to peanut antigens: modulation of sensitization and utility in a trun-cated immunotherapy regimen in mice. Mol Nutr Food Res 2013;57(5):906–15.

63. San Román B, Irache JM, Gómez S, et al. Co-delivery of ovalbumin and CpG mo-tifs into microparticles protected sensitized mice from anaphylaxis. Int Arch Al-lergy Immunol 2009;149(2):111–8.

64. Xu W, Tamura T, Takatsu K. CpG ODN mediated prevention from ovalbumin-induced anaphylaxis in mouse through B cell pathway. Int Immunopharmacol 2008;8(2):351–61.

65. Creticos PS, Schroeder JT, Hamilton RG, et al. Immunotherapy with a ragweed-toll-like receptor 9 agonist vaccine for allergic rhinitis. N Engl J Med 2006; 355(14):1445–55.

66. Tulic MK, Fiset PO, Christodoulopoulos P, et al. Amb a 1-immunostimulatory oligo-deoxynucleotide conjugate immunotherapy decreases the nasal inflammatory response. J Allergy Clin Immunol 2004;113(2):235–41.

67. Patel P, Holdich T, Fischer von Weikersthal-Drachenberg KJ, et al. Efficacy of a short course of specific immunotherapy in patients with allergic rhinoconjunctivi-tis to ragweed pollen. J Allergy Clin Immunol 2014;133(1):121–9.e1-2.

68. Pfaar O, Barth C, Jaschke C, et al. Sublingual allergen-specific immunotherapy adjuvanted with monophosphoryl lipid A: a phase I/IIa study. Int Arch Allergy Im-munol 2011;154(4):336–44.

69. Rosewich M, Schulze J, Fischer von Weikersthal-Drachenberg KJ, et al. Ultra-short course immunotherapy in children and adolescents during a 3-yrs post-marketing surveillance study. Pediatr Allergy Immunol 2010;21(1 Pt 2):e185–9.

70. Liu MA. DNA vaccines: an historical perspective and view to the future. Immunol Rev 2011;239(1):62–84.

71. Su Y, Connolly M, Marketon A, et al. CryJ-LAMP DNA vaccines for japanese red cedar allergy induce robust Th1-type immune responses in murine model. J Immunol Res 2016;2016:4857869.

72. Wood RA, Sicherer SH, Burks AW, et al. A phase 1 study of heat/phenol-killed, E. coli-encapsulated, recombinant modified peanut proteins Ara h 1, Ara h 2, and Ara h 3 (EMP-123) for the treatment of peanut allergy. Allergy 2013;68(6):803–8.

73. Stephen-Victor E, Crestani E, Chatila TA. Dietary and microbial determinants in food allergy. Immunity 2020;53(2):277–89.

74. Rachid R, Chatila TA. The role of the gut microbiota in food allergy. Curr Opin Pediatr 2016;28(6):748–53.

75. Zhao W, Ho HE, Bunyavanich S. The gut microbiome in food allergy. Ann Allergy Asthma Immunol 2019;122(3):276–82.

76. Abdel-Gadir A, Stephen-Victor E, Gerber GK, et al. Microbiota therapy acts via a regulatory T cell MyD88/RORγt pathway to suppress food allergy. Nat Med 2019; 25(7):1164–74.

77. Berni Canani R, Nocerino R, Terrin G, et al. Effect of Lactobacillus GG on tolerance acquisition in infants with cow's milk allergy: a randomized trial. J Allergy Clin Immunol 2012;129(2):580–2, 582.e1-5.

78. Hol J, van Leer EH, Elink Schuurman BE, et al. The acquisition of tolerance toward cow's milk through probiotic supplementation: a randomized, controlled trial. J Allergy Clin Immunol 2008;121(6):1448–54.

79. Zhang GQ, Hu HJ, Liu CY, et al. Probiotics for Prevention of Atopy and Food Hypersensitivity in Early Childhood: A PRISMA-Compliant Systematic Review and Meta-Analysis of Randomized Controlled Trials. Medicine (Baltimore) 2016; 95(8):e2562.

80. Tang ML, Ponsonby AL, Orsini F, et al. Administration of a probiotic with peanut oral immunotherapy: A randomized trial. J Allergy Clin Immunol 2015;135(3): 737–44.e8.

81. van Nood E, Vrieze A, Nieuwdorp M, et al. Duodenal infusion of donor feces for recurrent Clostridium difficile. N Engl J Med 2013;368(5):407–15.

82. Youngster I, Russell GH, Pindar C, et al. Oral, capsulized, frozen fecal microbiota transplantation for relapsing Clostridium difficile infection. JAMA 2014;312(17): 1772–8.

83. Feehley T, Plunkett CH, Bao R, et al. Healthy infants harbor intestinal bacteria that protect against food allergy. Nat Med 2019;25(3):448–53.

The Infant Microbiome and Its Impact on Development of Food Allergy

Kylie N. Jungles, MD[a,b,1], Kassidy M. Jungles, BS[c,1],
Leah Greenfield, BS[b,d], Mahboobeh Mahdavinia, MD, PhD[b,*,1]

KEYWORDS

- Food allergy (FA) • Gut microbiome • Mediterranean diet • *Prevotella copri (P copri)*

KEY POINTS

- Infant gut microbiome influences the development of food allergy (FA).
- The gut microbiome begins developing during gestation and is influenced heavily by environmental factors during gestation and early infancy.
- Gut microbiome is impacted by infant feeding method, probiotics, infant diet, and maternal diet during lactation.
- Diet has been linked to the commensal gut microbiota, which can be associated with the risk of inflammation and FA.

INTRODUCTION

Food allergies (FAs) have become a growing public health problem, especially in the United States and other industrialized Western nations. The prevalence of FA has been increasing steadily over the past 2 decades to 3 decades.[1] Moreover, it is more common in pediatric populations, with 8% of children impacted compared with 3% of adults.[1] Of those with diagnosed FAs, approximately 3% experience severe or life-threatening reactions and 2.4% have an FA to multiple foods.[1,2]

There currently are no cures available for the treatment of FA, with avoidance the primary measure for preventing an acute allergic reaction. A great deal of research has aimed to help better explain which individuals are at risk for the development of

[a] Department of Pediatrics, University of Michigan C.S. Mott Children's Hospital, 1540 E Hospital Dr #4204, Ann Arbor, MI 48109, USA; [b] Department of Internal Medicine, Allergy and Immunology Division, Rush University Medical Center, 1725 West Harrison Street, Suite 117, Chicago, IL 60612, USA; [c] Department of Pharmacology, University of Michigan, 1150 W Medical Center Dr, Ann Arbor, MI 48109, USA; [d] Rush Medical College, 600 S Paulina St Suite 524, Chicago, IL 60612, USA
[1] Have contributed equally.
* Corresponding author. Allergy and Immunology Division, Internal Medicine Department, Rush University Medical Center, 1725 West Harrison Street, Suite 117, Chicago, IL 60612.
E-mail address: Mahboobeh_mahdavinia@rush.edu

Immunol Allergy Clin N Am 41 (2021) 285–299
https://doi.org/10.1016/j.iac.2021.01.004
0889-8561/21/© 2021 Elsevier Inc. All rights reserved.
immunology.theclinics.com

FA and whether the individual's microbiota may play a role in this risk. Race and ethnicity are major risk factors for the development of FAs and other atopic conditions.[1,3] Additionally, there is an abundance of modifiable risk factors that have been shown to increase an individual's risk for developing FA, including mode of delivery (vaginal delivery vs cesarean section), infant feeding method (breastfeeding vs formula feeding), use of antibiotics in pregnancy, rural versus urban living, and diet (consumption of dietary fats, antioxidants, and vitamin D).[4] This abundance of FA-associated risk factors calls into question whether they individually increase a person's risk for development of FA, or, if perhaps, it is a culmination of these factors that modifies an individual's immune system, making that individual more susceptible for FA development. Current research suggests that it likely is a combination of risk factors, and together these modifiable and nonmodifiable risk factors influence the composition of an individual's gut microbiome.[4]

Studies suggest that an individual's gut microbiota begins developing during gestation and is influenced heavily by factors in early infant life. Environmental factors, such as mode of delivery, infant feeding, and various environmental exposures, influence the development of gut microbiota and can lead to disruption of the original gut microbiota composition.[5] Research suggests that this gut dysbiosis can have an impact on an individual's immune system and lead to the development of FA.[5] This article discusses how alterations to the gut microbiome may influence the development of FA.

HISTORY
The Crucial Role of the Gut Microbiome in Tolerance or Allergy

In understanding FA, the gut microbiota and the potential role of the gut immune response in oral tolerance first must be understood. The gut microbiome is essential to an individual's immune system function. Trillions of microbes colonize sites within the human body, with a majority of those microbes localized to the gastrointestinal tract.[5] Studies suggest that these microbes are essential for the health of the gastrointestinal mucosa, which is responsible for producing the majority of antibodies within the human body.[6] The gut-associated lymphoid tissue (GALT) refers to the inductive sites of the immune system that contain various structures, including lymphoid follicles, mesenteric lymph nodes, and Peyer patches.[6,7] GALT contains more than half of the peripheral lymphocytes of the body and functions in recognizing foreign food particles.[7]

Oral tolerance refers to the immune system's ability to not respond to orally administered harmless antigens, such as those found in food.[6] GALT plays a role in oral tolerance by recognizing antigens found within the mucosal surface that covers the intestinal epithelium of the gut.[7] The intestinal system typically breaks down ingested food antigens via digestive enzymes, and GALT contains structures responsible for properly presenting food antigens to T cells.[5] The follicle-associated epithelium refers to the collection of the GALT lymphoid follicles and contains microfold (M) cells.[7] M cells are intestinal epithelial cells that phagocytose antigens from the lumen of the gut and deliver them to dendritic cells (DCs) of the submucosa.[7,8] Although GALT is considered the inductive region of the intestinal immune system, the effector immune site of the intestine consists of DCs, macrophages, and lymphocytes.[7] In this complex, stepwise process, stromal cells help with activating these T cells into Foxp3[+] regulatory T cells (Tregs) and/or interleukin (IL)-10–secreting type 1 regulatory cells.[5] and deficiency in these processes can lead to inflammation and allergy.[5]

Studies show that the microbiota plays a critical role in the integrity of the mucosal epithelial barrier, thus being a critical factor in the regulation of the immune system and allergy.[5,8] In the intestine, mucus is produced by goblet cells and antimicrobial peptides are secreted by Paneth cells to help maintain the integrity of the intestinal epithelium and maintain a barrier between the external environment and internal environment of the body.[7,8] The amount of mucus and antimicrobial peptides produced correlates to the amount and types of microorganisms present in the gut microbiota, such as *Clostridia*.[8] Dysbiosis of the gut microbiota triggers the secretion of alarmin molecules, such as IL-33, thymic stromal lymphopoietin, and IL-25 at epithelial barrier surfaces.[8] These alarmins trigger lymphoid cells to create type 2 helper T (T_H2) cell cytokines, and, consequently, promote B cells to carry out class switching to IgE.[8] FA typically is associated with the production of IgE antibodies, and, by understanding the role of the gut microbiota in the development of these antibodies, this perhaps can provide important insight in treating allergic disease.[8,9]

The Evolution of the Hygiene Hypothesis

The hygiene hypothesis first was introduced in 1989 and stated that an increased prevalence of allergies was occurring across populations due to enhanced sanitation practices that decreased exposure to microorganisms.[5] Some of the enhanced sanitation and public health measures that correlated to this increase in allergy include the pasteurization of food products, vaccination against disease, prescription of antibiotics against bacterial infections, and sanitation of water.[10] Under this hypothesis, the reason for the development of allergy was linked to a shift in allergic responses due to type 1 helper T (T_H1) cells and T_H2 cells. T_H1 cells produce the cytokines, tumor necrosis factor β, Il-1, interferon-γ, and IL-2, and interact with B cells to product immunoglobulins. Unlike T_H1 cells, however, T_H2 cells produce the cytokines, IL-4, IL-5, IL-9, and IL-13, which cause B cells to produce IgE immunoglobulins that are involved in allergy by triggering the production and activation of mast cells and eosinophils.[11] In respect to the hygiene hypothesis, it initially was asserted that when individuals are not exposed to microbes at an early age, this favors T_H2 cell development that causes allergic responses.[10] Consequently, it was hypothesized that when individuals are exposed to microorganisms at an early age, this favors a T_H1 cell response and does not cause a similar predisposition for allergy.[10] Recent studies examining autoimmune diseases, endotoxins, and parasites suggest, however, that this type of helper T-cell interaction not always is the sole explanation for allergy susceptibility.[10,12] Further studies emphasize the importance of Tregs in allergy risk and more work must be done to understand the role of Tregs in allergy predisposition.[11]

Although the hygiene hypothesis offers important insights into the susceptibility to allergy, this hypothesis is more simplistic than initially believed. Current studies highlight the importance of understanding both the microbiota found in the external environment and internal environment of those with allergies.[5] A plethora of studies emphasizes the importance of the gut microbiota as playing a critical role in the development of allergy and exposure to microorganisms—often as early as birth—contributing significantly to the predisposition for developing allergy.[12]

DISCUSSION
Relationship Between the Infant Microbiome and Food Allergy

The gut microbiome is a dynamic environment that constantly is being influenced and modified by external factors. The composition of gut microbiota is impacted by various environmental factors, such as diet, lifestyle, and pathogen exposure. These exposures begin as early as gestation and continue throughout the course of an individual's lifetime, as the gut and immune system are educated on which exposures require the body to mount an immune response against foreign invaders.[5] Disruptions occurring throughout this process may result in a malfunctioning or hyperactive immune system, resulting in inappropriate immune responses to innocuous targets, such as harmless food proteins. The immune response against food proteins also has been linked to other comorbid conditions.[13] Disruptions in this educational process and dysbiosis of an individual's original gut microbiome are associated with the development of FA.[5]

The gut microbiome is established in early gestation and continues to be heavily influenced by external factors throughout infancy and early childhood.[14] Infants are exposed to microbiota via the placenta, meconium, and vaginal canal during gestation and birth, which influence the colonization of their gut microbiome.[5,15] A significant difference in microbiota composition exists between the neonatal period and infancy. The gut microbiome of a fetus is influenced first by the maternal gut microbiome, diet, and health and consists mainly of *Proteobacteria* species.[5,15] When infants are born, their microbiome is changed significantly in accordance with the mode of delivery and also changes based on diet during infancy.[15] Another major change occurs between infancy and childhood, when children begin to consume solid food and have an increased diversity of bacteria species, including *Enterococci, Enterobacteria, Clostridium, Streptococcus,* and *Bacteroides* species.[15] At 3 years to 4 years of age, children have a more stable microbiome that is, representative of the adult microbiome; however, the microbiome still can change based on diet, health, and medical treatments.[15] These changes that occur with aging also are indicative of an increase in *Bacteroidaceae* species and decrease in *Enterobacteriaceae* species throughout life—also known as an *Enterobacteriaceae/ Bacteroidaceae* ratio[5] (**Fig. 1**).

Previous studies have shown that early infancy, specifically between 3 months and 6 months of age, is a crucial time where gut microbiota has an impact on the development of FA.[15,16] Specifically, Azad and colleagues[16] found that a low species richness of gut microbiota in children at 3 months of age is associated with increased likelihood of food sensitization by 1 year of age. The Canadian Healthy Infant Longitudinal Development study found that each quartile increase in species richness at 3 months old reduced the risk of them developing food sensitization at 1 year of age by 55%.[15] Additionally, this study found that each quartile increase in the ratio of *Enterobacteriaceae/Bacteroidaceae*, or the greater the abundance of *Bacteroidaceae* species, increased a child's risk of developing food sensitization twofold.[15] Numerous studies have found that individuals with a higher relative abundance of *Bacteroides* and

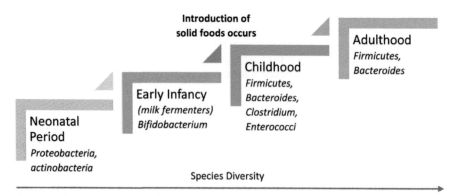

Fig. 1. Predominant gut microbiota throughout the stages of childhood development.

Clostridium clusters have an increased risk of developing atopic dermatitis (AD) and other atopic comorbidities.[17] On the other hand, *Prevotella* species have been found to serve a protective role in the gut against the development of AD, which often is associated with FA in children.[18] Current research suggests that environmental exposures during infancy, including breastfeeding, and both infant and maternal diets may influence gut microbiome development in neonates.

Breastfeeding and Infant Microbiome

Breastfeeding in infancy has many positive effects for both mother and baby, one of which potentially is serving as a protective factor against the development of food sensitization. Breastfeeding currently is recommended for multiple reasons, including but not limited to possible prevention of allergic diseases, including FA.[19] The current scientific basis for this recommendation, however, is based on cohort studies and is not understood completely due to research limitations, because it is unethical to have randomized controlled studies where mothers are asked to refrain from breastfeeding.[20] One study found that exclusive breastfeeding demonstrated a protective effect on the development of cow's milk allergy in pediatric patients during early childhood.[19] Goldsmith and colleagues,[21] however, performed a population-based study of approximately 5000 infants and found that duration of exclusive breastfeeding and use of partially hydrolyzed formula were not associated with development of food sensitization at 1 year of age. Additionally, studies have found that maternal avoidance of the top 8 food allergens during breastfeeding is ineffective in prevention of food sensitization in infants.[22]

Although the association between food sensitization and infant feeding still is unclear, there have been confirmed correlations between infant feeding and the development of the infant gut microbiome. One study found that early feeding patterns in infants have a significant effect on the composition of a child's gut microbiome.[23] Breastfeeding has been associated with a higher diversity of gut microbiota in infants compared with infants who are formula-fed.[24] Additionally, cohort study findings, including the Wayne County Health, Environment, Allergy, and Asthma Longitudinal Study (see article by Eapen and Kim, in this issue), have found that breastfeeding is a major source of beneficial bacterial species, including *Bifidobacteria*, *Lactobacilli*, and *Enterobacteriaceae*.[19] Conversely, formula-fed infants have been found to have significantly higher concentrations of *Clostridium*, *Streptococcus*, and *Bacteroides*[25–27] which, when present in high quantities, have been associated with the development of food sensitization.[15,17] A study by Levin and colleagues[23] found that exclusive breastfeeding was associated with a decreased abundance of taxa from *Clostridia*, *Faecalibacterium*, and *Ruminococcus* genera. These findings are supported further by studies suggesting that once cessation of breastfeeding occurs, the gut microbiota of breastfed infants, which was dominated by *Bifidobacteria*, *Lactobacilli*, and *Enterobacteriaceae* species, is surpassed by *Clostridium* and *Bacteroides* species.[19,28] A significant change in gut microbiota composition occurs with the cessation of breastfeeding and is seen in most children approximately 9 months to 18 months of age, once they transition from breastfeeding to introduction of solid foods.[28] In coordination with infant feeding method, there is evidence suggesting that maternal diet during gestation and lactation has an impact on a child's risk of developing FA.

Infant/Maternal Diet and Infant Microbiome

There are some studies on the association between maternal diet and infant's health and microbiota. The Mediterranean diet is widely recognized as a healthy dietary pattern that focuses on intake of fruits, vegetables, legumes, nuts, and whole grains, while largely avoiding saturated fats, meats, sweets, and dairy products.[29] A maternal Mediterranean diet during gestation has been associated with a lower risk of asthma and atopy development[30–32] and elements of the Mediterranean diet, such as high maternal intake of fruits, vegetables, fish oil, and vitamin D, may confer protection against atopic disease.[33–35]

Netting and colleagues[33] conducted a systematic review of 42 studies examining the relationship between maternal diet and atopic disease of the offspring that included more than 40,000 children. Higher adherence to a Mediterranean diet was one of the few consistent associations that could be made between maternal diet during gestation or lactation and protection from subsequent development of allergic disease in the child. In contrast, a maternal diet during gestation consisting of high levels of vegetable oils, margarine, nuts, and fast food frequently, although not universally, were found to increase a child's risk of developing atopic disease.[33] In terms of FA specifically, some studies demonstrated that inclusion of common food allergens in the maternal diet during gestation and lactation may confer protection against development of FA, but others were inconclusive.[33] No studies associated maternal Mediterranean diet with an increased risk of atopy in the child, and, considering its well-demonstrated health benefits,[36] it is a safe and advisable dietary pattern during gestation and lactation.[37] Another systematic review evaluating 32 studies on maternal diet in relation to atopic disease in offspring largely was inconclusive, demonstrating only a possible protective effect of vitamin D, vitamin E, and zinc against wheeze, and of copper against FA.[38] Both reviews cite inconsistent dietary questionnaires and heterogeneity in the outcome measurements of included studies as limitations and suggest cautious interpretation of their results given the considerable potential for confounding.[33–38]

There also is evidence for an association between infant diet in early life and protection against atopic symptoms.[39–41] A prospective cohort study including 123 infants was conducted to evaluate the relationship between early life diet and the development of FA.[40] The results show that an infant diet rich in fruits, vegetables, and homemade foods is associated with lower rates of FA by 2 years of age. It was theorized that higher fruit and vegetable intake is protective because of the beneficial anti-inflammatory effects of nutrients found in these foods, such as β-carotenes, folate, oligosaccharides, and vitamin C. The benefit of homemade foods was attributed to higher overall micronutrient content, because food processing is known disrupt this. These effects were not allergen-specific, because the differences were significant regardless of the food that the child was sensitized to.[40] In older children, adherence to a Mediterranean diet also has been shown to reduce wheeze and hay fever symptoms,[42,43] suggesting that the protection of a healthy diet against atopy is not limited to the first few years of life. Importantly, delayed introduction or avoidance of potentially allergenic foods no longer is recommended to decrease the risk of FA because the efficacy of this strategy is not well supported.[44] Taking the opposite approach by early introduction of potentially allergenic food into the infant diet has proved effective in reducing the risk of peanut allergy, but further research on other common allergens is needed.[22]

High-sugar and high-fat diets also have been associated with an increased risk of atopic disease in both children and adults.[18,45] This association may be moderated by the gut microbiome, epigenetic changes, or interaction of both. A case-control study, which linked atopic disease to high-sugar and high-fat intake in children, also found that atopic disease risk was associated with significant differences in the gut microbiome.[18] Recent literature review provides further evidence of the modulatory role of the gut in allergic disease, concluding that the gut microbiome is 1 likely factor to explain the protective effect of breastfeeding against FA.[19] These findings suggest that mediators, such as the gut microbiome, are important in explaining the link between diet and FA. Epigenetic changes also may be an important explanation of the link between high-sugar and high-fat diets and FA. It has been demonstrated that diet can activate epigenetic changes directly in early life, which can result in modifications of gut mucosal immunity.[46,47] These early-life modifications might be a causal factor in the development of atopic disease because, once induced, epigenetic changes can have long-term consequences. For example, transiently high glucose levels have been implicated in causing persistent glucose intolerance via epigenetic changes in the nuclear factor (NF)-κB gene.[48] The NF-κB gene regulates gene expression in the immune system, and its specific relationship to atopic disease is still being elucidated.[5] Similar mechanisms of epigenetic dysregulation in this or other genes induced by dietary intake could underlie the development of FA.

Epigenetic mechanisms and the gut microbiome may influence the development of atopic disease both separately and through interaction with one another. A review by Paparo and colleagues[46] explains that dietary differences have been associated with differences in the metabolic outputs of the gut microbiome and that these metabolic outputs then go on to influence epigenetic changes in host immune cells, such as macrophages and DCs. A focus on multistep causal pathways, such as this one, will be important as more work is done to further clarify the pathogenesis of FA and other atopic conditions.

Some of the most influential gut microbial outputs to be identified are short-chain fatty acids (SCFAs), which may help explain how the microbes in the gut interact with diet to modulate allergic responses. SCFAs are produced by commensal bacteria in the gut through fermentation of undigested dietary carbohydrates.[49] Higher adherence to the Mediterranean diet is associated with higher levels of fecal SCFA,[50] which can be attributed the Mediterranean diet's high levels of undigestible complex carbohydrates and fiber.[51] SCFAs are used by colonic epithelial cells for energy, having epigenetic influence on immune tolerance in the gut by modulating tight junction proteins, mucus production, and several types of adaptive (T cells and B cells) and innate (macrophages, neutrophils, and DCs) immune cells.[52–67]

The 4 major SCFA groups are acetate, propionate, butyrate, and valerate. Butyrate has been well documented as playing a modulatory role in the gut by strengthening epithelial barrier function[49] and promoting numerous immune tolerance mechanisms.[4] In a murine model, higher acetate and butyrate levels observed in mice fed a high-fiber diet were associated with increased numbers of CD103[+] DCs, which promote the growth of Tregs, protecting against FA.[51] A prospective cohort study of 139 children in Sweden demonstrated a consistent association between SCFA levels and FA.[58,59] They found that lower fecal butyrate and valerate levels at 1 year were associated with both current FA at 1 year and development of FA by 4 years.[58,59] In addition to explaining the mechanisms by which the diet has an impact on risk of atopy, SCFAs show early promise as a treatment of allergic disease, because oral butyrate supplementation can inhibit allergic responses in mice.[4] Taken together, these findings support that SCFAs, butyrate in particular, may be 1 link to explain associations between dietary intake and FA development, helping to elucidate why Mediterranean diet–like, fiber-rich diets confer protection against FA.[40,51,60]

Link Between Diet and Colonization of Protective Bacterial Species Within the Gut

Genetically similar individuals living in different environments have been demonstrated to have significantly different rates of atopic disease, including higher rates of atopic disease in African American children compared with African children living in African countries.[61] This emphasizes the importance of environmental factors, such as diet and urbanization, in the development of atopic disease. There is evidence that the protective effect of living in Africa may be explained by the beneficial effect of high-fiber diets and rural living on the gut microbiome. For example, the abundance of the *Prevotella* genus in the gut has been associated with agrarian diets rich in fruits and vegetables, whereas westernized diets abundant in fat and protein tend to be dominated by *Bacteroides*.[62] *Prevotella* abundance also positively correlates with living in rural environments, and this association has been attributed to higher dietary intake of complex carbohydrates in rural populations.[63] Although these findings have begun to explain the association between environmental factors and atopic disease, members of the *Prevotella* genus have been associated with both inflammatory conditions[66,67] and health-promoting, anti-inflammatory effects.[50,63,68–71] These inconsistencies highlight the necessity of species and strain specific analysis in fully understanding the effects of this genus on the gut microbiome and atopic disease.[67] Evidence of a link to atopic disease at lower taxonomic levels may offer more clarity, and it is already available in some cases, like *Prevotella copri*.

P copri is a species within the *Prevotella* genus that is necessary for the breakdown of complex polysaccharides.[72] There is evidence that diet influences *P copri* at both the species and strain levels. De Filippis and colleagues[62] demonstrated that different strains of *P copri* are found in individuals with different dietary patterns. *P copri* strains from vegans and individuals with agrarian-like diets demonstrated higher potential for complex fiber breakdown than the *P copri* strains found in individuals with high-fat and high-protein diets. In short, the high-fiber–consuming people had high-fiber–consuming *P copri*.[62] Another study in young children had similar results, demonstrating an inverse association between levels of *P copri* in the gut and dietary intake of sugar and saturated fat.[18] This same study found significantly reduced levels of *P copri* in children with atopic disease compared with healthy children,[18] and another showed that succinate, a metabolite of *P copri*, is present at lower levels in infants who go on to develop atopic disease.[73] Maternal *P copri* during gestation also may be protective, because 1 study demonstrated significantly lower levels of this species in mothers whose infants later have FA.[74] Taken together, these results suggest that it is possible that the diet and the environment select the gut microbes and that the gut microbes go on to select the disease. *P copri*, and the most protective strains within it, appear to thrive in the settings of a healthy diet and closer contact with natural environments, where they can in turn protect against atopic disease, such as FA. Conversely, poor diet and altered microbial exposure in urban settings, combined with a lack of protective factors from *P copri*, may result in poor control of sugar metabolism, setting the stage for atopic disease.[18]

Other bacterial genera and species in the gut also have been implicated in the development of atopic disease. A study in 38 South African toddlers aged 12 months to 36 months found no significant differences in the gut microbiota of healthy children compared with those with FA.[75] Investigation of a larger sample (n = 83) from the same population of toddlers, however, found many significant differences in the gut microbiota between healthy children and those AD.[18] This is notable when discussing FA because it so often is comorbid with AD, with evidence that up to a third of children with AD also suffer from FA.[76,77] Another study examining 79 Chinese infants 2 months to 11 months old did find significant differences in the gut microbiota of healthy infants compared with those with FA.[78] Both studies found that the gut microbiota of healthy infants/toddlers have increased *Streptococcus* and decreased *Faecalibacterium* and *Clostridium cluster XIVa* compared with those with AD[18] or FA.[78] Toddlers with AD, however, had decreased *Prevotella* and increased *Blautia*, *Bacteroides*, *Lachnospiraceae*, and *Clostridium cluster XI*.[18,78] Although the conflicts in these findings could be attributed to any number of factors, they may indicate that the gut microbiome exerts its influence on FA differently in the first year of life while the immune system is forming.

Role of Probiotics in Modulating Gut Microbiome and Preventing Food Allergy

Resolution of allergic disease has been described on reintroduction of commensal microbes to the gut microbiome, but the role of probiotics in FA is incompletely understood.[5] Probiotic supplements most commonly include the *Lactobacillus* and *Bifidobacterium* phyla, which are found at higher levels in nonallergic children.[79] Their presence also has been shown to confer protection against atopic disease and correct gut dysbiosis in both animals and humans.[5,80–83]

There are many mechanisms by which probiotics interact with the gut microbiome that may confer protection against allergic disease. These include direct interactions with the gut epithelial cells to strengthen the epithelial barrier, competition with pathogenic microbes via depletion of nutrients, production of acid, creation of antimicrobial metabolites, and interactions with the immune system to promote tolerogenic responses.[5,83,84] By adhering strongly to the gut epithelium and taking up space and nutrients, probiotics block adhesion of pathogenic bacteria and strengthen barrier function to prevent pathogen invasion.[85–87] Probiotics containing lactic acid bacteria, such as species contained within *Lactobacillus* and *Bifidobacterium*, also have been demonstrated to harm pathogens directly through secretion of antimicrobial substances and signaling peptides that promote further colonization of antipathogenic bacteria.[88,89] Probiotics also can be immunomodulatory, with evidence of bacterial metabolites, such as SCFAs and biotransformed bile acids acting as ligands in cell signaling mechanisms.[90] Although the precise nature of probiotics in inducing immune tolerance is not well understood, it has been demonstrated that effective probiotics tend to reduce the allergenic T_H2 profile to restore T_H1/T_H2 balance.[5]

Probiotic supplementation shows early promise as a safe and effective strategy for both treatment and prevention of atopic disease, including FA. *Lactobacillus* species, in particular, have been demonstrated to mitigate FA.[5] Despite considerable variation in the species, strains, and combinations used during these investigations, the benefits of *Lactobacillus* on improving allergic symptoms have been fairly consistent.[5] For example, a randomized controlled trial of 62 children with peanut allergy demonstrated that concurrent administration of a *Lactobacillus* probiotic with peanut oral immunotherapy (OIT) resulted in sustained unresponsiveness to peanut allergens in 82.1% of the treated group versus 3.6% of patients receiving a placebo.[91] The trial did not include groups treated with probiotic or OIT alone, so it is not possible to conclusively determine their individual impact. The results of a similar study that administered OIT alone, however, showed only a 50% sustained unresponsiveness rate,[92] suggesting that the probiotic may have significantly boosted efficacy. Although there is some literature that proposes solutions like the inclusion of probiotics in foods to combat allergic disease,[79] Paparo and colleagues argue that the evidence is not yet robust enough to recommend probiotics for treatment or prevention of atopy.[93] Further investigation is needed to determine the most beneficial probiotic dose, delivery, and types of bacteria, but such research has significant potential to create actionable solutions for FA.

CLINICS CARE POINTS

- A low species richness of gut microbiota at 3 months of age is associated with increased likelihood of FA by 1 year of age.[15]

- Each quartile increase in the ratio of *Enterobacteriaceae/Bacteroidaceae* increases a child's risk of developing food sensitization 2-fold.[15]
- Breastfeeding currently is recommended for the possible prevention of allergic diseases, including FA.[19]
- Early infant feeding patterns have a significant effect on the composition of the infant gut microbiome.[23]
- Breastfeeding is a major source of beneficial bacterial species, including *Bifidobacteria*, *Lactobacilli*, and *Enterobacteriaceae*.[19]
- Adherence to a Mediterranean diet during lactation and gestation has been found to protect against the subsequent development of allergic disease and FA.[33]
- An infant diet rich in fruits, vegetables, and homemade foods is associated with lower rates of FA by 2 years of age.[40]
- In older children, adherence to a Mediterranean diet also has been shown to reduce wheeze and hay fever symptoms.[42,43]
- High-sugar and high-fat diets also have been associated with an increased risk of atopic disease in both children and adults.[18,45]
- Lower levels of SCFA groups (specifically, butyrate, and valerate) at 1 year of age are associated with development of FA by 4 years of age.[58,59]
- Certain bacterial species, including *Prevotella* have been found to protect against the development of FA and are associated with diets rich in fruits and vegetables.[62]
- Resolution of allergic disease has been described on reintroduction of commensal microbes to the gut microbiome.[5]

SUMMARY

In conclusion, the infant gut microbiome has a significant impact on a child's overall gut health and predisposition for FA. The development of an individual's gut microbiome begins as early as gestation. Environmental factors contributing to gut dysbiosis from that time forward can exert influence over microbiota composition and overall species richness. Although breastfeeding is not correlated directly with lower risk for FA development, infants who are breastfed have been found to have a higher diversity of gut microbiota and possess particular bacterial species that serve a protective role against the development of FA.[19,24] Additionally, studies suggest that when lactating mothers and table-fed infants adhere to a Mediterranean diet, there is a lower risk of developing atopic disease, including FA.[33] Diet also has been correlated with a higher abundance of *Prevotella* species of bacteria, which has been shown to serve as a protective factor against inflammation and the development of atopic disease.[63] Recent studies suggest that reintroducing commensal microbes via probiotics potentially can confer protection against atopic disease when these commensal bacteria are lost during gut dysbiosis.[5] Further research is necessary to better understand the timeline for gut dysbiosis in early infancy and the commensal microbes necessary to protect against FA. This area of research is promising for the development of therapeutic targets for protection against FA in early infancy.

DISCLOSURE

None of the authors have any conflict of interest related to this research. M. Mahdavinia is supported by NIH and Brinson Foundation for research in FA.

REFERENCES

1. Seth D, Poowutikul P, Pansare M, et al. Food allergy: a review. Pediatr Ann 2020; 49(1):50–8.
2. Sicherer SH, Sampson HA. Food allergy: Epidemiology, pathogenesis, diagnosis, and treatment. J Allergy Clin Immunol 2014;133(2):291–304.
3. Mahdavinia M, Fox SR, Smith BM, et al. Racial differences in food allergy phenotype and health care utilization among US Children. J Allergy Clin Immunol In Pract 2017;5(2):352–7.
4. Canani B, Paparo L, Nocerino R, et al. Gut microbiome as target for innovative strategies against food allergy. Front Immunol 2019;191(10):1–15.
5. Shu S, Yuen AWT, Woo E, et al. Microbiota and Food Allergy. Clin Rev Allergy Immunol 2019;57:83–97.
6. Pabst O, Mowat AM. Oral tolerance to food protein. Nature 2012;5(3):232–9.
7. Ohno H. Intestinal M cells. J Biochem 2016;159(2):151–60.
8. Iweala OI, Nagler CR. The microbiome and food allergy. Annu Rev Immunol 2019; 37:377–403.
9. Koboziev I, Karlsson F, Grisham MB. Gut-associated lymphoid tissue, T cell trafficking, and chronic intestinal inflammation. Ann N Y Acad Sci 2010;1207:E86–93.
10. Okada H, Kuhn C, Feillet H, et al. The 'hygiene hypothesis' for autoimmune and allergic diseases: an update. Br Soc Immunol Clin Exp Immunol 2010;160:1–9.
11. Romagnani S. The increased prevalence of allergy and the hygiene hypothesis: missing immune deviation, reduced immune suppression, or both. Immunology 2004;112:352–63.
12. Bendiks M, Kopp MV. The relationship between advances in understanding the microbiome and the maturing hygiene hypothesis. Curr Allergy Asthma Rep 2013;13:487–94.
13. Karakula-Juchnowicz H, Gałęcka M, Rog J, et al. The food-specific serum igg reactivity in major depressive disorder patients, irritable bowel syndrome patients and healthy controls. Nutrients 2018;10:1–16.
14. Kumbhare SV, Patangia DV, Patil RH, et al. Factors influencing the gut microbiome in children: from infancy to childhood. Indian Acad Sci 2019;44(49):1–19.
15. Bunyavanich S, Shen N, Grishin A, et al. Early-life gut microbiome composition and milk allergy resolution. J Clin Immunol 2016;138(4):1122–9.
16. Azad MB, Konya T, Guttman DS, et al. Infant gut microbiota and food sensitization: associations in the first year of life. Clin Exp Allergy 2015;45:632–43.
17. Nylund L, Satokari R, Nikkila J, et al. Microarray analysis reveals marked intestinal microbiota abherrancy in infants having eczema compared to healthy children at-risk for atopic disease. BMC Microbiol 2013;13:12.
18. Mahdavinia M, Rasmussen HE, Botha M, et al. Effects of diet on the childhood gut microbiome and its implications for atopic dermatitis. J Allergy Clin Immunol 2018;143(4):1636–7.
19. Jarvinen KM, Martin H, Oyoshi MK. Immunomodulatory effects of breast milk on food allergy. Ann Allergy Asthma Immunol 2019;123(2):133–43.
20. Netting MJ, Allen KJ. Reconciling breast-feeding and early food introduction guidelines in the prevention and management of food allergy. J Allergy Clin Immunol 2019;144(2):397–400.
21. Goldsmith AJ, Koplin JJ, Lowe AJ, et al. Formula and breast feeding in infant food allergy: a population-based study. J Pediatr Child Health 2016;52:377–84.
22. Comberiati P, Costagliola G, D'Elios S, et al. Prevention of food allergy: the significance of early introduction. Medicina 2019;55(7):323.

23. Levin AM, Sitarik AR, Havstad SL, et al. Joint effects of pregnancy, sociocultural, and environmental factors on early life gut microbiome structure and diversity. Sci Rep 2016;6:31775.

24. Cong X, Xu W, Janton S, et al. Gut microbiome developmental patterns in early life of preterm infants: Impacts of feeding and gender. PLoS One 2016;11:1–19.

25. Penders J, Thijs C, Vink C, et al. Factors influencing the composition of the intestinal microbiota in early infancy. Pediatrics 2006;118:511–21.

26. Adlerberth I, Wold AE. Establishment of the gut microbiota in Western infants. Acta Paediatr 2009;98:229–38.

27. Timmerman HM, Rutten NBMM, Boekhorst J, et al. Intestinal colonization patterns in breastfed and formula-fed infants during the first 12 weeks of life reveal sequential microbiota signatures. Sci Rep 2017;7:1–10.

28. Begstrom A, Hjort Skov T, Iain Bahl M, et al. Establishment of intestinal microbiota during early life: a longitudinal, explorative study of a large cohort of danish infants. Appl Environ Microbiol 2014;80(9):2889–900.

29. Davis C, Bryan J, Hodgson J, et al. Definition of the mediterranean diet; a literature review. Nutrients 2015;7(11):9139–53.

30. Castro-Rodriguez JA, Garcia-Marcos L. What are the effects of a mediterranean diet on allergies and asthma in children? Front Pediatr 2017;5:72.

31. Chatzi L, Torrent M, Romieu I, et al. Mediterranean diet in pregnancy is protective for wheeze and atopy in childhood. Thorax 2008;63(6):507–13.

32. Zhang Y, Lin J, Fu W, et al. Mediterranean diet during pregnancy and childhood for asthma in children: A systematic review and meta-analysis of observational studies. Pediatr Pulmonol 2019;54(7):949–61.

33. Netting MJ, Middleton PF, Makrides M. Does maternal diet during pregnancy and lactation affect outcomes in offspring? A systematic review of food-based approaches. Nutrition 2014;30(11–12):1225–41.

34. Garcia-Larsen V, Ierodiakonou D, Jarrold K, et al. Diet during pregnancy and infancy and risk of allergic or autoimmune disease: A systematic review and meta-analysis. PLoS Med 2018;15(2):e1002507.

35. Barker DJP. Sir Richard Doll Lecture. Developmental origins of chronic disease. Public Health 2012;126(3):185–9.

36. Sofi F, Cesari F, Abbate R, et al. Adherence to Mediterranean diet and health status: meta-analysis. BMJ 2008;337:a1344.

37. Amati F, Hassounah S, Swaka A. The impact of mediterranean dietary patterns during pregnancy on maternal and offspring health. Nutrients 2019;11(5):1098.

38. Beckhaus AA, Garcia-Marcos L, Forno E, et al. Maternal nutrition during pregnancy and risk of asthma, wheeze, and atopic diseases during childhood: a systematic review and meta-analysis. Allergy 2015;70(12):1588–604.

39. Pellegrini-Belinchón J, Lorente-Toledano F, Galindo-Villardón P, et al. Factors associated to recurrent wheezing in infants under one year of age in the province of Salamanca, Spain: Is intervention possible? A predictive model. Allergol Immunopathol (Madr) 2016;44(5):393–9.

40. Grimshaw KE, Maskell J, Oliver EM, et al. Diet and food allergy development during infancy: birth cohort study findings using prospective food diary data. J Allergy Clin Immunol 2014;133(2):511–9.

41. Papamichael MM, Itsiopoulos C, Susanto NH, et al. Does adherence to the Mediterranean dietary pattern reduce asthma symptoms in children? A systematic review of observational studies. Public Health Nutr 2017;20(15):2722–34.

42. De Batlle J, Garcia-Aymerich J, Barraza-Villarreal A, et al. Mediterranean diet is associated with reduced asthma and rhinitis in Mexican children. Allergy 2008; 63(10):1310–6.

43. Chatzi L, Apostolaki G, Bibakis I, et al. Protective effect of fruits, vegetables and the Mediterranean diet on asthma and allergies among children in Crete. Thorax 2007;62(8):677–83.

44. Agostoni C, Decsi T, Fewtrell M, et al. Complementary Feeding: A Commentary by the ESPGHAN Committee on Nutrition. J Pediatr Gastroenterol Nutr 2008; 46(1):99–110.

45. Barros R, Moreira A, Padrão P, et al. Dietary patterns and asthma prevalence, incidence and control. Clin Exp Allergy 2015;45(11):1673–80.

46. Paparo L, di Costanzo M, di Scala C, et al. The influence of early life nutrition on epigenetic regulatory mechanisms of the immune system. Nutrients 2014;6(11): 4706–19.

47. Canani RB, Costanzo MD, Leone L, et al. Epigenetic mechanisms elicited by nutrition in early life. Nutr Res Rev 2011;24(2):198–205.

48. El-Osta A, Brasacchio D, Yao D, et al. Transient high glucose causes persistent epigenetic changes and altered gene expression during subsequent normoglycemia. J Exp Med 2008;205(10):2409–17.

49. Canani RB, Costanzo MD, Leone L, et al. Potential beneficial effects of butyrate in intestinal and extraintestinal diseases. World J Gastroenterol 2011;17(12): 1519–28.

50. De Filippis F, Pellegrini N, Vannini L, et al. High-level adherence to a Mediterranean diet beneficially impacts the gut microbiota and associated metabolome. Gut 2016;65(11):1812–21.

51. Tan J, McKenzie C, Vuillermin PJ, et al. Dietary fiber and bacterial SCFA enhance oral tolerance and protect against food allergy through diverse cellular pathways. Cell Rep 2016;15(12):2809–24.

52. Peng L, Li Z-R, Green RS, et al. Butyrate enhances the intestinal barrier by facilitating tight junction assembly via activation of AMP-activated protein kinase in caco-2 cell monolayers. J Nutr 2009;139(9):1619–25.

53. Kim M, Kim CH. Regulation of humoral immunity by gut microbial products. Gut Microbes 2017;8(4):392–9.

54. Kasubuchi M, Hasegawa S, Hiramatsu T, et al. Dietary gut microbial metabolites, short-chain fatty acids, and host metabolic regulation. Nutrients 2015;7(4): 2839–49.

55. Ohira H, Fujioka Y, Katagiri C, et al. Butyrate attenuates inflammation and lipolysis generated by the interaction of adipocytes and macrophages. J Atheroscler Thromb 2013;20(5):425–42.

56. Nastasi C, Candela M, Bonefeld CM, et al. The effect of short-chain fatty acids on human monocyte-derived dendritic cells. Sci Rep 2015;5:16148.

57. Fontenelle B, Gilbert KM. n-Butyrate anergized effector CD4+ T cells independent of regulatory T cell generation or activity. Scand J Immunol 2012;76(5): 457–63.

58. Sandin A, Bråbäck L, Norin E, et al. Faecal short chain fatty acid pattern and allergy in early childhood. Acta Paediatr 2009;98(5):823–7.

59. Böttcher MF, Nordin EK, Sandin A, et al. Microflora-associated characteristics in faeces from allergic and nonallergic infants. Clin Exp Allergy 2000;30(11): 1590–6.

60. McKenzie C, Tan J, Macia L, et al. The nutrition-gut microbiome-physiology axis and allergic diseases. Immunological Rev 2017;278(1):277–95.

61. Odhiambo JA, Williams HC, Clayton TO, et al. Global variations in prevalence of eczema symptoms in children from ISAAC Phase Three. J Allergy Clin Immunol 2009;124(6):1251–8.e23.

62. De Filippis F, Pasolli E, Tett A, et al. Distinct genetic and functional traits of human intestinal prevotella copri strains are associated with different habitual diets. Cell Host Microbe 2019;25(3):444–53.e3.

63. De Filippo C, Cavalieri D, Di Paola M, et al. Impact of diet in shaping gut microbiota revealed by a comparative study in children from Europe and rural Africa. Proc Natl Acad Sci U S A 2010;107(33):14691–6.

64. Scher JU, Sczesnak A, Longman RS, et al. Expansion of intestinal Prevotella copri correlates with enhanced susceptibility to arthritis. Elife 2013;2:e01202.

65. Maeda Y, Kurakawa T, Umemoto E, et al. Dysbiosis contributes to arthritis development via activation of autoreactive T cells in the intestine. Arthritis Rheumatol 2016;68(11):2646–61.

66. Lozupone CA, Rhodes ME, Neff CP, et al. HIV-induced alteration in gut microbiota: driving factors, consequences, and effects of antiretroviral therapy. Gut Microbes 2014;5(4):562–70.

67. Pedersen HK, Gudmundsdottir V, Nielsen HB, et al. Human gut microbes impact host serum metabolome and insulin sensitivity. Nature 2016;535(7612):376–81.

68. Kovatcheva-Datchary P, Nilsson A, Akrami R, et al. Dietary fiber-induced improvement in glucose metabolism is associated with increased abundance of prevotella. Cell Metab 2015;22(6):971–82.

69. De Vadder F, Kovatcheva-Datchary P, Zitoun C, et al. Microbiota-produced succinate improves glucose homeostasis via intestinal gluconeogenesis. Cell Metab 2016;24(1):151–7.

70. De Angelis M, Montemurno E, Vannini L, et al. Effect of whole-grain barley on the human fecal microbiota and metabolome. Appl Environ Microbiol 2015;81(22):7945–56.

71. Vitaglione P, Mennella I, Ferracane R, et al. Whole-grain wheat consumption reduces inflammation in a randomized controlled trial on overweight and obese subjects with unhealthy dietary and lifestyle behaviors: role of polyphenols bound to cereal dietary fiber. Am J Clin Nutr 2015;101(2):251–61.

72. Dodd D, Mackie RI, Cann IK. Xylan degradation, a metabolic property shared by rumen and human colonic Bacteroidetes. Mol Microbiol 2011;79(2):292–304.

73. Kim HK, Rutten NB, Besseling-van der Vaart I, et al. Probiotic supplementation influences faecal short chain fatty acids in infants at high risk for eczema. Benef Microbes 2015;6(6):783–90.

74. Vuillermin PJ, O'Hely M, Collier F, et al. Maternal carriage of Prevotella during pregnancy associates with protection against food allergy in the offspring. Nat Commun 2020;11(1):1452.

75. Mahdavinia M, Rasmussen HE, Engen P, et al. Atopic dermatitis and food sensitization in South African toddlers: Role of fiber and gut microbiota. Ann Allergy Asthma Immunol 2017;118(6):742–3.e3.

76. Mavroudi A, Karagiannidou A, Xinias I, et al. Assessment of IgE-mediated food allergies in children with atopic dermatitis. Allergol Immunopathol (Madr) 2017;45(1):77–81.

77. Cartledge N, Chan S. Atopic dermatitis and food allergy: a paediatric approach. Curr Pediatr Rev 2018;14(3):171–9.

78. Ling Z, Li Z, Liu X, et al. Altered fecal microbiota composition associated with food allergy in infants. Appl Environ Microbiol 2014;80(8):2546–54.

79. Ozdemir O. Various effects of different probiotic strains in allergic disorders: an update from laboratory and clinical data. Clin Exp Immunol 2010;160(3):295–304.
80. Hoarau C, Lagaraine C, Martin L, et al. Supernatant of Bifidobacterium breve induces dendritic cell maturation, activation, and survival through a Toll-like receptor 2 pathway. J Allergy Clin Immunol 2006;117(3):696–702.
81. Song S, Lee SJ, Park DJ, et al. The anti-allergic activity of Lactobacillus plantarum L67 and its application to yogurt. J Dairy Sci 2016;99(12):9372–82.
82. Xiao JZ, Kondo S, Yanagisawa N, et al. Effect of probiotic Bifidobacterium longum BB536 [corrected] in relieving clinical symptoms and modulating plasma cytokine levels of Japanese cedar pollinosis during the pollen season. A randomized double-blind, placebo-controlled trial. J Investig Allergol Clin Immunol 2006; 16(2):86–93.
83. Castellazzi AM, Valsecchi C, Caimmi S, et al. Probiotics and food allergy. Ital J Pediatr 2013;39:47.
84. Sarowska J, Choroszy-Król I, Regulska-Ilow B, et al. The therapeutic effect of probiotic bacteria on gastrointestinal diseases. Adv Clin Exp Med 2013;22(5): 759–66.
85. Servin AL. Antagonistic activities of lactobacilli and bifidobacteria against microbial pathogens. FEMS Microbiol Rev 2004;28(4):405–40.
86. O'Toole PW, Cooney JC. Probiotic bacteria influence the composition and function of the intestinal microbiota. Interdiscip Perspect Infect Dis 2008;2008: 175285.
87. Bermudez-Brito M, Plaza-Díaz J, Muñoz-Quezada S, et al. Probiotic mechanisms of action. Ann Nutr Metab 2012;61(2):160–74.
88. Musikasang HSN, Tani A, Maneerat S. Bacteriocin-producing lactic acid bacteria as a probiotic potential from Thai indigenous chickens. Czech J Anim Sci 2012; 57:137–49.
89. Dobson A, Cotter PD, Ross RP, et al. Bacteriocin production: a probiotic trait? Appl Environ Microbiol 2012;78(1):1–6.
90. Rizzetto L, Fava F, Tuohy KM, et al. Connecting the immune system, systemic chronic inflammation and the gut microbiome: The role of sex. J Autoimmun 2018;92:12–34.
91. Tang ML, Ponsonby AL, Orsini F, et al. Administration of a probiotic with peanut oral immunotherapy: A randomized trial. J Allergy Clin Immunol 2015;135(3): 737–44.e8.
92. Vickery BP, Scurlock AM, Kulis M, et al. Sustained unresponsiveness to peanut in subjects who have completed peanut oral immunotherapy. J Allergy Clin Immunol 2014;133(2):468–75.
93. Paparo L, Nocerino R, Di Scala C, et al. Targeting Food Allergy with Probiotics. Adv Exp Med Biol 2019;1125:57–68.

Genetics of Food Allergy

Elisabet Johansson, PhD, Tesfaye B. Mersha, PhD*

KEYWORDS

- Food allergy • genetics • epigenetics • human leukocyte antigen complex • filaggrin
- ancestry • single nucleotide polymorphism (SNP)
- genome-wide association study (GWAS)

KEY POINTS

- Food allergy (FA) is a growing clinical and public health problem in the United States and worldwide.
- The development of FA likely results from complex interactions between multiple environmental and genetic factors.
- Although the genetics of FA are somewhat understudied, advances have been made in recent years using candidate-gene association studies and agnostic genome-wide approaches.
- Most genes found to be associated with FA are involved either in immune responses or in skin/epithelial barrier functioning, with filaggrin and genes in the HLA complex being among the most studied.

What is food to one is bitter poison to another.
—Lucretius (ca. 96 bc–55 bc), based on his observation of individual variations
in adverse reactions caused by food allergy[1]

INTRODUCTION

Food allergy (FA) is a complex disease of substantial public health concern; it affects ~8% of the pediatric population, and is the common cause of anaphylaxis in children, affecting up to 15 million people including 5 million children.[2–4] FA accounts for 3 million doctor visits, 125,000 to emergency rooms, 2000 hospitalizations, and about 150 deaths annually. The economic cost of FAs is nearly $25 billion per year.[5] FA is an adverse reaction to food (food hypersensitivity) occurring in susceptible individuals, which is mediated by a classical immune mechanism specific for the food itself. The best established mechanism in FA is caused by the presence of IgE antibodies against the offending food. Food intolerance (FI) is nonimmune-mediated adverse reactions to food. The subgroups of FI are enzymatic (eg, lactose intolerance cause by lactase

Division of Asthma Research, Department of Pediatrics, Cincinnati Children's Hospital Medical Center, University of Cincinnati, 3333 Burnet Avenue, Cincinnati, OH 45229-3026, USA
* Corresponding author.
E-mail address: tesfaye.mersha@cchmc.org

Immunol Allergy Clin N Am 41 (2021) 301–319
https://doi.org/10.1016/j.iac.2021.01.010   immunology.theclinics.com
0889-8561/21/© 2021 Elsevier Inc. All rights reserved.

deficiency), pharmacologic (reactions against biogenic amines, histamine intolerance), and undefined FI (eg, against some food additives). The diagnosis of an IgE-mediated FA (IgE-FA) is made by a carefully taken case history, supported by the demonstration of an IgE sensitization either by skin prick tests (SPTs) or by in vitro tests, and confirmed by positive oral provocation. For scientific purposes the only accepted test for the confirmation of FA/FI is a properly performed double-blind, placebo-controlled food challenge. A panel of recombinant allergens, produced as single allergenic molecules, may in future improve the diagnosis of IgE-FA. Because of a lack of causal treatment possibilities, the elimination of the culprit "food allergen" from the diet is the only therapeutic option for patients with real FA. The basic immunopathology underlying FA is divided into non-IgE-mediated (ie, cell-mediated slow onset) and IgE-mediated (acute immediate reactions) FA.[6] The non-IgE-mediated food hypersensitivity encompasses nonimmune-mediated adverse reaction with delayed hypersensitivity whose mechanisms are less clear.[7] Such reactions include cell-mediated reactions that involve sensitized lymphocytes in tissues rather than antibodies.[8] The overall prevalence of cell-mediated reactions remains uncertain.[9,10] The most common non-IgE-mediated hypersensitivity reactions affecting all age groups of the population are celiac disease, also known as gluten-sensitive enteropathy, and lactose intolerance caused by histamine intolerance.[11] IgE-FA is the most common and life-threatening type of food allergic disorder.[12] It is also called immediate hypersensitivity reaction because of the short onset time between the ingestion of the offending food and the onset of symptoms.[3,8,13] Oral exposure to potential food allergens early in life is believed to promote tolerance, whereas cutaneous exposure through an impaired skin barrier promotes sensitization.[14] Tolerance is mediated by CD103[+] dendritic cells in the gastrointestinal tract that bind to food allergens and migrate to mesenteric lymph nodes where regulatory T cells are induced. In IgE-FA, the induction and functioning of regulatory T cells is believed to be compromised and the immune response is shifted toward the generation of T helper 2 (Th2) cells, leading to IgE class-switching in B cells.[15,16] The most common symptoms associated with IgE-mediated reactions involve the skin and may lead to anaphylaxis.[17,18] IgE-mediated mechanisms are also responsible for allergic reactions to pollens, mold spores, animal danders, insect venoms, and other environmental stimuli.[19] Anaphylaxis is a severe and life-threatening systemic allergic reaction characterized by fall of blood pressure, upper airway obstruction, and difficulty breathing. IgE-mediated immunologic reactions are the most important type of FA because these reactions involve a wide variety of different foods.[20] More than 170 foods are known to cause IgE-FAs. In the United States, eight foods account for 90% of serious allergic reactions: milk, eggs, fish, shellfish, wheat, soy, peanuts, and tree nuts.[21,22] Hence, federal law requires food labels to clearly identify the food allergen source of all foods and ingredients that contain any protein derived from these common allergens (Food Allergen Labeling and Consumer Protection Act of 2004, Public L No. 108–282). To date, except strict avoidance, there are no effective curative treatments for IgE-FAs.[23,24] This article primary addresses the genetics of IgE-FA.

FOOD ALLERGY AND THE ATOPIC MARCH

The role of FA in the atopic march (progression of allergic diseases starting from infancy and typically includes atopic dermatitis [AD], FA, allergic rhinitis, and asthma) is not well understood, but a strong association between FA and AD has been established.[25] Although the causal nature of this association has been debated, it is now generally accepted that cutaneous sensitization to food allergens is an important step in the development of FA, whereas exposure to food allergens through the oral route seems to promote tolerance.[26–28] Although FA sometimes precedes AD,[29] sensitization through an impaired nonlesional skin barrier before manifestation of AD has developed is likely a common route for food allergens. Indeed, skin barrier impairment at birth as measured by transepidermal water loss predicts FA at age 2,[30] and one study found FLG genotype to be associated with sensitization to peanut allergen regardless of the presence of eczema.[31] Several rare monogenic disorders that are caused by genes involved in skin barrier formation and maintenance have been linked to FA. A well-known example is Netherton syndrome, caused by autosomal-recessive mutations in the serine protease inhibitor Karzal type 5 (SPINK5).[32] The gene product of SPINK5, LEKTI, is involved in the regulation of desquamation. Netherton syndrome is characterized by defective cornification, chronic skin inflammation, impaired skin barrier, and multiple allergies, including FA.[33] Furthermore, the desmoglein 1 gene (DSG1) is involved in maintaining the structure of the epidermis, and loss-of-function mutations in this gene are the cause of severe dermatitis, multiple allergies, and metabolic wasting syndrome. In addition to skin conditions, such as severe psoriasiform dermatitis, ichthyosis, and keratosis, elevated IgE levels and multiple FAs have been observed in patients with severe dermatitis, multiple allergies, and metabolic wasting syndrome.[34,35]

The link between FA and monogenic inherited skin disorders further strengthens the case for cutaneous food sensitization through an impaired skin barrier as a causative event in the development of FA.[36] There are, however, several monogenic diseases associated with FA that have been shown to be caused by mutations in genes involved in immune system responses. Immunodysregulation, polyendocrinopathy, enteropathy, X-linked syndrome is a rare disorder caused by mutations in the FOXP3 gene that leads to impaired development of $CD4^+CD25^+$ regulatory T cells. In addition to autoimmunity conditions, patients with immunodysregulation, polyendocrinopathy, enteropathy, X-linked syndrome have a high risk of FAs, AD, and elevated IgE levels.[37,38] Another example is the connective tissue disorder Loeys-Dietz syndrome, which is usually caused by mutations in TGFBR1 or TGFBR2. The resulting upregulation of transforming growth factor-β signaling seems to skew naive $CD4(^+)$ T cells toward Th2 cytokine-producing cells, and patients have a strongly increased risk of all major allergic diseases, including FA.[39]

FOOD ALLERGY AND RACIAL VARIATION

Pediatric FA has increased tremendously over the past two decades and it is on the rise among all demographic groups.[40] However, its prevalence rates differ across ethnic groups.[41] Results from the National Health and Nutrition Examination Survey indicated that the prevalence of FA is four times higher in African Americans (AA) than European Americans (EA).[42] AA children are reported to have an eightfold increase in the prevalence of peanut allergy as compared with the general US pediatric population. AA individuals with FA have elevated levels of IgE, peripheral eosinophilia, Th2 cytokines, and epithelial dysfunction as compared with EAs.[43–45] Recent studies showed that variants in several cytokine candidate genes that encode Th2-related molecules, such as interleukin (IL)-4 and IL-13, show higher allele frequency in AA, suggesting that these alleles have been conserved to combat parasitic infections in Africans but not in Europeans.[46] This unique evolutionary trajectory might be the reason for high prevalence of allergic disorders in AAs.[47] Although AAs experience higher rates of FA prevalence and mortality than any other racial or ethnic group in America, few studies of FA have focused on this population, and almost all studies have predominantly used EA samples. A PubMed search demonstrated that EAs are mentioned five times more often in various FA-related literature as compared with AAs. Bringing AA families into research will help to compare their results with those of other groups and to better understand the basis of FA disparities.[48,49] It might help to unravel population-specific disease risk in the context of environmental exposure factors.[50]

GENETICS AND FOOD ALLERGY

Investigators study the genetics of FA for many reasons. First, some investigators study it to understand the evolutionary basis of the current population distribution of FA and its genetic architecture. For others, such information provides insights into how malleable FA may be and what type of interventions may be most effective in altering population levels of FA. A second reason is the hope of identifying genes associated with increased risk of FA that can be used as prognostic factors to indicate who is likely to become allergic so that they can be given preventive therapy. A third reason is to identify genes that moderate the safety and/or efficacy of treatments. If we can identify such genes, then we are on our way to personalized medicine.[51] Finally, among most biomedical researchers, the most common reason for wishing to identify genes that confer variations in FA is to identify physiologic pathways through which FA develops so that such pathways can then be further studied and made targets for potential pharmaceutical intervention. Several experimental designs, including family, twin, and cohort studies, and analytical approaches, such as linkage analysis, candidate gene, genome-wide association study (GWAS), DNA methylation, and microbiome analysis, have been used to study important questions, such as: Why do some individuals develop FA and others do not? How do environmental and genetics factors interact to increase the risk of FA? A brief history of the search for genetic causes of FA is presented in **Fig. 1**. Investigators screen the genome to locate regions contributing to variance (**Box 1**) in FA-related outcomes.

FAMILY-BASED STUDIES

Family studies can address whether a disease aggregates in families. Such studies typically compare the prevalence of the disorder among first-degree relatives of affected cases with the prevalence in the population or among relatives of unaffected control subjects. A higher risk among relatives of cases indicates that the disease may

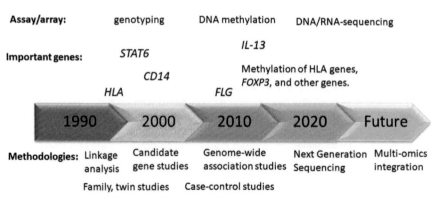

Fig. 1. A brief history of the search for genetic causes of food allergy (FA).

Box 1
Definitions of genetic and genetic-related terminology

Variance: A measure of statistical dispersion indicating how far values typically are from the distribution's mean.

Genome: Complete set of genetic information for an individual.

Epistatic variance: Variance caused by interaction among alleles at different loci (gene-gene interactions).

Heritability: The proportion of population variance in a trait attributable to segregation of a gene or genes (overall phenotypic variation/risk that is attributable to genetic factors).

Gene-gene interaction: When 2 or more DNA variations interact either directly (DNA-DNA or DNA-mRNA interactions), to change transcription or translation levels, or indirectly by way of their protein products, to alter disease risk separate from their independent effects.

Gene-environment interaction: When a DNA variation interacts with an environmental factor, such that their combined effect is distinct from their independent effects. An interaction is indicated when the presence of one factor (eg, diet) affects the influence of the second factor (eg, genetic) on disease risk.

Epigenetics: changes in gene function that are heritable and that are not attributed to alterations of the DNA sequence.

Trait heterogeneity: When a trait has been defined with insufficient specificity such that it represents at least 2 distinct underlying traits.

Genetic heterogeneity: The production of the same or similar phenotypes (observed biochemical, physiologic, and morphologic characteristics of a person determined by his/her genotype) by different underlying genetic mechanisms.

Race: Group based on physical attributes, a social construct; no biologic basis.

Ethnicity: Group based on culture, language, physical attributes, religion, country of origin.

Ancestry: Group based on DNA, line of decent.

Admixture: Interbreeding among different ancestry populations.

Candidate-gene association studies: Targeted studies of association between selected genes of interest and a phenotype.

Genome-wide association studies: Genetics research to associate specific genetic variations with particular trait.

GWAS Catalog: a curated human genome-wide association study.

Copy number variation: A sequence of bases within a genome differs in the number of copies among individuals or populations.

Population structure or population stratification: The presence of differences in allele frequencies between subpopulations in a population.

Admixture mapping: a method of gene mapping that uses a population of mixed ancestry (an admixed population) to find the genetic loci that contribute to differences in diseases or other phenotypes found between the different ancestral populations.

Next-generation sequencing: An entire genome is sequenced from fragmented DNA, producing short (less than 300 bp) sequencing reads at high speed and low cost.

Single-nucleotide variants: A single base within a read or genome differs from the base found at the same position in other individuals or populations.

Meta-analysis: A routine approach to combining smaller GWAS using summary statistics/results to overcome the smaller sample sizes of individual studies.

Fine mapping: A set of statistical and laboratory approaches to determine the causal genetic variant for associated genetic loci.

Multiomics analysis: biological analysis approach in which the data sets are multiple "omes", such as the genome, proteome, transcriptome, epigenome, metabolome, and microbiome.

be familial, but it does not necessarily mean that genes are involved; a disease may run in families for nongenetic reasons (ie, a shared environment). Although environmental factors play a significant role in the onset of FA, such as higher rate of food-related health problems in lower-income children than higher-income groups that might indicate the role of environmental exposure factors, the most widely used indicators of FA are familial aggregation and strong genetic component.[52–54]

TWIN-BASED STUDIES

Twin studies compare the concordance rates of a disease between identical/monozygotic (MZ) twins (siblings who are essentially genetically identical) and fraternal/dizygotic (DZ) twins (who share on average half of their genes). Assuming that shared environmental influences on MZ twins are not different from environmental influences on DZ twins (the equal environments assumption), significantly higher concordance rates in MZ twins reflect the action of genes. Nevertheless, an MZ concordance rate less than 100% means that environmental factors influence the phenotype. The importance of genetic variants in FA stems from twin studies. A child with a parent or sibling with peanut allergy, one of the most common forms of FA, has a seven times higher risk of having the condition than do children without familial risk factors.[55] Twin studies have demonstrated that the concordance rate of 82% among MZ twins in developing peanut allergy far exceeds the concordance rate of 20% observed among DZ twins.[56,57] In general, the heritability estimates for FA is as high as 81%.[58]

ASSOCIATION-BASED STUDIES

Successful association studies require adequate sample sizes, and this is difficult to achieve in GWAS studies in particular, where multiple testing corrections increases the number of participants required to reach significance. It is also important to have well-characterized study populations with regard to demographics, and when recruiting from ethnically or racially heterogenous populations, this needs to be adjusted for in the statistical analyses using population stratification.

Accurate and consistent phenotyping of FA is essential to the success of gene association studies because differences in FA definitions and diagnostic methods can have a considerable impact on the results. FA prevalence varies widely depending on the diagnostic criteria, as demonstrated in a systematic review of European studies,[59] which found that the point prevalence of self-reported FA was six to seven times higher than FA confirmed by oral food challenge (OFC). OFC in a clinical setting remains the gold standard for diagnosing FA, but although OFC is considered generally safe, it is not entirely risk-free, and is associated with considerable discomfort for the patient.[60] A positive SPT and elevated specific IgE levels have low predictive value on their own but can confirm the IgE component of possible FA in the presence of a convincing clinical history. Greater SPT wheal size or higher specific IgE levels are associated with increased risk of FA, and a careful evaluation of clinical history together with a positive SPT wheal size or IgE levels greater than suggested cutoff levels may reduce or eliminate the need for OFC.[61]

Compared with the genetics of asthma, the genetics of FA is still a somewhat underexplored area. Studies with large and well phenotyped cohorts are needed to confirm results from earlier studies and to identify additional genetic associations, and to explore interactions with environmental factors. The results can help increase the understanding of the mechanisms behind the FA, and lead to the development of biomarkers for prediction and monitoring of FA.

Candidate-gene studies

Until recently, studies of FA-gene associations were mainly performed on specific candidate genes based on their known biologic function. Hypothesis-driven studies of gene associations with FA have targeted well-known immune-related genes, some of which have previously been associated with other allergic diseases. A recent systematic review summarized results from candidate-gene association studies and genome-wide scans with different types of FA as outcomes.[62] In this section, some of the genes that have been associated with FA in more than one study are discussed.

The HLA system is important for the regulation the immune system and is encoded by a family of genes located in the major histocompatibility complex gene complex on chromosome 6p21. Several HLAs belonging to the major histocompatibility complex class II (DP, DM, DO, DQ, and DR), which present antigens from outside of the cell to T lymphocytes, have been associated with various forms of asthma in several studies.[63] Several class II genotypes have also been shown to be associated with FA, and peanut allergy in particular. In a small study based on peanut SPT and clinical history of peanut allergy, the genotypes DRB1*08, DRB1*08/12 tyr16, and DQB1*04 were found to be more frequent in peanut-allergic individual compared with control subjects.[64] The association between HLA DQB1 and peanut allergy was also demonstrated in a Canadian study that found associations between it and DQB1*02 and DQB1*06:03P in a study population of European ancestry.

CD14 plays an important role in the innate immunity system as part of the protein complex that binds to lipopolysaccharide, a bacterial cell wall component. Several studies have examined CD14 as a candidate gene for FA. The CD14 single-nucleotide polymorphism (SNP) rs2569190 was associated with general FA in a racially mixed study population, and the association was found to be stronger when the analysis was restricted to white participants.[65] In a study of 53 children with peanut allergy and their peanut-tolerant siblings, rs2569190 was significantly associated with peanut allergy.[66] By contrast, the same SNP was not associated with FA in a Japanese study population.[67]

IL-13 is a cytokine secreted by activated Th2 cells that plays a central role in allergic disease, and the association between the IL-13 gene and asthma is well established. The association between IL-13 and FA was explored in an Australian study of challenge-proven food-allergic infants of European ancestry. The IL-13 SNP rs1295686 was associated with FA in the discovery cohort and in an independent validation cohort and in a meta-analysis.[68] Moreover, the association seemed to be independent on the presence of eczema. There was no evidence that any of the variants tested increased the risk for FA when comparing food-allergic cases with food-sensitized tolerant children, and there was an association with increased plasma IgE levels, which suggests that the association between IL-13 and FA may be mediated by food sensitization. In a Japanese study of associations between FA and 26 loci previously linked to AD and eosinophilic esophagitis, an association between rs1295686 was seen regardless of eczema comorbidity.[69]

Several studies have found associations between FA and signal transducer and activator of transcription 6 (STAT6), a gene encoding a transcription factor that plays a role in IL-4-mediated responses. STAT6 genotype has been shown to be associated with general nut allergy in a study using participants of European ancestry,[70] and the association was later validated at the gene level in a Japanese population. The STAT6 SNPs rs324015 and rs1059513 were found to be associated with challenge-proven FA and peanut allergy in a family study of 369 trios that included 262 children with FA. Both SNPs were also associated with more severe FA symptoms. In a recent case-control study of a West Bengal Indian population the STAT6 SNP rs3024974 was not significantly associated with FA. There was, however, an association with food-specific IgE levels in individuals with childhood onset, but not adult onset, of FA.[71]

Entry through an impaired skin barrier is believed to be a common route of sensitizing food allergens, and genes involved in maintenance of the skin barrier have been investigated for associations with FA. The barrier gene filaggrin (FLG), in particular, has been investigated as a candidate gene and found to be significantly associated with peanut allergy[72] and general FA.[73] In the latter study, path analysis indicated that the effect of FLG-LOF mutations on FA risk was indirect and mediated by eczema and allergic sensitization to foods, suggesting that the association between FLG and FA is explained by the increased risk of sensitization through a faulty skin barrier in individuals with FLG mutations. Similarly, in a study of peanut allergy, the association between FLG-LOF mutations and FA-sensitized but tolerant children was similar to the association between FLG-LOF mutations and food-sensitized children with FA, although the power to detect a difference was somewhat limited.[74]

The gene product of SPINK5, LEKTI, is involved in the maintenance of the skin barrier, and several mutations in the SPINK5 gene have been associated with Netherton syndrome. In addition, the SPINK5 variant rs9325071 has been found to be associated with challenge-proven FA in an Australian candidate-gene study of 12-month-old infants, and the association was replicated in an independent study population.[75] The association remained in both study populations when the analysis was restricted to children without eczema.

Genome-wide association studies

The strength of genome-wide agnostic approaches is the ability to identify novel loci without an a priori biologic hypothesis. Corrections for testing high numbers of loci can, however, make it difficult to reach statistical significance, and necessitates large study populations. Recently, several GWAS of FA have confirmed some associations with genes previously identified using candidate-gene studies, and in addition, novel candidate loci have been discovered. The first GWAS to specifically investigate FA, and peanut, milk, and egg allergy, confirmed the association with HLA-DR and HLA-DQ in peanut allergy and identified specific loci in a region at 6p21.32 tagged by rs7192 and rs9275596.[76] These associations were replicated in individuals of European, but not non-European, ancestry. In a genome-wide scan of DNA methylation differential DNA methylation at 72 different loci were associated with one or both of rs7192 and rs9275596, and there was a difference in methylation levels between peanut allergy cases and control subjects at 18 of the differentially methylated positions. Further evidence of a role for HLA-DQ in peanut allergy came from a German GWAS of FA diagnosed by OFC in 497 cases and 2387 control subjects of European ancestry.[77] FA was stratified by food-specific allergy (egg, peanut, and milk), and loci centered on rs9273440 in the HLA-DQB untranslated 3'-region was specifically associated with peanut allergy. By contrast, loci in the epidermal differentiation near the filaggrin genes on 1q21.3 was associated with any FA unstratified for type, and the association was shown to be caused by known LOF mutations in FLG. Loci in Serpin Family B Member 7 (SERPINB7), a region centered on rs11949166 between the IL4 gene and the kinesin family member 3a gene (KIF3A), and the locus were also associated with risk for any FA. All three loci have previously been implicated in allergic disease. The association with FA was observed regardless of the presence of eczema in all five loci identified in the study except C11orf30/LRRC32.

To explore novel gene associations with peanut allergy, Asai and colleagues[78,79] recently performed a GWAS on a Canadian group of patients and a meta-analysis of seven studies from Canadian, American, Australian, German, and Dutch populations of varied ethnicity. In the main GWAS analysis, only HLA SNPs and rs115218289, an imputed SNP located close to Integrin α6 (ITGA6), reached genome-wide significance. Conditioning on the top HLA SNP located upstream of HLA-DQB1, rs3134976, identified additional SNPs near the T-cell adapter protein Src Kinase Associated Phosphoprotein 1 (SKAP1) and Catenin Alpha 3 (CTNNA3). In the meta-analysis of any FA, rs7936434 near *C11orf30* reached genome-wide significance. Loci that were suggestive of significance with FA and peanut allergy in the meta-analyses included rs115218289, rs523865 in Angiopoietin-4 (ANGPT4), rs144897250 near Matrix metalloproteinase-12 (MMP12) and Matrix metalloproteinase-13 (MMP13), and rs78048444 near Coiled-Coil-Helix-Coiled-Coil-Helix Domain Containing 3 (CHCHD3) and Exocyst complex component 4 (EXOC4). There were variations in phenotype definition ranging from self-report to food challenges among the studies included in the meta-analyses. The results differed between populations, and the association between FA and rs7936434 when the study using an FA definition based on self-report was excluded.

One genome-wide study of FA associations made use of copy number variations, which are common genomic alterations, as molecular markers.[80] Copy number variations in the cell adhesion gene Catenin Alpha 3 (*CTNNA3*) were significantly associated FA in a discovery cohort of 357 cases with confirmed FA and 3980 control subjects, and the association was confirmed in an independent replication cohort. Copy number variations in Fox-1 homolog A (*RBFOX1*) were significantly associated FA in a meta-analysis of participants of European ancestry. **Fig. 2** lists variants and genes for which statistically significant (or suggestive) association has been found in several independent studies with FAs, yet the truth of whether these studies are associated with, let alone cause, FA still remains questionable in most cases.

EPIGENETICS AND CONTRIBUTIONS FROM THE ENVIRONMENT IN FOOD ALLERGY

The dramatic rise in FA cases over the past 50 years is more likely caused by alterations in the environment rather than by changes in the gene pool. Environmental factors, such as the physical environment, the social environment, and the economic environment, have all presumably contributed to an increase in the prevalence of FA. The association of putatively influential environment factors on FA has been demonstrated in studies on twins with a high genetic predisposition to FA. Further evidence of environmental effects has come from studies showing that emigrants to the United States usually showed marked differences in the incidence of allergy compared with their counterparts who remained in their native countries. These observations also show the relationship between genes and the environment.

Among environmental factors implicated in FA are dietary habits; vitamin D intake; exposure to food allergens; pollution; and hygiene-related factors, including pet exposure.[60,81] The gut microbiota is part of the total exposome, and is influenced by components in the external environment, such as diet and the environmental microbiome. Early life dysbiosis has been associated with FA.[82] Environmental factors can modify risk of disease in genetically predisposed individuals, and gene-environment (GxE) interactions are believed to be important for the risk of allergic disease (**Fig. 3**). Although GxE interactions have been studied extensively in asthma,[83,84] the literature is sparser for other allergic diseases, and few studies on interactions between genes and environmental factors in FA have been published to date. The association between challenge-proven FA and low serum 25-hydroxyvitamin D_4 levels has been shown

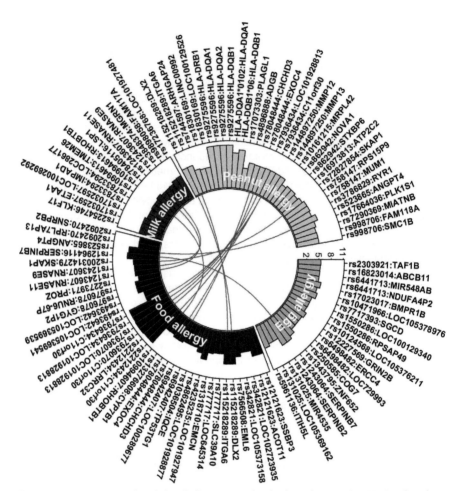

Fig. 2. Variants associated with food allergies. Circle plot based on NHGRI-EBI Catalog shows genome-wide association studies variants associated with food allergies. SNPs and the corresponding mapped genes are shown along the *outer circle*. The *rectangles* show the log transformed *P* value from the SNP-trait association. y-axis is the −log10(*P* value), x-axis is the SNP-gene pair for each disease. *Red lines* connect the shared gene (regardless of SNP) between traits.

to be modified by a polymorphism in the vitamin D–binding protein (DBP) in such a way that the association was only found in the genotype associated with higher serum DBP levels.[85] Because high DBP levels decrease the vitamin D bioavailability, the results are consistent with vitamin D deficiency as a risk factor for FA. Another example of an interaction between genotype and an environmental variable is a study of peanut allergy, which demonstrated a modifying effect of peanut allergen levels in dust on the association between FLG and peanut sensitization and allergy.[86] The interaction was significant when adjusted for AD.

In recent years, evidence has accumulated indicating that environmentally induced epigenetic changes in the DNA of target genes is an important mechanism mediating GxE interactions. In particular, DNA methylation at loci of genetic variation can lead to a variable response to an environmental exposure depending on genotype. Although

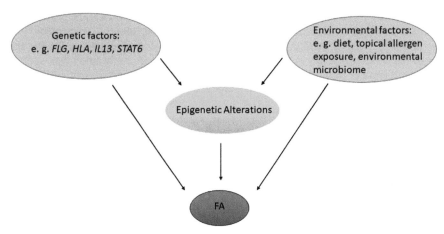

Fig. 3. Overview of possible pathways to food allergy (FA), based on genetic and environmental risk factors.

there are few demonstrated examples of associations between FA and genotypes being modified by environmental factors, several studies have linked DNA methylation to the risk of FA. Two SNPs in the *HLA-DQ* and *-DR* genomic region significantly associated with peanut allergy in a GWAS were also found to be associated with differential methylation at multiple CpG sites.[76] In an epigenome-wide association study of methylation in CD4$^+$ T cells from 12 children with FA to egg or peanut and 12 age-matched control subjects, 153 CpG loci differentially methylated at birth and 179 differentially methylated at 12 months of age were identified.[87] A total of 136 loci were common to both time points. Of these, 44 loci were located within 10 base pairs of SNPs, and these loci were annotated to *HLA-DQB1*. Differentially methylated loci that were not associated with SNPs were annotated to 49 different genes. These were subjected to pathways enrichment analysis, which suggested enrichment of the KEGG pathway "MAPK signaling pathway," a proinflammatory pathway with many different roles, including T-cell development and differentiation.

A recent study explored transcriptomic and CD4$^+$ T-cell epigenetic associations with reaction severity in 21 children allergic to peanut during double-blinded peanut challenges.[88] Among genes for which expression changes during challenge was significantly associated with reaction severity, 318 were replicated in an independent cohort of 19 children allergic to peanut. Gene ontology analysis on the 318 genes found them to be associated with regulation of nitric oxide processes, neutrophil activation, and macrophage activation, among other processes. Moreover, the association between reaction severity and 203 differentially methylated CpG sites was replicated in the independent cohort, and these CpG sites mapped to 197 unique genes. Four of the severity-associated CpG sites were located within 10 Mb of a gene with severity-associated expression, and causal mediation analysis indicated that expression of PHACTR1 and ZNF121 mediates the association between reaction severity and methylation of the associated CpGs. Interaction networks with the differentially expressed genes and the severity associated CpGs identified *NFKBIA* and *ARG1* as key hubs.

DNA methylation has been shown to be associated with immune tolerance in children undergoing oral immunotherapy for peanut allergy. In a study of 23 patients with peanut allergy undergoing oral immunotherapy and 20 control subjects with peanut allergy receiving standard of care and abstaining from peanut, participants who were immune tolerant to peanut 3 months after therapy withdrawal had decreased methylation of *FOXP3* CpG sites in antigen-induced regulatory T cells relative to the baseline before immunotherapy.[89] No change in methylation was seen in control subjects or participants who remained nontolerant after the treatment period. The changes in methylation in immune-tolerant participants were accompanied by increased expression of *FOXP3* in antigen-induced regulatory T cells. The results add support to previous studies showing a role for regulatory T cells in the response to immunotherapy.[90]

Genome-wide DNA methylation profiling has also been used to develop signatures that can predict clinical outcomes of FA. Using DNA from peripheral blood mononuclear cells in whole blood, a signature of 96 CpG sites was found to predict response to OFC better than SPT and allergen-specific IgE levels in 58 food-sensitized children aged 11 to 15 months and 13 control subjects without allergy.[91] The results were validated using CD4$^+$ T cells from an independent cohort. Studies of epigenetic changes in FA can contribute to the understanding of the pathways involved in the development of FA, and the interplay between genes, epigenetics, and environmental factors. More studies are needed to validate and replicate earlier results, and to explore the role of environmental factors in triggering changes in methylation patterns and other epigenetic alterations.

Genomic information is measurable and well established, whereas phenotyping and environmental exposures are less well standardized. Moving forward, deep phenotyping (eg, OFC) will be limiting. In the future, multilayer and longitudinal data, detailed measures of environmental exposures, detailed and standardized clinical information, combined genetic, race, clinical and environmental information, and GxE interactions in risk prediction and leveraging big genomic data in racially diverse population could pave the way to cost-effective personalized genomic medicine.[92] Precision medicine in FA requires precise inference of genetic ancestry.

FUTURE RESEARCH AND DIRECTIONS

Rapid progress in molecular genetics has increased the knowledge of the genomes of humans and other organisms and led to more detailed research into the genetic elements of allergy. Common human diseases, such as FA, are complicated by multiple factors (see **Box 1**): phenocopies, genetic heterogeneity (locus heterogeneity and allelic heterogeneity), trait heterogeneity, gene-gene interactions, GxE interactions, and such factors as admixture.[93–95] Future research into FA is expected to include analyses of gene-gene and GxE interactions and transcriptome-wide expression studies that estimate the differences in the expression of genes under diverse environmental conditions. Gene-gene interactions, also known as epistasis, refers to the expression of phenotypes only when specific alleles of two or more genes are present. Additionally, genomic studies have been expanded to include variations in DNA structure (see **Box 1**).

Admixture Mapping

It is well known that disease does not affect populations equally. This is because different populations are subject to distinct environmental exposure. Natural selection during the out-of-Africa expansion[96] may produce population-specific allele frequencies. Assessing variation in the rates of disease according to demographic factors, such as race or ethnicity, is the basis of epidemiologic research and affects clinical and public health practice.[97] The association between increased FA risk and

African ancestry and the admixed nature of the AA population suggests that admixture mapping might be an important FA gene-finding strategy to study directly genetically heterogeneous populations of AA nature.[98] Admixture mapping involves screening the genome of individuals of mixed ancestry who have a disease for chromosomal regions that have a greater percentage of alleles from the parental population with the higher disease risk.

Multiomics Approach

With the advent of omics-based big data–driven and unbiased approaches to define and characterize endotypes, including more accessible tools for human immunophe-notyping, detailed molecular information can now be gathered to deconvolute and identify patterns from the data, and gather further insights into the biology of diseases and health states of individual patients.[99,100] Statistical methods to integrate multio-mics data are emerging to provide important insights into disease pathophysiology of allergic diseases.[101] For example, machine learning approach uses computer algo-rithms to identify patterns from the systematically collected large molecular profile data, and along with clinical metadata, can assist personalized treatments for effective management of FAs with similar molecular subtypes.[102,103] The increasing focus on multiomics is expected to play an important role in the development of personalized medicine approaches that takes racial ancestry into account. It needs to be stressed, however, that any racial differences identified using proteomics, transcriptomics, or epigenetics are expected to be modified or confounded by environmental factors associated with ancestry, given the profound influence of the environment on epige-netics and gene regulation.[104] Genomics can provide deep insights into the genetic drivers of FA; transcriptomics sheds light on dysregulated gene regulation; and prote-ome provides deeper insight into what is going on at the molecular, tissue, and whole-body level.

Although racial disparities have been noted in the prevalence of FA, determining the relative contribution of ancestry-specific genetic risk factors from environmental fac-tors has proved to be challenging because of the limited number of studies performed on AA and other minority populations.[105] The delineation and deconstruction of shared and unique biologic and genetic pathways among atopic disorders and ancestry-specific GxE interactions can help resolve the clinical complexity and better inform the development of novel therapies.

Future research should include deep phenotyping of diverse ancestral popula-tions, better characterization of environmental determinants, and the application of new technologies using -omics tools. These include next-generation sequencing, epigenetics, and eQTL approaches in appropriate tissues/cells along with publicly available bioinformatics and ancestry tools. Systematic integration of "big data" coming from providers (eg, electronic medical records), from omics (eg, genomic, proteomic, epigenomic, metabolomic), and from multiethnic patients and nonpro-viders (eg, smart phone, monitoring tools for environmental triggers) can thus pro-vide valuable insights to resolve the clinical complexity and ancestry-specific (or shared) cause of FA.[106–109]

CLINICS CARE POINTS

- Food allergies are increasing and are a global health problem.
- IgE-mediated food allergies are the most common type of allergic reaction to food.

- Multiple studies suggest higher rate of food allergen sensitization in African American than European American children.
- Risk factors for the development of food allergy include parental history and atopic diseases, particularly atopic dermatitis (AD), which can lead to the development of the atopic march through mechanisms of cutaneous sensitization.

ACKNOWLEDGMENT

This work was supported by the National Institutes of Health (NIH) grant R01HL132344.

DISCLOSURE

The authors have nothing to disclose.

REFERENCES

1. Taylor SL. Review of the development of methodology for evaluating the human allergenic potential of novel proteins. Mol Nutr Food Res 2006;50(7): 604–9.
2. Gupta RS, Springston EE, Warrier MR, et al. The prevalence, severity, and distribution of childhood food allergy in the United States. Pediatrics 2011;128(1): e9–17.
3. Sicherer SH, Sampson HA. 9. Food allergy. J Allergy Clin Immunol 2006;117(2 Suppl Mini-Primer):S470–5.
4. Sicherer S. Understanding and managing your child's food allergies. Baltimore, MD: The Johns Hopkins University Press; 2006.
5. Gupta R, Holdford D, Bilaver L, et al. The economic impact of childhood food allergy in the United States. JAMA Pediatr 2013;167(11):1026–31.
6. Sicherer SH. Clinical implications of cross-reactive food allergens. J Allergy Clin Immunol 2001;108(6):881–90.
7. Nowak-Wegrzyn A, Sampson HA. Adverse reactions to foods. Med Clin North Am 2006;90(1):97–127.
8. Sampson HA. Peanut anaphylaxis. J Allergy Clin Immunol 1990;86(1):1–3.
9. Burks AW, Sampson H. Food allergies in children. Curr Probl Pediatr 1993;23(6): 230–52.
10. Burks AW, Sampson HA, Buckley RH. Anaphylactic reactions after gamma globulin administration in patients with hypogammaglobulinemia. Detection of IgE antibodies to IgA. N Engl J Med 1986;314(9):560–4.
11. Strober W. Gluten-sensitive enteropathy: a nonallergic immune hypersensitivity of the gastrointestinal tract. J Allergy Clin Immunol 1986;78(1 Pt 2):202–11.
12. Madsen C. Prevalence of food allergy: an overview. Proc Nutr Soc 2005;64(4): 413–7.
13. Sampson HA. Update on food allergy. J Allergy Clin Immunol 2004;113(5): 805–19 [quiz: 820].
14. Tordesillas L, Berin MC. Mechanisms of oral tolerance. Clin Rev Allergy Immunol 2018;55(2):107–17.
15. Noval Rivas M, Chatila TA. Regulatory T cells in allergic diseases. J Allergy Clin Immunol 2016;138(3):639–52.
16. Tordesillas L, Berin MC, Sampson HA. Immunology of food allergy. Immunity 2017;47(1):32–50.

17. Taylor SL. Food allergies and sensitivities. J Am Diet Assoc 1986;86(5):599–600.
18. Chehade M. IgE and non-IgE-mediated food allergy: treatment in 2007. Curr Opin Allergy Clin Immunol 2007;7(3):264–8.
19. Bruijnzeel-Koomen C, Ortolani C, Aas K, et al. Adverse reactions to food. European Academy of Allergology and Clinical Immunology Subcommittee. Allergy. 1995;50(8):623–35.
20. Werfel T. Epicutaneous allergen administration: a novel approach for allergen-specific immunotherapy? J Allergy Clin Immunol 2009;124(5):1003–4.
21. Boyce JA, Assa'ad A, Burks AW, et al. Guidelines for the diagnosis and management of food allergy in the United States: summary of the NIAID-sponsored expert panel report. Nutr Res 2011;31(1):61–75.
22. Boyce JA, Assa'ad A, Burks AW, et al. Guidelines for the Diagnosis and Management of Food Allergy in the United States: Summary of the NIAID-Sponsored Expert Panel Report. J Allergy Clin Immunol 2010;126(6):1105–18.
23. Woods RK, Stoney RM, Raven J, et al. Reported adverse food reactions overestimate true food allergy in the community. Eur J Clin Nutr 2002;56(1):31–6.
24. Miles S, Fordham R, Mills C, et al. A framework for measuring costs to society of IgE-mediated food allergy. Allergy. 2005;60(8):996–1003.
25. Tsakok T, Marrs T, Mohsin M, et al. Does atopic dermatitis cause food allergy? A systematic review. J Allergy Clin Immunol 2016;137(4):1071–8.
26. Du Toit G, Sayre PH, Roberts G, et al. Effect of avoidance on peanut allergy after early peanut consumption. N Engl J Med 2016;374(15):1435–43.
27. Schmiechen ZC, Weissler KA, Frischmeyer-Guerrerio PA. Recent developments in understanding the mechanisms of food allergy. Curr Opin Pediatr 2019;31(6):807–14.
28. Brough HA, Nadeau KC, Sindher SB, et al. Epicutaneous sensitization in the development of food allergy: what is the evidence and how can this be prevented? Allergy. 2020;75(9):2185–205.
29. Paller AS, Spergel JM, Mina-Osorio P, et al. The atopic march and atopic multimorbidity: many trajectories, many pathways. J Allergy Clin Immunol 2019;143(1):46–55.
30. Kelleher MM, Dunn-Galvin A, Gray C, et al. Skin barrier impairment at birth predicts food allergy at 2 years of age. J Allergy Clin Immunol 2016;137(4):1111–6.e8.
31. Johansson EK, Bergstrom A, Kull I, et al. IgE sensitization in relation to preschool eczema and filaggrin mutation. J Allergy Clin Immunol 2017;140(6):1572–9.e5.
32. Chavanas S, Bodemer C, Rochat A, et al. Mutations in SPINK5, encoding a serine protease inhibitor, cause Netherton syndrome. Nat Genet 2000;25(2):141–2.
33. Hannula-Jouppi K, Laasanen SL, Heikkila H, et al. IgE allergen component-based profiling and atopic manifestations in patients with Netherton syndrome. J Allergy Clin Immunol 2014;134(4):985–8.
34. Samuelov L, Sarig O, Harmon RM, et al. Desmoglein 1 deficiency results in severe dermatitis, multiple allergies and metabolic wasting. Nat Genet 2013;45(10):1244–8.
35. Has C, Jakob T, He Y, et al. Loss of desmoglein 1 associated with palmoplantar keratoderma, dermatitis and multiple allergies. Br J Dermatol 2015;172(1):257–61.
36. Carter CA, Frischmeyer-Guerrerio PA. The genetics of food allergy. Curr Allergy Asthma Rep 2018;18(1):2.

37. Park JH, Lee KH, Jeon B, et al. Immune dysregulation, polyendocrinopathy, enteropathy, X-linked (IPEX) syndrome: a systematic review. Autoimmun Rev 2020; 19(6):102526.

38. Torgerson TR, Linane A, Moes N, et al. Severe food allergy as a variant of IPEX syndrome caused by a deletion in a noncoding region of the FOXP3 gene. Gastroenterology 2007;132(5):1705–17.

39. Frischmeyer-Guerrerio PA, Guerrerio AL, Oswald G, et al. TGFbeta receptor mutations impose a strong predisposition for human allergic disease. Sci Transl Med 2013;5(195):195ra194.

40. Arias K, Waserman S, Jordana M. Management of food-induced anaphylaxis: unsolved challenges. Curr Clin Pharmacol 2009;4(2):113–25.

41. Celedon JC, Sredl D, Weiss ST, et al. Ethnicity and skin test reactivity to aeroallergens among asthmatic children in Connecticut. Chest. 2004;125(1):85–92.

42. Liu AH, Jaramillo R, Sicherer SH, et al. National prevalence and risk factors for food allergy and relationship to asthma: results from the National Health and Nutrition Examination Survey 2005-2006. J Allergy Clin Immunol 2010;126(4): 798–806.e3.

43. Vergara C, Caraballo L, Mercado D, et al. African ancestry is associated with risk of asthma and high total serum IgE in a population from the Caribbean Coast of Colombia. Hum Genet 2009;125(5–6):565–79.

44. Cardoso BA, Martins LR, Santos CI, et al. Interleukin-4 stimulates proliferation and growth of T-cell acute lymphoblastic leukemia cells by activating mTOR signaling. Leukemia 2009;23(1):206–8.

45. Wegienka G, Sitarik A, Bassirpour G, et al. The associations between eczema and food and inhalant allergen-specific IgE vary between black and white children. J Allergy Clin Immunol Pract 2017;6(1):292–4.e2.

46. Le Souef PN, Candelaria P, Goldblatt J. Evolution and respiratory genetics. Eur Respir J 2006;28(6):1258–63.

47. Stevenson LA, Gergen PJ, Hoover DR, et al. Sociodemographic correlates of indoor allergen sensitivity among United States children. J Allergy Clin Immunol 2001;108(5):747–52.

48. Mahdavinia M, Fox SR, Smith BM, et al. Racial differences in food allergy phenotype and health care utilization among US children. J Allergy Clin Immunol Pract 2017;5(2):352–7.e1.

49. Hartman H, Dodd C, Rao M, et al. Parental timing of allergenic food introduction in urban and suburban populations. Ann Allergy Asthma Immunol 2016;117(1): 56–60.e2.

50. Muers M. Human disease: edges, nodes and networks. Nat Rev Genet 2010; 11(1):4.

51. Kalow W. Pharmacogenetics and pharmacogenomics: origin, status, and the hope for personalized medicine. Pharmacogenomics J 2006;6(3):162–5.

52. Luccioli S, Ross M, Labiner-Wolfe J, et al. Maternally reported food allergies and other food-related health problems in infants: characteristics and associated factors. Pediatrics 2008;122(Suppl 2):S105–12.

53. Bonini S, Ruffilli A. Genetics of food allergy. Environ Toxicol Pharmacol 1997; 4(1–2):71–8.

54. Tsai HJ, Kumar R, Pongracic J, et al. Familial aggregation of food allergy and sensitization to food allergens: a family-based study. Clin Exp Allergy 2009; 39(1):101–9.

55. Hourihane JO, Dean TP, Warner JO. Peanut allergy in relation to heredity, maternal diet, and other atopic diseases: results of a questionnaire survey, skin prick testing, and food challenges. BMJ 1996;313(7056):518–21.

56. Sicherer SH, Furlong TJ, Maes HH, et al. Genetics of peanut allergy: a twin study. J Allergy Clin Immunol 2000;106(1 Pt 1):53–6.

57. Liu X, Zhang S, Tsai HJ, et al. Genetic and environmental contributions to allergen sensitization in a Chinese twin study. Clin Exp Allergy 2009;39(7): 991–8.

58. Ober C, Yao TC. The genetics of asthma and allergic disease: a 21st century perspective. Immunol Rev 2011;242(1):10–30.

59. Muraro A, Werfel T, Hoffmann-Sommergruber K, et al. EAACI food allergy and anaphylaxis guidelines: diagnosis and management of food allergy. Allergy. 2014;69(8):1008–25.

60. Sicherer SH, Sampson HA. Food allergy: a review and update on epidemiology, pathogenesis, diagnosis, prevention, and management. J Allergy Clin Immunol 2018;141(1):41–58.

61. Calvani M, Bianchi A, Reginelli C, et al. Oral food challenge. Medicina (Kaunas). 2019;55(10):651–76.

62. Suaini NHA, Wang Y, Soriano VX, et al. Genetic determinants of paediatric food allergy: a systematic review. Allergy. 2019;74(9):1631–48.

63. Kontakioti E, Domvri K, Papakosta D, et al. HLA and asthma phenotypes/endo-types: a review. Hum Immunol 2014;75(8):930–9.

64. Howell WM, Turner SJ, Hourihane JO, et al. HLA class II DRB1, DQB1 and DPB1 genotypic associations with peanut allergy: evidence from a family-based and case-control study. Clin Exp Allergy 1998;28(2):156–62.

65. Woo JG, Assa'ad A, Heizer AB, et al. The -159 C-->T polymorphism of CD14 is associated with nonatopic asthma and food allergy. J Allergy Clin Immunol 2003;112(2):438–44.

66. Dreskin SC, Ayars A, Jin Y, et al. Association of genetic variants of CD14 with peanut allergy and elevated IgE levels in peanut allergic individuals. Ann Allergy Asthma Immunol 2011;106(2):170–2.

67. Campos E, Shimojo N, Inoue Y, et al. No association of polymorphisms in the 5' region of the CD14 gene and food allergy in a Japanese population. Allergol Int 2007;56(1):23–7.

68. Ashley SE, Tan HT, Peters R, et al. Genetic variation at the Th2 immune gene IL13 is associated with IgE-mediated paediatric food allergy. Clin Exp Allergy 2017;47(8):1032–7.

69. Hirota T, Nakayama T, Sato S, et al. Association study of childhood food allergy with genome-wide association studies-discovered loci of atopic dermatitis and eosinophilic esophagitis. J Allergy Clin Immunol 2017;140(6):1713–6.

70. Amoli MM, Hand S, Hajeer AH, et al. Polymorphism in the STAT6 gene encodes risk for nut allergy. Genes Immun 2002;3(4):220–4.

71. Laha A, Ghosh A, Moitra S, et al. Association of the STAT6 rs3024974 (C/T) poly-morphism with IgE-mediated food sensitization among West Bengal population in India. Int Arch Allergy Immunol 2020;181(3):200–10.

72. Brown SJ, Asai Y, Cordell HJ, et al. Loss-of-function variants in the filaggrin gene are a significant risk factor for peanut allergy. J Allergy Clin Immunol 2011; 127(3):661–7.

73. Venkataraman D, Soto-Ramirez N, Kurukulaaratchy RJ, et al. Filaggrin loss-of-function mutations are associated with food allergy in childhood and adoles-cence. J Allergy Clin Immunol 2014;134(4):876–82.e4.

74. Tan HT, Ellis JA, Koplin JJ, et al. Filaggrin loss-of-function mutations do not predict food allergy over and above the risk of food sensitization among infants. J Allergy Clin Immunol 2012;130(5):1211–3.e3.

75. Ashley SE, Tan HT, Vuillermin P, et al. The skin barrier function gene SPINK5 is associated with challenge-proven IgE-mediated food allergy in infants. Allergy. 2017;72(9):1356–64.

76. Hong X, Hao K, Ladd-Acosta C, et al. Genome-wide association study identifies peanut allergy-specific loci and evidence of epigenetic mediation in US children. Nat Commun 2015;6:6304.

77. Marenholz I, Grosche S, Kalb B, et al. Genome-wide association study identifies the SERPINB gene cluster as a susceptibility locus for food allergy. Nat Commun 2017;8(1):1056.

78. Asai Y, Eslami A, van Ginkel CD, et al. A Canadian genome-wide association study and meta-analysis confirm HLA as a risk factor for peanut allergy independent of asthma. J Allergy Clin Immunol 2018;141(4):1513–6.

79. Asai Y, Eslami A, van Ginkel CD, et al. Genome-wide association study and meta-analysis in multiple populations identifies new loci for peanut allergy and establishes C11orf30/EMSY as a genetic risk factor for food allergy. J Allergy Clin Immunol 2018;141(3):991–1001.

80. Li J, Fung I, Glessner JT, et al. Copy number variations in CTNNA3 and RBFOX1 associate with pediatric food allergy. J Immunol 2015;195(4):1599–607.

81. Lieberman JA, Greenhawt M, Nowak-Wegrzyn A. The environment and food allergy. Ann Allergy Asthma Immunol 2018;120(5):455–7.

82. Stephen-Victor E, Crestani E, Chatila TA. Dietary and microbial determinants in food allergy. Immunity 2020;53(2):277–89.

83. Johansson H, Mersha TB, Brandt EB, et al. Interactions between environmental pollutants and genetic susceptibility in asthma risk. Curr Opin Immunol 2019;60: 156–62.

84. Morales E, Duffy D. Genetics and gene-environment interactions in childhood and adult onset asthma. Front Pediatr 2019;7:499.

85. Koplin JJ, Suaini NH, Vuillermin P, et al. Polymorphisms affecting vitamin D-binding protein modify the relationship between serum vitamin D (25[OH]D3) and food allergy. J Allergy Clin Immunol 2016;137(2):500–6.e4.

86. Brough HA, Simpson A, Makinson K, et al. Peanut allergy: effect of environmental peanut exposure in children with filaggrin loss-of-function mutations. J Allergy Clin Immunol 2014;134(4):867–75.e1.

87. Martino D, Joo JE, Sexton-Oates A, et al. Epigenome-wide association study reveals longitudinally stable DNA methylation differences in CD4+ T cells from children with IgE-mediated food allergy. Epigenetics. 2014;9(7):998–1006.

88. Do AN, Watson CT, Cohain AT, et al. Dual transcriptomic and epigenomic study of reaction severity in peanut-allergic children. J Allergy Clin Immunol 2020; 145(4):1219–30.

89. Syed A, Garcia MA, Lyu SC, et al. Peanut oral immunotherapy results in increased antigen-induced regulatory T-cell function and hypomethylation of forkhead box protein 3 (FOXP3). J Allergy Clin Immunol 2014;133(2):500–10.

90. Ozdemir C, Kucuksezer UC, Akdis M, et al. Specific immunotherapy and turning off the T cell: how does it work? Ann Allergy Asthma Immunol 2011;107(5): 381–92.

91. Martino D, Dang T, Sexton-Oates A, et al. Blood DNA methylation biomarkers predict clinical reactivity in food-sensitized infants. J Allergy Clin Immunol 2015;135(5):1319–28.e1–2.

92. Coulson E, Rifas-Shiman SL, Sordillo J, et al. Racial, ethnic, and socioeconomic differences in adolescent food allergy. J Allergy Clin Immunol Pract 2020;8(1): 336–8.e3.

93. Savage JH, Lee-Sarwar KA, Sordillo J, et al. A prospective microbiome-wide association study of food sensitization and food allergy in early childhood. Allergy. 2018;73(1):145–52.

94. Lee TD, Gimenez G, Grishina G, et al. Profile of a milk-allergic patient who tolerated partially hydrolyzed whey formula. J Allergy Clin Immunol Pract 2015;3(1): 116–8.

95. Jin H, Sifers T, Cox AL, et al. Peanut oral food challenges and subsequent feeding of peanuts in infants. J Allergy Clin Immunol Pract 2020. https://doi. org/10.1016/j.jaip.2020.11.045.

96. Young JH, Chang YP, Kim JD, et al. Differential susceptibility to hypertension is due to selection during the out-of-Africa expansion. PLoS Genet 2005;1(6):e82.

97. Risch N. Dissecting racial and ethnic differences. N Engl J Med 2006;354(4): 408–11.

98. Mersha TB. Mapping asthma-associated variants in admixed populations. Front Genet 2015;6:292.

99. Holzinger A, Dehmer M, Jurisica I. Knowledge discovery and interactive data mining in bioinformatics–state-of-the-art, future challenges and research directions. BMC Bioinformatics 2014;15(Suppl 6):I1.

100. Yu KH, Snyder M. Omics profiling in precision oncology. Mol Cell Proteomics 2016;15(8):2525–36.

101. Reinke SN, Gallart-Ayala H, Gomez C, et al. Metabolomics analysis identifies different metabotypes of asthma severity. Eur Respir J 2017;49(3):1601740.

102. Greene CS, Tan J, Ung M, et al. Big data bioinformatics. J Cell Physiol 2014; 229(12):1896–900.

103. Alag A. Machine learning approach yields epigenetic biomarkers of food allergy: a novel 13-gene signature to diagnose clinical reactivity. PLoS One. 2019;14(6):e0218253.

104. Watson CT, Cohain AT, Griffin RS, et al. Integrative transcriptomic analysis reveals key drivers of acute peanut allergic reactions. Nat Commun 2017;8(1): 1943.

105. Barnes KC. Genomewide association studies in allergy and the influence of ethnicity. Curr Opin Allergy Clin Immunol 2010;10(5):427–33.

106. Zhao W, Ho HE, Bunyavanich S. The gut microbiome in food allergy. Ann Allergy Asthma Immunol 2019;122(3):276–82.

107. Irizar H, Kanchan K, Mathias RA, et al. Advancing food allergy through omics sciences. J Allergy Clin Immunol Pract 2020;9(1):119–29.

108. Ho HE, Bunyavanich S. Role of the microbiome in food allergy. Curr Allergy Asthma Rep 2018;18(4):27.

109. Fazlollahi M, Chun Y, Grishin A, et al. Early-life gut microbiome and egg allergy. Allergy. 2018;73(7):1515–24.

The Unmet Needs of Patients with Food Allergies

Melissa L. Engel, MA[a], Bryan J. Bunning, MS(c)[b],*

KEYWORDS

- Food allergy • Anxiety • Developmental psychology • Adolescence • PRO
- Oral immunotherapy

KEY POINTS

- Food allergy–related anxiety is prevalent among pediatric patients and their caregivers.
- The current treatment paradigm, involving only strict allergen avoidance, is associated with anxiety-related symptoms. An appropriate level of anxiety is protective to the patient. However, in excess, anxiety may decrease quality of life.
- As pediatric patients transition into adolescence and adulthood, responsibility of care must shift from caregiver to patient. The anxiety that often co-occurs with food allergies among both patients and caregivers may make this transition difficult.
- A great deal of uncertainty surrounds daily self-management, leaving patients and caregivers to frequently crowdsource guidance, which is of variable utility.
- Managing treatment expectations and addressing psychological concerns regarding exposure will be increasingly important as various forms of allergen immunotherapy become available.

Food allergies present patients with a unique set of psychosocial challenges. As others have reviewed, many of these challenges involve elements of anxiety, which can be defined as anticipation of future threat.[1–3] From a psychological perspective, this is expected. As a protective measure, individuals with food allergies have been conditioned, often from a very young age, to associate their allergens with danger. They have learned through experiencing an allergic reaction, or, in the case of a young child, through parental modeling, that exposure to their allergens is a severe threat to bodily integrity. Although variants of immunotherapy are on the clinical horizon, only peanut-specific oral immunotherapy has approval in the United States; thus, allergen avoidance and emergency epinephrine administration remain the current food allergy treatment for most of the allergic population.[4] Patients have been explicitly directed by physicians to strictly avoid their allergens. Although such allergen avoidance is critical,

[a] Department of Psychology, Emory University, 36 Eagle Row, Atlanta, GA 30322, USA;
[b] Department of Biostatistics, Mailman School of Public Health, Columbia University, 722 West 168th Street, FL R6, New York, NY 10032, USA
* Corresponding author.
E-mail address: Bjb2178@columbia.edu

Immunol Allergy Clin N Am 41 (2021) 321–330
https://doi.org/10.1016/j.iac.2021.01.005
immunology.theclinics.com
0889-8561/21/© 2021 Elsevier Inc. All rights reserved.

from a cognitive-behavioral perspective, avoidance is precisely what may fuel anxiety. Others have argued that a certain level of anxiety is adaptive for individuals living with food allergies.[5] The authors take this 1 step further, suggesting that anxiety should be considered a side effect of the recommended food allergy management strategy of avoidance.

This article reviews psychosocial challenges faced by individuals with food allergies through both daily self-management and through treatment (**Box 1**). Next, it addresses the allergy-anxiety relationship as an unmet need for the patients or their caregivers, in part because of a lack of clear guidance and the heterogeneity of food allergy severity and management. Then, it highlights the dearth of research on the transition to adulthood and calls for an increased focus on the psychosocial needs of individuals with food allergies across children's development. As more and more pediatric food-allergic patients become adult food-allergic patients, this is a critical direction for future research. In addition, this article highlights the conflict that may arise as patients switch from the previous paradigm of avoidance to one involving avoidance, including a therapy with constant and measured exposure. With an increasing number of exposure-based food allergy therapies on the horizon, this will be a growing issue.

THE ANXIETY OF DAILY MANAGEMENT: ARE THERE PEANUTS ON THE PREMISES?

Traditionally, to be labeled clinically significant, anxious thoughts and/or avoidant behaviors must be deemed out of proportion to the degree of threat.[3] Cognitive-behavior therapy to treat anxiety may generally focus on altering cognitive misappraisals of danger and preventing avoidant behaviors.[6] This focus presents a challenge when it comes to food allergies, in which allergen exposure may be life threatening and allergen avoidance is paramount. Furthermore, many behaviors that are associated with anxiety and are considered maladaptive, such as perfectionism, repeated checking, leaving social situations, and hypervigilance, may be adaptive in the context of food allergies.[6,7] Interestingly, longitudinal epidemiologic research has identified that youth with food allergies are at increased risk for symptoms of anxiety, as well as depression and anorexia nervosa, but not actual psychiatric disorders.[1,8] These anxious symptoms tend to be specific to food allergies, as opposed to general fear or anxiety. Although such symptoms may be subthreshold from a psychiatric perspective and reflect reasonable adaptations to living with food allergies, they may also negatively affect quality of life.[9] For instance, youth with food allergies report increased rates of anxious coping, as well as symptoms of separation anxiety, social anxiety, and panic disorder.[10]

It is easy to see how anxiety is an inherent part of food allergy management; fear of allergen exposure is what motivates allergen avoidance and prevents potentially life-threatening risky behavior. Patterns of increased anxiety and reduced quality of life are

---

Box 1
Summary of unmet needs in food-allergic patients discussed in this article

- Establishing and promoting practices for the safe transition of care from caregiver to patient
- Understanding the impact of transition of allergy-related care on a family unit
- Creating and disseminating patient-centered psychoeducational information
- Psychosocial difficulties in adults with food allergies
- Preventing and treating patient and parent anxiety related to desensitization treatments

common among families of children with food allergies.[11] However, it is difficult to determine what level of avoidance constitutes adaptive versus excessive. Allergen avoidance can range from simply not eating buckets of peanuts to approaching every life activity by first detecting whether there is even the slightest chance that there have been any peanuts on the premises. Although the latter approach may reduce reaction risk, such paralyzing fear may also lead to an overly restricted diet and avoidance of social situations, which have serious consequences for child and adolescent growth and development.[12] Furthermore, 1 study of children with seafood allergy found that parental over-restriction of children's diet was not associated with decreased risk of accidental reactions. In fact, over-restriction was associated with increased anxiety and decreased quality of life.[13] Thus, at a certain level, heightened anxiety, avoidance, and restriction may exert significant psychosocial cost with little physical benefit. It has been suggested that pediatric allergists are not well prepared to identify clinically significant anxiety among patients.[14] Perhaps this is because there is little consensus as to what an appropriate so-called Goldilocks, or just-right, level of anxiety looks like.[5] At what point should food allergy worries, checking, restrictions, and avoidance be considered excessive? Patients with food allergies, and perhaps allergists as well, need guidance as to what constitutes helpful versus harmful anxiety. Without such guidance, overly anxious individuals may simply be labeled adherent, with no detection of anxious distress or opportunities for behavioral interventions.

Importantly, how food allergy–related anxiety manifests changes across development. Younger children show fear of going places without their primary caregivers, whereas older children and adolescents experience fear surrounding uncertain social situations, negative social evaluation, and bullying.[15,16] Beyond adolescence, there is remarkably little research on anxiety in adults with food allergies,[2] perhaps because the food allergy epidemic has increased only in the past few decades, mostly affecting children.[17] Given that many children currently with food allergies will become adults with food allergies, prospective longitudinal research following allergy-related anxiety across development is critical.

The limited existing research suggests that adults with food allergies indeed experience anxiety. Adults with food allergies have reported experiencing anxiety related to food safety and social situations, and young adults with food allergies who rated themselves high in health competence reported experiencing anxiety from maintaining constant vigilance.[18] Although this research is in its infancy, there is far more literature devoted to the psychosocial issues faced by adults in relation to parenting a child with food allergies. Mothers of children with food allergies experience greater rates of stress, anxiety, and depression, and these symptoms have each been linked to children's food-related anxiety, emotional functioning, and social limitations.[19] However, little is known about exactly how these dynamics shift across development.

ALL GROWN UP?

Throughout childhood, food allergy management is often in the hands of the primary caregivers. As mentioned earlier, caring for a child with a life-threatening condition is an enormous responsibility and thus often comes with a burden of stress and anxiety.[19] In addition to keeping a child with food allergies physically safe, caregivers carry the additional responsibility of teaching the child skills to manage the allergies autonomously and develop independence before reaching adulthood. Across medical conditions, health care transitions from pediatric, parent-supervised care to adult, patient-centered care are rife with vulnerability, and transitions in food allergy management are no exception.[20] Caregivers who teach too much vigilance set the stage for anxiety, whereas those who do not teach enough vigilance predispose the risky behavior that is already common in adolescence, resulting in an increased potential for life-threatening reactions.[5] However, caregivers have insufficient guidance when it comes to scaffolding children through such developmental transitions. Clarity and guidance are made difficult by the vast heterogeneity, at both the individual and population levels, that characterizes food allergens as well as the degree of severity of the reactions they provoke.[21] However, patients with food allergies and their families are in need of more structured developmental recommendations. Although individual circumstances call for unique timelines, creating a centralized, vetted template of food allergy–specific developmental milestones may be a worthwhile endeavor. At what age should the average child with food allergies be reading labels, speaking with a chef on their own, or independently carrying their epinephrine? Creating such guidelines may instill caregiver confidence and alleviate stress while simultaneously giving allergists developmental benchmarks to routinely assess.

Pediatric patients with food allergy and their caregivers need assistance in navigating this transition safely while maximizing quality of life, especially given that mental health disorders, such as anxiety and depression, are highly prevalent and persistent among adolescents, with less favorable trajectories among those with chronic illness.[22,23] As previously discussed, there is little research examining the long-term outcomes of youth who experience food allergy–related anxiety. However, the developmental psychopathology literature suggests that there is reason for concern. Child and adolescent anxiety may not be a transient phenomenon that disappears over time but may be the root of psychological distress across the lifespan. Children and adolescents who experience anxiety are more likely to experience anxiety, depression, and substance use as adults.[24] Developmental psychologists have argued that properly managing child anxiety may prevent a future of diverse mental health problems, and this advice may be applicable to youth with food allergy–related anxiety.[24] Developmental psychologists have also highlighted the intergenerational transmission of anxiety from parents to children, and research indicates that such anxiety is directly transmitted through the environment, rather than genetically.[25] When applied to food allergies, this suggests that some young patients may model their parents' anxious behaviors and subsequently grow to experience psychological distress themselves. Thus, in order to prevent young people with food allergies from developing future psychological challenges, routine screening and monitoring of anxiety among children and adolescents with food allergies is warranted. This monitoring may be especially important when transitioning the responsibility of care from caregiver to patient, an ambiguous and highly variable period of time that may be fertile ground for anxiety. As others have reported, the lack of availability of mental health services for patients with food allergies is a major unmet need, and integrating mental health professionals into allergy clinics is a priority.[26]

IN SEARCH OF CERTAINTY

Regardless of who holds the burden of responsibility, stress among patients and caregivers with food allergies remains high. Perceived stress generally depends on how unpredictable or uncontrollable individuals interpret their circumstances to be.[27] Given that uncertainty is a core feature of allergic reactions, and that intolerance of uncertainty is a key component of emotional distress, it is rational that individuals with food allergies, or their caregivers, feel a high degree of stress and a need to reduce this distress by feeling in control.[6,21] As Feng and Kim[1] (2019) have asserted, "the stress from having a food allergy may be more burdensome than the food allergy itself"

(p. 77). Qualitative research suggests that parents of children with food allergies sense that they are perpetually on guard and feel a strong need to control every aspect of their children's daily lives.[2,28,29] Such need for control may explain why many parents of children with food allergies have been found to avoid dining out or to repeatedly visit the same safe restaurant; limit travel based on perceived risk of airplanes and overnight stays; and restrict children's participation in play dates, sports teams, camp, birthday parties, and even school.[1,7,28,30,31] Likewise, it may explain why stakeholders in the food allergy community place a high priority on the area of product labeling, rating it far more important than researchers perceive.[32] Current precautionary allergen labeling is inconsistent, and patients with food allergy and their parents report a need for greater clarity.[33] In the absence of such clarity, patients and caregivers need tools to manage the stress associated with daily uncertainties.

A dearth of clear information with regard to food allergy management, aside from allergen avoidance and epinephrine administration, leads many patients and parents to make decisions rooted in fear rather than facts.[34] For instance, despite little evidence supporting the efficacy of peanut-free schools, tables, or airplanes, such policies often give parents a greater perception of control.[34] Likewise, despite little evidence of the smell of peanut butter, aerosolizing peanut dust on airplanes, or minor skin contact with peanut butter causing a reaction in most patients with peanut allergy, many individuals endorse these beliefs and mold their behaviors around these potential situations.[34–38] Messages delivered by the media, as well as by providers, tend to emphasize worst-case scenarios, such as fatality, setting the stage for anxiety-driven thoughts, feelings, and behaviors, which some patients describe as paralyzing.[34,39]

Clarity, education, and support are major unmet needs in the food allergy community, leaving many to find this information through whatever means necessary. Many patients and caregivers now turn to the Internet, where they may find supplemental information from large food allergy organizations and local support groups.[40] In addition, individuals managing food allergies may also look to crowdsourcing for lifestyle guidelines or advice. This tendency is evident by quickly searching through the preponderance of Facebook groups, Instagram pages, and apps geared toward individuals with food allergies and their families. In addition, individuals who were recently diagnosed with food allergy have been shown to be more likely to use social media for allergy-related purposes.[41] As of September 2020, membership in the Dining Out With Food Allergies Facebook group exceeded 29,000, the No Nuts Moms Group exceeded 32,000, and the Food Allergy Adventurers Club: Managing Food Allergies at Disney exceeded 12,000. That patients and caregivers with food allergies are seeking help is undeniable; however, less known is the effectiveness of such unvetted crowdsourced information. One study noted that individuals generally report finding online resources and social media helpful, and another study found that the top reasons for online engagement included searching for information about food allergies, asking questions, and looking for safe restaurants.[40,41] It is important to recognize that the Internet is full of misinformation, including when it comes to food allergies.[1] Although parents have reported valuing information offered by consumer organizations, certain aspects have been found to be unhelpful, such as advice that was not applicable to their unique experiences, and anxiety contagion from interaction with anxious parents.[42] The potential for an iatrogenic effect from online resources, such as social media groups for parents of children with food allergies, is further supported by a study identifying new information regarding potential risk as a key contributor to renewed parental anxiety.[5] It is possible that frequent exposure to anxiety from other parents of children with food allergies, whether it be through articles about severe allergic reactions or posts about excessive social restrictions, may serve to increase parental anxiety rather than provide reputable, evidence-based information. This area is important for future research to explore.

To complement this crowdsourced information, the authors suggest that allergy researchers, clinicians, and educators continue to create and promote patient-centered psychoeducational materials. To reduce anxiety and improve quality of life, patients and families need practical guidance for navigating daily life and the development process while managing food allergies. Research suggests that a food allergy management curriculum may simultaneously educate parents, model adaptive coping, and empower them with a sense of control.[43] Furthermore, many parents have identified lack of knowledge among other parents and the school system as major contributors to anxiety, suggesting that allergy education efforts on a population level are critical.[2,28,29] Education in schools has also been suggested as a method to decrease social anxiety among children.[44] Such education may simultaneously decrease stigma and bullying while increasing safety in the event of an emergency.

THE ANXIETY OF TREATMENT: YOU ARE EXPOSING ME TO MY KILLER?

As clinicians move toward the next generation of therapy, it is important to remember where patients are coming from psychologically. Patients' were taught strict avoidance and have developed a framework to manage it and then suddenly have an option for a desensitization-based therapy. Some may have trouble adapting to the therapy at a psychological level. Anxiety and stress are heterogeneous between patients and their caregivers.[11] Adapting and helping high-stress-level families will only become more important as desensitization treatments become more widely available. It is important to provide support and acknowledge the confusing situations treatment may put pediatric patients and/or their caregivers in. The patient's and caregiver's mental state is one of many factors that should be taken into account on an individual basis. The first iteration of oral immunotherapy is not a 1-treatment-fits-all situation. It is well established that immunotherapy is not a therapy for everyone, because it requires strict compliance and high time investment.[45] Further, it is a treatment with both benefits and risks, including adverse events associated with therapy.[45–47] Although research into sustained unresponsiveness is ongoing, compliance is essential for the up-dosing and maintenance phases of oral immunotherapy.[45] Looking ahead, there is hope that combination therapies, including those using biologics, may lessen the burden of desensitization-based therapies on the patients and their families.[48]

When initiating immunotherapy, allergists may consider drawing from the child anxiety literature on exposure therapy. Exposure therapy for anxiety disorders such as specific phobia, obsessive-compulsive disorder, or posttraumatic stress disorder is conducted in a graded fashion. Rather than taking children who cannot swim and throwing them into the ocean, psychologists aim to get in the pool with the children and give them floaties.[24] In collaboration with the children, psychologists often create a fear hierarchy, in which patients may gradually work up to exposing themselves to feared stimuli. Each exposure is preceded by extensive preparation and followed by thoughtful processing. Adapted for patients with food allergies, this may begin with imaginal exposures, such as simply asking a patient to imagine seeing or touching a peanut, followed by looking at pictures of peanuts, smelling peanuts, and touching peanuts, all before ingestion. After ingestion, patients discuss how this experience made them feel, not only physically but also emotionally.

Acknowledging the anxiety and mental state of the patient and the caregivers, and further managing expectations, can remove uncertainty for the patient and family, reducing overall stress. This approach is especially relevant for pediatric patients and may have potential to improve outcomes and quality of life. A study by Howe and colleagues,[49] sought to use a mental framework as a method to improve patient quality of life during immunotherapy. In this randomized, blinded controlled trial, patients (n = 50) and their caregivers were randomized 1:1 and informed that non–life-threatening symptoms were either (1) unfortunate side effects of treatment or (2) a potential signal of the desensitization process. Those who were informed that symptoms signaled the desensitization process were significantly less likely to report being anxious and report experiencing a non–life-threatening adverse event.[49] Fostering and acknowledging the mindset of patients and using psychological tools to help them has potential to improve not only experiences and overall stress but potentially clinical outcomes as well.

SUMMARY

Patients with food allergies often experience anxiety because of the daily self-management and potential new desensitization treatments for food allergies. On one hand, anxiety can be seen as a necessary adaptation to remain vigilant and physically safe. In excess, however, anxiety can lead to significant psychological distress and impairments in quality of life. Little is known about food allergy anxiety across the lifespan, and patients and caregivers could benefit from guidance in developmental milestones, transitioning from parent to patient responsibility, and managing anxiety throughout this vulnerable period. In the absence of clear guidelines, patients and caregivers have turned to crowdsourced information with varying levels of utility. Patients are in need of reviewed guidelines from established knowledge sources. As more pediatric patients reach adulthood, this will be a critical target. Furthermore, as advanced therapeutic options become available, it will be important to provide individualized recommendations, considering and minimizing children's and caregivers' levels of anxiety, and draw from psychological research to best support the transition from a paradigm of avoidance to one of exposure through desensitization. Although improved therapeutics give hope for reduced overall patient and caregiver burden, it is important to ensure that the psychological burden of disease is acknowledged and minimized in the process.

CLINICS CARE POINTS

- An understanding of the psychosocial nature of food allergy and the relationship between allergic child and caregiver can improve outcomes.

DISCLOSURE

The authors have no financial or competing conflicts of interest.

REFERENCES

1. Feng C, Kim JH. Beyond avoidance: the psychosocial impact of food allergies. Clin Rev Allergy Immunol 2019;57(1):74–82.
2. Polloni L, Muraro A. Anxiety and food allergy: a review of the last two decades. Clin Exp Allergy 2020;50(4):420–41.
3. American Psychiatric Association. Anxiety disorders. In: Diagnostic and statistical manual of mental disorders, vol. 11. Washington, DC: American Psychiatric

Association; 2013. p. 1–992. https://doi.org/10.1176/appi.books.9780890425596. dsm05.

4. Muraro A, Halken S, Arshad SH, et al. EAACI food allergy and anaphylaxis guidelines. Primary prevention of food allergy. Allergy 2014;69(5):590–601.

5. Mandell D, Curtis R, Gold M, et al. Anaphylaxis: how do you live with it? Health Soc Work 2005;30(4):325–35.

6. Barlow DH. Clinical handbook of psychological disorders: a step-by-step treatment manual. New York, NY: Guilford Publications; 2014.

7. Cummings AJ, Knibb RC, King RM, et al. The psychosocial impact of food allergy and food hypersensitivity in children, adolescents and their families: a review. Allergy 2010;65(8):933–45.

8. Shanahan L, Zucker N, Copeland WE, et al. Are children and adolescents with food allergies at increased risk for psychopathology? J Psychosom Res 2014; 77(6):468–73.

9. Friedman AH, Morris TL. Allergies and anxiety in children and adolescents: a review of the literature. J Clin Psychol Med Settings 2006;13(3):323–36.

10. King RM, Knibb RC, Hourihane JOB. Impact of peanut allergy on quality of life, stress and anxiety in the family. Allergy 2009;64(3):461–8.

11. Fedele DA, McQuaid EL, Faino A, et al. Patterns of adaptation to children's food allergies. Allergy 2016;71(4):505–13.

12. Klinnert MD, Robinson JL. Addressing the psychological needs of families of food-allergic children. Curr Allergy Asthma Rep 2008;8(3):195–200.

13. Ng IE, Turner PJ, Kemp AS, et al. Parental perceptions and dietary adherence in children with seafood allergy. Pediatr Allergy Immunol 2011;22(7):720–8.

14. Rubes M, Podolsky AH, Caso N, et al. Utilizing physician screening questions for detecting anxiety among food-allergic pediatric patients. Clin Pediatr (Phila) 2014;53(8):764–70.

15. DunnGalvin A, Gaffney A, Hourihane JO. Developmental pathways in food allergy: a new theoretical framework. Allergy 2009;64(4):560–8.

16. Muraro A, Polloni L, Lazzarotto F, et al. Comparison of bullying of food-allergic versus healthy schoolchildren in Italy. J Allergy Clin Immunol 2014;134(3):749–51.

17. Keet C. Getting to the root of the food allergy "epidemic". J Allergy Clin Immunol Pract 2018;6(2):449–50.

18. Herbert LJ, Dahlquist LM. Perceived history of anaphylaxis and parental overprotection, autonomy, anxiety, and depression in food allergic young adults. J Clin Psychol Med Settings 2008;15(4):261–9.

19. Birdi G, Cooke R, Knibb R. Quality of life, stress, and mental health in parents of children with parentally diagnosed food allergy compared to medically diagnosed and healthy controls. J Allergy 2016;2016:1497375.

20. White PH, Cooley WC. Supporting the health care transition from adolescence to adulthood in the medical home. Pediatrics 2018;142(5):20182587.

21. Pettersson ME, Koppelman GH, Flokstra-de Blok BMJ, et al. Prediction of the severity of allergic reactions to foods. Allergy 2018;73(7):1532–40.

22. Ferro MA, Gorter JW, Boyle MH. Trajectories of depressive symptoms during the transition to young adulthood: the role of chronic illness. J Affect Disord 2015;174: 594–601.

23. Kessler RC, Avenevoli S, Costello EJ, et al. Prevalence, persistence, and sociodemographic correlates of DSM-IV disorders in the National Comorbidity Survey Replication Adolescent Supplement. Arch Gen Psychiatry 2012;69(4):372–80.

24. Kendall PC. Working with anxious youth: strategies within empirically supported treatment. In: Annual Meeting of the Association for Behavioral and Cognitive

Therapies. Atlanta, GA: Association for Behavioral and Cognitive Therapies; 2019.

25. Eley TC, McAdams TA, Rijsdijk FV, et al. The intergenerational transmission of anxiety: a children-of-twins study. Am J Psychiatry 2015;172(7):630–7.

26. Herbert LJ, Marchisotto MJ, Sharma H, et al. Availability of mental health services for patients with food allergy. J Allergy Clin Immunol Pract 2019;7(8):2904–5.

27. Cohen S, Kamarck T, Mermelstein R. A global measure of perceived stress. J Health Soc Behav 1983;24(4):385–96.

28. Lagercrantz B, Persson Å, Kull I. "Healthcare seems to vary a lot": a focus group study among parents of children with severe allergy. J Asthma 2017;54(7):672–8.

29. Akeson N, Worth A, Sheikh A. The psychosocial impact of anaphylaxis on young people and their parents. Clin Exp Allergy 2007;37(8):1213–20.

30. Walkner M, Warren C, Gupta RS. Quality of life in food allergy patients and their families. Pediatr Clin North Am 2015;62(6):1453–61.

31. Bollinger ME, Dahlquist LM, Mudd K, et al. The impact of food allergy on the daily activities of children and their families. Ann Allergy Asthma Immunol 2006;96(3):415–21.

32. Bilaver LA, Sharma HP, Gupta RS, et al. Food allergy research priorities: results from a patient-centered study. J Allergy Clin Immunol Pract 2019;7(7):2431–3.e4.

33. DunnGalvin A, Chan C-H, Crevel R, et al. Precautionary allergen labelling: perspectives from key stakeholder groups. Allergy 2015;70(9):1039–51.

34. Chan ES, Dinakar C, Gonzales-Reyes E, et al. Unmet needs of children with peanut allergy: aligning the risks and the evidence. Ann Allergy Asthma Immunol 2020;124(5):479–86.

35. Greenhawt M. Environmental exposure to peanut and the risk of an allergic reaction. Ann Allergy Asthma Immunol 2018;120(5):476–81.e3.

36. Perry TT, Conover-Walker MK, Pomés A, et al. Distribution of peanut allergen in the environment. J Allergy Clin Immunol 2004;113(5):973–6.

37. Venter C, Sicherer SH, Greenhawt M. Management of peanut allergy. J Allergy Clin Immunol Pract 2019;7(2):345–55.e2.

38. Weinberger T, Annunziato R, Riklin E, et al. A randomized controlled trial to reduce food allergy anxiety about casual exposure by holding the allergen: TOUCH study. J Allergy Clin Immunol Pract 2019;7(6):2039–42.e14.

39. Waggoner MR. Parsing the peanut panic: the social life of a contested food allergy epidemic. Soc Sci Med 2013;90:49–55.

40. Strong BD, Ross J, Fishman J, et al. Patient use online resources and social media for food allergy information. J Allergy Clin Immunol 2016;137(2):AB84.

41. Lee YM, Chen H. An exploration of activities, reasons, and barriers of using social media for food allergy management. Vol 8. 2019. Available at: https://thejsms.org/index.php/TSMRI/article/view/501. Accessed October 1, 2020.

42. Hu W, Loblay R, Ziegler J, et al. Attributes and views of families with food allergic children recruited from allergy clinics and from a consumer organization. Pediatr Allergy Immunol 2008;19(3):264–9.

43. Vargas PA, Sicherer SH, Christie L, et al. Developing a food allergy curriculum for parents. Pediatr Allergy Immunol 2011;22(6):575–82.

44. Goodwin RD, Rodgin S, Goldman R, et al. Food allergy and anxiety and depression among ethnic minority children and their caregivers. J Pediatr 2017;187:258–64.e1.

45. Patrawala M, Shih J, Lee G, et al. Peanut oral immunotherapy: a current perspective. Curr Allergy Asthma Rep 2020;20(5):14.

46. Vickery BP, Vereda A, Casale TB, et al. AR101 oral immunotherapy for peanut allergy. N Engl J Med 2018;379(21):1991–2001.
47. Chinthrajah RS, Purington N, Andorf S, et al. Sustained outcomes in oral immunotherapy for peanut allergy (POISED study): a large, randomised, double-blind, placebo-controlled, phase 2 study. Lancet 2019;394(10207):1437–49.
48. Andorf S, Purington N, Block WM, et al. Anti-IgE treatment with oral immunotherapy in multifood allergic participants: a double-blind, randomised, controlled trial. Lancet Gastroenterol Hepatol 2018;3(2):85–94.
49. Howe LC, Leibowitz KA, Perry MA, et al. Changing patient mindsets about non–life-threatening symptoms during oral immunotherapy: a randomized clinical trial. J Allergy Clin Immunol Pract 2019;7(5):1550–9.

Food Allergy
Catering for the Needs of the Clinician

Sami L. Bahna, MD, DrPH[a], Amal H. Assa'ad, MD[b],*

KEYWORDS

- Food allergy • Food allergy prevention • Food allergy diagnosis • Serum IgE
- Skin test • Oral food challenge • Oral immunotherapy

KEY POINTS

- Clinicians are caring for an increasing number of patients with food allergy of different ages, gender and ethnic/racial background. This is due to an increased prevalence of the disorder and in part due to increased awareness.
- Early food introduction for the prevention of peanut allergy and oral immunotherapy with peanut have generated a change in paradigm in the approach of the clinician to prevention and management of food allergy. Use of biologics for food allergy is highly anticipated.
- Clinicians have been given much welcomed national and international guidelines for the diagnosis of food allergy and for the prevention of peanut allergy.
- Clinicians continue to be faced with the high sensitivity but low specificity of the available skin tests and serum IgE tests for food allergy, even with the availability of component resolved diagnostics.
- The oral food challenge remains the most reliable confirmatory test for food allergy. Clinicians will welcome novel tests that may avoid the oral food challenge or ameliorate its potential side effects.

A HISTORIC PERSPECTIVE

Other than the rising prevalence of food allergy (FA), as discussed by Warren, Brewer, Grobman et al: Racial/Ethnic Differences in Food Allergy[1] in this issue, over the past decade, several events have led to the heightened awareness of FA in the scientific community and in the population (**Boxes 1** and **2**. These have included guidelines on FA and novel research on prevention and therapy in addition to advocacy efforts.

A landmark event that ushered the changes seen today in the field of FA and those anticipated in the near future is the National Institute of Allergy and Infectious Diseases (NIAID) of the National Institutes of Health (NIH) assembling a coordinating committee

[a] Allergy and Immunology Section, Louisiana State University Health Sciences Center in Shreveport, 1501 Kings Highway Rm 5-323 Shreveport, Louisiana 71130-3832, USA; [b] Division of Allergy and Immunology, Cincinnati Children's Hospital Medical Center, 3333 Burnet Avenue, Cincinnati, OH 45229
* Corresponding author.
E-mail address: amal.assaad@cchmc.org

Immunol Allergy Clin N Am 41 (2021) 331–345
https://doi.org/10.1016/j.iac.2021.02.002
0889-8561/21/© 2021 Elsevier Inc. All rights reserved.
immunology.theclinics.com

Box 1
Events during the past decade that resulted in a large impact on the field of food allergy in the United States

- NIAID/NIH expert panel guidelines on food allergy
- Publication of the LEAP study results
- NIAID/NIH expert panel guidelines supplement on the prevention of peanut allergy
- Epidemiologic surveys that demonstrate the widespread diagnosis
- Completion of the clinical trials of peanut oral immunotherapy and the receipt of FDA approval for Palforzia

---

made up of 35 professional and lay organization stakeholders, which named an expert panel to draft the first guidelines on FA in the United States.[2] The guidelines were published in 2010 within the same timeframe as other international guidelines, as reviewed by Mennini, Arasi, Fiocchi et al: Developing National and International Guidelines[3] in this issue. An important part of the evidence-based guidelines is the segment on the gaps in knowledge, which demonstrated to the NIH, the most reliable funding organization for research, that there are many areas in FA that need to be investigated.

On the prevention front, initial recommendations for prevention of FA by avoiding highly allergenic foods in the first 3 years of life published in 2000 were reversed in 2008, citing no or little evidence that delaying timing of the introduction of complementary foods beyond 4 months to 6 months of age prevents the occurrence of atopic disease. Despite evidence-based publications to promote the reversal of recommendations, it was not universally accepted or implemented, as shown in a study examining the knowledge and implementation differences between urban and suburban populations.[4,5] It was not until the primary prevention study that has come to be known by its acronym, the Learning Early About Peanut Allergy (LEAP) study, was published and received large publicity, that a change in paradigm occurred.[6] This was followed by another NIAID/NIH expert panel supplement to the guidelines, this time for the prevention of peanut allergy.[7] For the first time, the practice of allergists started seeing infants at a very young age, either because parents wanted guidance on implementing the guidelines or for the evaluation of reactions related to early introduction of allergenic food in infants at risk. Using Current Procedural Terminology (CPT) codes to categorize the diagnosis in the authors' practice shows that FA diagnosis has reached 44% and, along with eczema, which constitutes 7% and commonly accompanies FA, makes for patients with FA constituting half the number of patients in the practice (**Fig. 1**).

On the therapy front, in 2012, the first of the Consortium of Food Allergy Research (CoFar) studies of oral immunotherapy for egg was published, followed by several other results of maintenance therapy and sustained unresponsiveness.[8–12] Studies of oral immunotherapy for peanut were launched soon after by the CoFar centers and reported

---

Box 2
Events that are expected to impact in the near future the field of food allergy in the United States

- FDA review of the data on the effect of epicutaneous immunotherapy on peanut allergy
- Completion of multiple clinical trials of biologics in patients with FA
- The Food Allergy Research and Education patient advocacy organization assembling more than 50 centers of excellence in clinical care and research around the country

---

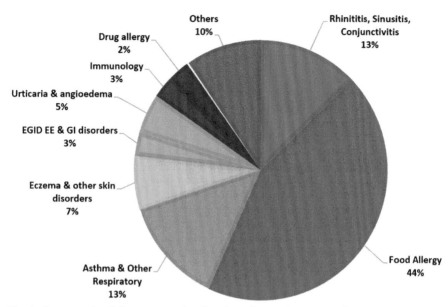

Fig. 1. An example of the current mix of patient diagnosis in an academic allergy practice showing that FA diagnosis and the related eczema diagnosis constitute more than half of the diagnoses. EE, Eosinophilic Esophagitis; EGID, Eosinophilic Gastrointestinal Disorder; GI, Gastrointestinal.

on sublingual immunotherapy for peanuts and moved on to epicutaneous immunotherapy.[9] Around the same time, 2 pharmaceutical companies launched clinical trials for peanut oral immunotherapy (Allergen Research Corporation, which later became Aimmune, Brisbane, CA, USA) and for epicutaneous immunotherapy by DBV Technologies, Montrouge, France. This was another paradigm change where exposure to the allergen, albeit in small gradually increasing amounts and under strict medical supervision, rather than avoidance, became an optional therapeutic modality. Several publications chronicled the progress and successes of these forms of therapy.[13–18] The clinical trials led to the approval by the US Food and Drug Administration (FDA) of AR101, now Palforzia, for the treatment of peanut allergy in 4-year olds to 17-year olds. Oral immunotherapy became another reason that patients with FA flocked to allergists practices. This due to the fact that oral immunotherapy has been conducted with foods in their natural form in practices and under research protocols. The controversy over the practice led to the publication of a white paper by leaders of various national organizations and stake holders.[19]

With the rise of numbers of patients with FA seen by clinicians come more questions about the epidemiology of the disorder, the accuracy of the diagnostic tools, and the benefits and potential side effects of the therapies. Besides the topics discussed later, clinicians can avail themselves of collaborations with dietitians, as discussed by Durban, Groetch, Meyer et al: Dietary Management of Food Allergy in this issue,[20] and with psychologists, as discussed by Rubeiz and Ernst: Psychosocial Aspects of Food Allergy in this issue.[21]

EPIDEMIOLOGY
Prevalence

Published figures on the prevalence of FA are estimates and vary widely.[2,22–26] They are influenced by multiple factors, including definitions, foods studied, diagnostic methods, age of subjects, infant feeding methods, and geographic dietary habits.[27] In recent years, survey estimates of the prevalence of food allergy have been 1 in 13 children and 1 and 10 in adults.[26,28] What is more important is the rising trend that has been well documented by many studies in different countries.[29–37] Such a trend seems to be more real than due to improved diagnosis and is more conspicuous in Western countries. The prevalence over-estimates, based on self-diagnosis reported on surveys or on positive allergy skin or serum testing that reflect sensitization that may or may not be clinically relevant, still translate to FA. This led to FA patients becoming the largest number of patients seen in an allergy clinic today, patients with asthma and allergic rhinitis and other atopic conditions. (see **Fig. 1**).

Figures based on FA confirmed by appropriate challenge testing are scarce and cannot be generalized. Several studies have shown that when food challenges are performed in the office, only approximately a third result in an allergic reaction consistent with FA.[38] On the other hand, the patients who are given a diagnosis of an FA, whether clinically significant or not, live the life of patients with FA, with all the stresses and the needs, as discussed by Engel and Bunning: The Unmet Needs of Patients with Food Allergies in this issue.[39] This makes the prevalence that may be based on self-reports, even if an over-estimate, still significant. The prevalence of FA among various ethnic and racial backgrounds in the United States and the current state of knowledge and research are discussed in the article by Warren, Brewer, Grobman et al: Racial/Ethnic Differences in Food Allergy[1] in this issue. There are some ethnic groups in the United States, however, who are not yet studied. Attention recently has been drawn to the Asian population in the United States by the authors' research that examined scores for anxiety over FA from a questionnaire. The research found that the Asian population in the United States is highest in anxiety scores compared with whites, blacks, and Latinex.[40]

Causative Foods

Knowledge of the common food allergens can guide a clinician's approach to the diagnosis, even though, theoretically, any food can cause allergy. The most allergenic foods are those with high protein content, with multiplicity of allergenic components, and that are consumed frequently. The NIAID/NIH expert panel guidelines published in 2010 reviewed the evidence-based literature that addressed FA in the United States. At that time, the common food allergens were cow milk, eggs and peanuts, fish, and crustaceans in all ages both by self-report and by self-report combined with skin tests and/or serum IgE. Cow milk allergy was stated to be more common in children than adults.[2] The guidelines also stated that allergy to fruits, vegetables, nonpeanut legumes, wheat, and soy were much less common compared with the 5 food groups listed. The Food Allergen Labeling and Consumer Protection Act of 2004 listed the top 8 foods as peanut, cow milk, hen egg, shellfish, tree nuts, wheat, fish, and soy.[41] Recently, the US Senate passed the Food Allergy Safety, Treatment, Education, and Research Act, which directs the Centers for Disease Control and Prevention to expand data collection of information related to food allergies and specific allergens and revises the definition of major allergen to specifically include sesame.

FA varies by ethnicity and geographic location. Thus, in the absence of diagnostic modalities with high sensitivity and specificity, clinicians need to be aware of the common food allergies in their communities and in the age range that they serve.

Clinical Manifestations

The clinician usually is presented with 1 or a set of symptoms. IgE-mediated FA can cause symptoms in the skin, the gastrointestinal tract, the respiratory tract, or in multiple systems simultaneously, that is, anaphylaxis[42] (**Fig. 2**). The symptoms of IgE-mediated FA can coexist or overlap with symptoms of other disorders in the same organ system. Multiple manifestations can be caused by a single food or 1 manifestation be caused by multiple foods. The latter may or may not be cross-reactive. The oral allergy syndrome (pollen-FA syndrome) typically is caused by certain food allergens that cross-react with certain pollen allergens.[43,44] Allergy to galactose-alpha-1,3-galactose (alpha-gal) is a late IgE-mediated hypersensitivity that occurs a couple of hours after eating red mammalian meat in subjects sensitized through the bite of the tick *Ixodes racinus*.[45]

DIAGNOSIS

A diagnosis of FA has 2 main stages. First is a patient's illness an allergic disease? Depending on information from the medical history and findings from the physical examination, a differential diagnosis can be formulated. Second, if FA seems to be the most likely diagnosis, what is (are) the causative food(s)? The latter may be suspected through the medical history and allergy tests.

Medical History

The general population often attribute various symptoms to FA, may not be confirmed in some cases. In a few cases, the relationship between ingesting a certain food and the recurrence of symptoms is so convincing that further testing may not be necessary. Skillful history taking may narrow down the list of suspected foods.

Skin Testing

Percutaneous testing has been well established as the most common allergy testing procedure for IgE-mediated reactions. It is an in vivo test in which the allergen extract (1:10 wt/vol or 1:20 wt/vol) is brought in contact with the cutaneous mast cells using skin prick (or skin puncture) test (SPT). If IgE antibodies specific to the allergen are on the mast cell, histamine and other mediators are released, causing local

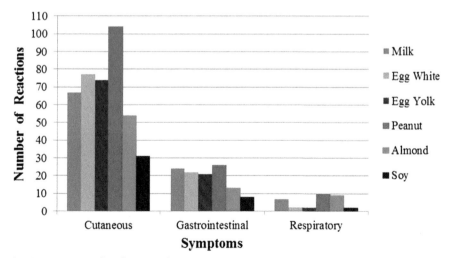

Fig. 2. Frequency distribution of presenting symptoms in patients with FA. Figure from Amin, Khoury and Assa'ad. Food-specific serum immunoglobulin E measurements in children presenting with food allergy. Ann Allergy Asthma Immunol 2014; 112(2):121-5.

vasodilatation, erythema, wheal formation, and irritation of the nerve endings. The area of the reaction is compared with the negative control (diluent) and the positive control (histamine). The larger the reaction, the more likely the allergen is the culprit. The test in patients with eczema and high serum total IgE level usually is positive to many foods, most of which are not clinically relevant. SPT has several advantages and a few disadvantages (**Table 1**). Because the allergenicity of extracts can be different from the consumed food, testing with the actually ingested food (prick-by-prick) may be done.[46] Some investigators reported SPT wheal size cutoff values that showed high correlation with positive challenge testing. Not surprisingly, such cutoff values vary among different studies because of the variability in the patient populations studied, the age, and the symptoms and their severity. They thus are difficult to generalize or be applied to individual patients in clinical practice.[47–54]

The general consensus is that a large positive SPT to a food is an indication that the test is a definite positive and an indication of the presence of sensitization to the food, but is not an indication of clinical allergy or the severity of a reaction. The NIH expert panel supplement to the Guidelines for the Prevention of Peanut Allergy, however, has utilized SPT size of the wheal to determine the risk of peanut clinical reactions in infants. The size of the wheal to a peanut SPT is used in the guidelines to determine whether the infant can have peanut introduced at home, introduced in the office through an observed feeding, introduced only after a graded oral challenge in the office determines tolerance to peanut, or avoided because the risk of clinical reaction is high.[7] These cutoffs were derived from the LEAP study, upon which the guidelines were based, with additional data from the HealthNuts study.[55] More recent further analysis of the LEAP data, with comparison of the SPT and the basophil activation test (BAT) performance regarding sensitivity, specificity, and prediction of reaction severity, reported that the SPT is best at detecting low threshold reactions to peanut.[56] The SPT remains one of the most used tests for FA in the allergist office, and intradermal testing, which has not been recommended because of its high false-positive result and potential risk in very sensitive subjects, has been studied and utilized in the diagnosis of red meat allergy produced by sensitization to the cross-reacting allergen alpha-gal.[57,58]

Patch testing is of little use for IgE-mediated FA. It can be useful in identifying the food causing allergic contact dermatitis in food handlers.

Serologic Testing

Specific IgE antibodies
Serum testing for allergen-specific IgE antibodies (sIgE) was developed in 1968, just a year after the discovery of IgE. The original assay was the radioallergosorbent test,

Table 1
Advantages and potential disadvantages of the skin test procedure for the diagnosis of food allergy

Advantages of Skin Prick Tests	Disadvantages of Skin Prick Tests
In-office procedure	Variation in test extracts
Easy to perform	Variation in devices
Immediate results	Variation in scoring
Low cost	Effect of skin disease
Large number of allergens can be applied	Suppression by many drugs
High specificity and sensitivity	Potential risk (minimal)
Visual reinforcement (to patient & clinician)	Requires trained personnel
In vivo biologic test mimicking type I reaction	Requires knowledge in interpretation

which went through several modifications by different laboratories that resulted in increasing the test's sensitivity and avoiding the use of radioisotopes. The results of test done by different methods do not correlate well.[59,60] At present, the ImmunoCAP assay (Thermo Fischer Scientific, Waltham, MA, USA) is the most commonly used in research and in clinical practice. There has been advances in the ImmunoCap measurement that has gotten the approval of the FDA, specifically, that the lower limit of the assay has been taken down to less than 0.1 KU/L.[42]

As in cases of SPT, the detection of sIgE merely indicates sensitization; the higher the level, the more likely to be clinically relevant. Whereas SPT is a biologic in vivo test, sIgE assay may be considered a passive test in the sense that it merely detects circulating IgE antibodies (**Table 2**).

In interpreting a sIgE level, several factors need to considered, in particular the total IgE level. The higher the latter, the less likely for slightly and moderately elevated sIgE to be clinically relevant. Serial follow-up measurement of sIgE level can be helpful in predicting the attainment of tolerance. In 1 study on children with milk or egg allergy, however, even when sIgE decreased to 1% of the initial level, milk was not tolerated in 6% and egg in 5% of children.[61] Several investigators reported cutoff sIgE levels that strongly correlated with positive challenge testing. As with studies on SPT, such levels varied from one study to another, obviously because were based on different patients' samples that varied in several ways. Hence, they cannot be generalized or applied to individual patients who are not seeking probabilities but expect a definite identification of the culprit food(s).[62–68]

Component-resolved diagnostic testing

Component-resolved diagnostic test (CRDT) has been developed recently. Whereas routine sIgE testing detects antibodies to the whole protein, CRDT measures the sIgE level to the food's major protein components. Such information was found to have high correlation with diagnostic precision, allergen cross-reactivity, and prognosis.[69,70] The test currently is available for several foods. It is costly and is not a substitute to conformation by challenge testing. In a study on sera of peanut allergy patients from 3 countries, the results revealed geographic/genetic differences. The most predictive antibodies in Americans were to Ara h 1, Ara h 2, and Ara h 3; in Swedes, to Ara h 8; and in the Spanish, to Ara h 9.[71]

Cellular Tests

Basophils, as the circulating cells bearing high-affinity receptors for IgE, have been explored for potential in vitro diagnosis of FA. Two main methods were tried, namely BAT and basophil histamine release (BHR) test.

Table 2
Advantages and potential disadvantages of food-specific, serum-specific IgE test procedure for the diagnosis of food allergy

Advantages of Food-specific, Serum-specific IgE Test	Disadvantages of Food-specific, Serum-specific IgE Test
Quantitative	High cost
Very safe	Delay in result
Unaffected by medications	Less impressive to patient
Provides results for protein components of a single food allergen	Variability among methods, laboratories, and allergens
	Requires knowledge in interpretation

A patient's basophils are incubated with various food allergens. If the cells are bearing IgE antibodies specific to that allergen, activation occurs (BAT) that can be measured by flow cytometry for the cell surface markers CD63 and CD203c.[72–75] Performing the test in microtiter plates, the basophils release their mediators, mainly histamine (BHR), that become adsorbed to the plate wells and can be measured.[73] Both tests have sound scientific basis. They require rapid processing of the blood samples as well as expensive equipment and special expertise. The few published studies showed promising results and work is in progress toward increasing the test's reproducibility and reliability. Although certain kits are marketed, these tests are not available in commercial laboratories and are considered investigational at this time.

Challenge Testing

Because FA commonly is over-diagnosed or misdiagnosed, depending on the diagnostic procedures discussed previously, verification of the offending food by the challenge test is required in most cases.[29] The procedure consists of safe administration of the food under supervision for accurate assessment and prompt treatment of any developing reaction.[76–78]

In patients with persistent symptoms, all suspected foods should be simultaneously strictly avoided to document definite improvement while on no or minimal symptomatic medications. The test material, one at a time, is administered in a titrated fashion. The start dose should be safe, and the cumulative dose should be at least equivalent to the usually consumed quantity. Depending on the degree of concern about bias by the patient or the observer, the procedure may be carried out in any of 3 ways: open, single-blind, or double-blind. A guideline on the oral food challenges was published in 2009 and recently updated in 2020.[78,79] Another guideline was published on conducting food challenges in infants.[80,81]

Challenge testing is essential particularly in evaluating reactions to food additives. They are thousands that increasingly are incorporated in foods yet are difficult for patients to suspect or to test reliably by skin or blood tests. Evaluation for suspected reactions to additives and spices require special approaches.[82,83]

Unproved Tests

Several procedures have been promoted in various countries over the years for FA diagnosis but without proved adequate reliability. They include, but are not limited to, specific IgG or IgG4 antibodies, cytotoxic test, change in leukocytes size, neutralization-provocation test, hair analysis, electrodermal Vega test, kinesiology, and iridiology.[84,85]

MANAGEMENT OF FOOD ALLERGY
Dietary Avoidance

Once the culprit food is identified, management basically is strict avoidance of that food, which can be difficult for patients allergic to multiple foods or to a food that commonly is incorporated in the usual diet. Patients should be provided with lists of foods that may contain that food allergen and be counseled on reading labels of commercially prepared foods, including unfamiliar names, such as casein, whey, ovalbumin, ovomucoid, and so forth. Highly sensitive patients may need to avoid exposure by skin contact, particularly if they have eczema, and by inhalation, particularly if they have asthma.[86,87]

Although some subjects allergic to milk or egg may tolerate these foods in baked goods, approximately 1 in 5 milk-allergic subjects may react to beef that is not well cooked.[88–90] Patients should be advised strongly against cross-reacting foods unless they are sorted out by challenge testing. For example, more than 90% of subjects allergic to bovine milk do not tolerate milks of sheep or goat.[91–93] A person allergic to a crustacean is unlikely to tolerate another crustacean. Hypoallergenic formulas are needed for infants who are allergic to milk or to multiple foods.[94] On the other hand, most fish-allergic subjects can tolerate one or more fish species.[95] Subjects with food-dependent, exercise-induced anaphylaxis should allow at least 4 hours between eating the offending food and exercise.[96,97] In certain cases, the reaction occurred only when a combination of multiple foods were eaten or when cofactors, such as hormonal changes, occur.[98,99]

Studies on using probiotics showed inconsistent findings possibly due to differences in study design, age of subjects, and the organism regarding type, dose, duration, and route of administration.[100–104]

Pharmacotherapy

Pharmacologic agents are used primarily for symptomatic treatment tailored to the clinical manifestation. Patients who had anaphylaxis or severe systemic reaction should be provided with an anaphylaxis treatment plan and epinephrine autoinjector.

New biologic agents have been studied and showed promising results in particular protocols. These are reviewed by Albuhairi and Rashid: Biologics and Novel Therapies for Food Allergy[105] in this issue. Although none is approved yet by the FDA for treating FA per se, a few are approved for certain allergic disorders that FA may be involved in. In a small series of peanut-allergic patients, omalizumab showed promising results in preventing reaction to small quantities of peanut protein.[106]

Immunotherapy

Several immunotherapy protocols for FA treatment have been studied over the past several years. Routes used were sublingual, oral,[107] and epicutaneous.[107–110] Various degrees of efficacy and safety have been reported, but at the time of preparing this article, only oral immunotherapy to one food is approved by the FDA. The expected benefit from immunotherapy is protection from accidental exposures to small amounts of the allergen and to not eat usual quantities.

In conclusion, several aspects of the care of patients with FA that clinicians can offer have had a breakthrough and a change in paradigms, whereas others have not changed and continue to rely on clinical acumen and tests. Clinicians are encouraged to continue to acquire expertise in the care of patients with FA, to apply the breakthroughs in the science and discoveries and to continue to be advocates for their patients.

CLINICS CARE POINTS

- Several recent advances in the care of patients with FA has led to an increase in the numbers of patients and families seeking care from clinicians for their FAs.

- Clinicians can make use of the advances in recommendations for prevention of peanut allergy and an approved therapy for peanut allergy to better the management of their patients.

- Diagnostic tools have not changed much and accurate diagnosis still relies on a combination of medical history, skin tests, serum IgE measurements, and food challenges.

DISCLOSURE

Dr Amal Assa'ad Received grants to my institution from NIH/NIAID, DBV Technologies, Aimmune Therapeutics, Astellas, ABBVIE, Sanofi, Food Allergy Research and Education (FARE).

REFERENCES

1. Warren CM, Brewer AG, Grobman B, et al. Racial/Ethnic differences in food allergy. Immunol Allergy Clin North Am 2021;41(2):xx.
2. Boyce JA, Assa'ad A, Burks AW, et al. Guidelines for the diagnosis and management of food allergy in the United States: summary of the NIAID-sponsored expert panel report. J Allergy Clin Immunol 2010;126(6):1105–18.
3. Mennini M, Arasi S, Fiocchi AG, et al. Developing national and international guidelines. Immunol Allergy Clin North Am 2021;41(2):xx.
4. Fleischer DM, Spergel JM, Assa'ad AH, et al. Primary prevention of allergic disease through nutritional interventions. J Allergy Clin Immunol Pract 2013;1(1):29–36.
5. Hartman H, Dodd C, Rao M, et al. Parental timing of allergenic food introduction in urban and suburban populations. Ann Allergy Asthma Immunol 2016;117(1):56–60.e2.
6. Du Toit G, Roberts G, Sayre PH, et al. Randomized trial of peanut consumption in infants at risk for peanut allergy. N Engl J Med 2015;372(9):803–13.
7. Togias A, Cooper SF, Acebal ML, et al. Addendum guidelines for the prevention of peanut allergy in the United States: report of the national institute of allergy and infectious diseases-sponsored expert panel. J Allergy Clin Immunol 2017;139(1):29–44.
8. Burks AW, Jones SM, Wood RA, et al. Oral immunotherapy for treatment of egg allergy in children. N Engl J Med 2012;367(3):233–43.
9. Fleischer DM, Burks AW, Vickery BP, et al. Sublingual immunotherapy for peanut allergy: a randomized, double-blind, placebo-controlled multicenter trial. J Allergy Clin Immunol 2013;131(1):119–27.e1-7.
10. Jones SM, Burks AW, Keet C, et al. Long-term treatment with egg oral immunotherapy enhances sustained unresponsiveness that persists after cessation of therapy. J Allergy Clin Immunol 2016;137(4):1117–27.e10.
11. Kim EH, Perry TT, Wood RA, et al. Induction of sustained unresponsiveness after egg oral immunotherapy compared to baked egg therapy in children with egg allergy. J Allergy Clin Immunol 2020;146(4):851–62.e10.
12. Wright BL, Kulis M, Orgel KA, et al. Component-resolved analysis of IgA, IgE, and IgG4 during egg OIT identifies markers associated with sustained unresponsiveness. Allergy 2016;71(11):1552–60.
13. Bird JA, Spergel JM, Jones SM, et al. Efficacy and safety of AR101 in oral immunotherapy for peanut allergy: results of ARC001, a randomized, double-blind, placebo-controlled phase 2 clinical trial. J Allergy Clin Immunol Pract 2018;6(2):476–85.e3.
14. Fleischer DM, Greenhawt M, Sussman G, et al. Effect of epicutaneous immunotherapy vs placebo on reaction to peanut protein ingestion among children with peanut allergy: the PEPITES randomized clinical trial. JAMA 2019;321(10):946–55.
15. Fleischer DM, Shreffler WG, Campbell DE, et al. Long-term, open-label extension study of the efficacy and safety of epicutaneous immunotherapy for peanut

allergy in children: PEOPLE 3-year results. J Allergy Clin Immunol 2020;146(4): 863–74.

16. Investigators PGoC, Vickery BP, Vereda A, et al. AR101 oral immunotherapy for peanut allergy. N Engl J Med 2018;379(21):1991–2001.

17. Sampson HA, Shreffler WG, Yang WH, et al. Effect of varying doses of epicutaneous immunotherapy vs placebo on reaction to peanut protein exposure among patients with peanut sensitivity: a randomized clinical trial. JAMA 2017;318(18):1798–809.

18. Scurlock AM, Burks AW, Sicherer SH, et al. Epicutaneous immunotherapy for treatment of peanut allergy: follow-up from the consortium for food allergy research. J Allergy Clin Immunol 2021;147(3):992–1003.e5.

19. Pepper AN, Assa'ad A, Blaiss M, et al. Consensus report from the food allergy research & education (FARE) 2019 oral immunotherapy for food allergy summit. J Allergy Clin Immunol 2020;146(2):244–9.

20. Durban R, Groetch M, Meyer R, et al. Dietary Management of Food Allergy. Immunol Allergy Clin North Am 2021;41(2):xx.

21. Rubeiz CJ, Ernst MM. Psychosocial aspects of food allergy: resiliency, challenges and opportunities. Immunol Allergy Clin North Am 2021;41(2):xx.

22. Sicherer SH, Warren CM, Dant C, et al. Food allergy from infancy through adulthood. J Allergy Clin Immunol Pract 2020;8(6):1854–64.

23. Nachshon L, Schwartz N, Elizur A, et al. The prevalence of food allergy in young Israeli adults. J Allergy Clin Immunol Pract 2019;7(8):2782–9.e4.

24. Lyons SA, Burney PGJ, Ballmer-Weber BK, et al. Food allergy in adults: substantial variation in prevalence and causative foods across Europe. J Allergy Clin Immunol Pract 2019;7(6):1920–8.e11.

25. Lee SC, Kim SR, Park KH, et al. Clinical features and culprit food allergens of Korean adult food allergy patients: a cross-sectional single-institute study. Allergy Asthma Immunol Res 2019;11(5):723–35.

26. Gupta RS, Warren CM, Smith BM, et al. Prevalence and severity of food allergies among US adults. JAMA Netw Open 2019;2(1):e185630.

27. Dunlop JH, Keet CA. Epidemiology of food allergy. Immunol Allergy Clin North Am 2018;38(1):13–25.

28. Gupta RS, Warren CM, Smith BM, et al. The public health impact of parent-reported childhood food allergies in the United States. Pediatrics 2018;142(6): e20181235.

29. Vierk KA, Koehler KM, Fein SB, et al. Prevalence of self-reported food allergy in American adults and use of food labels. J Allergy Clin Immunol 2007;119(6): 1504–10.

30. Zuberbier T, Edenharter G, Worm M, et al. Prevalence of adverse reactions to food in Germany - a population study. Allergy 2004;59(3):338–45.

31. Osterballe M, Hansen TK, Mortz CG, et al. The prevalence of food hypersensitivity in an unselected population of children and adults. Pediatr Allergy Immunol 2005;16(7):567–73.

32. Rance F, Grandmottet X, Grandjean H. Prevalence and main characteristics of schoolchildren diagnosed with food allergies in France. Clin Exp Allergy 2005; 35(2):167–72.

33. Steinke M, Fiocchi A, Kirchlechner V, et al. Perceived food allergy in children in 10 European nations. A randomised telephone survey. Int Arch Allergy Immunol 2007;143(4):290–5.

34. Venter C, Pereira B, Voigt K, et al. Prevalence and cumulative incidence of food hypersensitivity in the first 3 years of life. Allergy 2008;63(3):354–9.

35. Pereira B, Venter C, Grundy J, et al. Prevalence of sensitization to food allergens, reported adverse reaction to foods, food avoidance, and food hypersensitivity among teenagers. J Allergy Clin Immunol 2005;116(4):884–92.

36. Burks AW, Tang M, Sicherer S, et al. ICON: food allergy. J Allergy Clin Immunol 2012;129(4):906–20.

37. Sicherer SH, Sampson HA. Food allergy: a review and update on epidemiology, pathogenesis, diagnosis, prevention, and management. J Allergy Clin Immunol 2018;141(1):41–58.

38. Dang AT, Chundi PK, Mousa NA, et al. The effect of age, sex, race/ethnicity, health insurance, and food specific serum immunoglobulin E on outcomes of oral food challenges. World Allergy Organ J 2020;13(2):100100.

39. Engel M, Bunning BJ. The unmet needs of patients with food allergy. Immunol Allergy Clin North Am 2021;41(2):xx.

40. Rubeiz CSJ, Ernst M, Assa'ad A. Race/Ethnicity and socioeconomic status effect on food allergy-related quality of life in children and caregivers. Ann Allergy Asthma Immunol 2020;125(5):S8.

41. Food allergen labeling and consumer protection Act of 2004 (FALCPA). Available at: https://www.fda.gov/food/food-allergensgluten-free-guidance-documents-regulatory-information/food-allergen-labeling-and-consumer-protection-act-2004. Accessed Januray, 2021.

42. Amin MR, Khoury JC, Assa'ad AH. Food-specific serum immunoglobulin E measurements in children presenting with food allergy. Ann Allergy Asthma Immunol 2014;112(2):121–5.

43. Zuidmeer L, Goldhahn K, Rona RJ, et al. The prevalence of plant food allergies: a systematic review. J Allergy Clin Immunol 2008;121(5):1210–8.e4.

44. Brown CE, Katelaris CH. The prevalence of the oral allergy syndrome and pollen-food syndrome in an atopic paediatric population in south-west Sydney. J Paediatr Child Health 2014;50(10):795–800.

45. Platts-Mills TAE, Commins SP, Biedermann T, et al. On the cause and consequences of IgE to galactose-alpha-1,3-galactose: a report from the national institute of allergy and infectious diseases workshop on understanding IgE-mediated mammalian meat allergy. J Allergy Clin Immunol 2020;145(4):1061–71.

46. Rance F, Juchet A, Bremont F, et al. Correlations between skin prick tests using commercial extracts and fresh foods, specific IgE, and food challenges. Allergy 1997;52(10):1031–5.

47. Sporik R, Hill DJ, Hosking CS. Specificity of allergen skin testing in predicting positive open food challenges to milk, egg and peanut in children. Clin Exp Allergy 2000;30(11):1540–6.

48. Roberts G, Lack G. Diagnosing peanut allergy with skin prick and specific IgE testing. J Allergy Clin Immunol 2005;115(6):1291–6.

49. Hill DJ, Heine RG, Hosking CS. The diagnostic value of skin prick testing in children with food allergy. Pediatr Allergy Immunol 2004;15(5):435–41.

50. Verstege A, Mehl A, Rolinck-Werninghaus C, et al. The predictive value of the skin prick test weal size for the outcome of oral food challenges. Clin Exp Allergy 2005;35(9):1220–6.

51. Fiocchi A, Bouygue GR, Restani P, et al. Accuracy of skin prick tests in IgE-mediated adverse reactions to bovine proteins. Ann Allergy Asthma Immunol 2002;89(6 Suppl 1):26–32.

52. Nolan RC, Richmond P, Prescott SL, et al. Skin prick testing predicts peanut challenge outcome in previously allergic or sensitized children with low serum

peanut-specific IgE antibody concentration. Pediatr Allergy Immunol 2007; 18(3):224–30.

53. Klemans RJ, Broekman HC, Knol EF, et al. Ara h 2 is the best predictor for peanut allergy in adults. J Allergy Clin Immunol Pract 2013;1(6):632–8.e1.

54. Peters RL, Allen KJ, Dharmage SC, et al. Skin prick test responses and allergen-specific IgE levels as predictors of peanut, egg, and sesame allergy in infants. J Allergy Clin Immunol 2013;132(4):874–80.

55. Du Toit G, Roberts G, Sayre PH, et al. Identifying infants at high risk of peanut allergy: the learning early about peanut allergy (LEAP) screening study. J Allergy Clin Immunol 2013;131(1):135–43.e2.

56. Santos AF, Du Toit G, O'Rourke C, et al. Biomarkers of severity and threshold of allergic reactions during oral peanut challenges. J Allergy Clin Immunol 2020; 146(2):344–55.

57. Commins SP, Satinover SM, Hosen J, et al. Delayed anaphylaxis, angioedema, or urticaria after consumption of red meat in patients with IgE antibodies specific for galactose-alpha-1,3-galactose. J Allergy Clin Immunol 2009;123(2):426–33.

58. Platts-Mills TAE, Li RC, Keshavarz B, et al. Diagnosis and management of patients with the alpha-gal syndrome. J Allergy Clin Immunol Pract 2020;8(1): 15–23.e1.

59. Wang J, Godbold JH, Sampson HA. Correlation of serum allergy (IgE) tests performed by different assay systems. J Allergy Clin Immunol 2008;121(5): 1219–24.

60. Hamilton RG, Mudd K, White MA, et al. Extension of food allergen specific IgE ranges from the ImmunoCAP to the IMMULITE systems. Ann Allergy Asthma Immunol 2011;107(2):139–44.

61. Shek LP, Soderstrom L, Ahlstedt S, et al. Determination of food specific IgE levels over time can predict the development of tolerance in cow's milk and hen's egg allergy. J Allergy Clin Immunol 2004;114(2):387–91.

62. Sampson HA, Ho DG. Relationship between food-specific IgE concentrations and the risk of positive food challenges in children and adolescents. J Allergy Clin Immunol 1997;100(4):444–51.

63. Sampson HA. Utility of food-specific IgE concentrations in predicting symptomatic food allergy. J Allergy Clin Immunol 2001;107(5):891–6.

64. Garcia BE, Gamboa PM, Asturias JA, et al. Guidelines on the clinical usefulness of determination of specific immunoglobulin E to foods. J Investig Allergol Clin Immunol 2009;19(6):423–32.

65. Komata T, Soderstrom L, Borres MP, et al. The predictive relationship of food-specific serum IgE concentrations to challenge outcomes for egg and milk varies by patient age. J Allergy Clin Immunol 2007;119(5):1272–4.

66. Celik-Bilgili S, Mehl A, Verstege A, et al. The predictive value of specific immunoglobulin E levels in serum for the outcome of oral food challenges. Clin Exp Allergy 2005;35(3):268–73.

67. Niggemann B, Celik-Bilgili S, Ziegert M, et al. Specific IgE levels do not indicate persistence or transience of food allergy in children with atopic dermatitis. J Investig Allergol Clin Immunol 2004;14(2):98–103.

68. Skolnick HS, Conover-Walker MK, Koerner CB, et al. The natural history of peanut allergy. J Allergy Clin Immunol 2001;107(2):367–74.

69. Nicolaou N, Poorafshar M, Murray C, et al. Allergy or tolerance in children sensitized to peanut: prevalence and differentiation using component-resolved diagnostics. J Allergy Clin Immunol 2010;125(1):191–7.e1-13.

70. Santos AF, Brough HA. Making the most of in vitro tests to diagnose food allergy. J Allergy Clin Immunol Pract 2017;5(2):237–48.

71. Nicolaou N, Custovic A. Molecular diagnosis of peanut and legume allergy. Curr Opin Allergy Clin Immunol 2011;11(3):222–8.

72. Santos AF, Douiri A, Becares N, et al. Basophil activation test discriminates between allergy and tolerance in peanut-sensitized children. J Allergy Clin Immunol 2014;134(3):645–52.

73. Hamilton RG, Franklin Adkinson N Jr. In vitro assays for the diagnosis of IgE-mediated disorders. J Allergy Clin Immunol 2004;114(2):213–25 [quiz 226].

74. Ocmant A, Mulier S, Hanssens L, et al. Basophil activation tests for the diagnosis of food allergy in children. Clin Exp Allergy 2009;39(8):1234–45.

75. Sanz ML, Gamboa PM, Mayorga C. Basophil activation tests in the evaluation of immediate drug hypersensitivity. Curr Opin Allergy Clin Immunol 2009;9(4):298–304.

76. Bahna SL. Food challenge procedure: optimal choices for clinical practice. Allergy Asthma Proc 2007;28(6):640–6.

77. Niggemann B, Beyer K. Diagnosis of food allergy in children: toward a standardization of food challenge. J Pediatr Gastroenterol Nutr 2007;45(4):399–404.

78. Nowak-Wegrzyn A, Assa'ad AH, Bahna SL, et al. Work Group report: oral food challenge testing. J Allergy Clin Immunol 2009;123(6 Suppl):S365–83.

79. Bird JA, Leonard S, Groetch M, et al. Conducting an oral food challenge: an update to the 2009 adverse reactions to foods committee work group report. J Allergy Clin Immunol Pract 2020;8(1):75–90.e17.

80. Bird JA, Fleischer DM, Groetch M, et al. Additional oral food challenge considerations. J Allergy Clin Immunol 2018;141(6):2322.

81. Bird JA, Groetch M, Allen KJ, et al. Conducting an oral food challenge to peanut in an infant. J Allergy Clin Immunol Pract 2017;5(2):301–11.e1.

82. Bahna SL, Burkhardt JG. The dilemma of allergy to food additives. Allergy Asthma Proc 2018;39(1):3–8.

83. Chen JL, Bahna SL. Spice allergy. Ann Allergy Asthma Immunol 2011;107(3):191–9 [quiz 199, 265].

84. Beyer K, Teuber SS. Food allergy diagnostics: scientific and unproven procedures. Curr Opin Allergy Clin Immunol 2005;5(3):261–6.

85. Sampson HA, Aceves S, Bock SA, et al. Food allergy: a practice parameter update-2014. J Allergy Clin Immunol 2014;134(5):1016–25.e43.

86. Bahna SL. Adverse food reactions by skin contact. Allergy 2004;59(Suppl 78):66–70.

87. Ramirez DA Jr, Bahna SL. Food hypersensitivity by inhalation. Clin Mol Allergy 2009;7:4.

88. Nowak-Wegrzyn A, Bloom KA, Sicherer SH, et al. Tolerance to extensively heated milk in children with cow's milk allergy. J Allergy Clin Immunol 2008;122(2):342–7, 347.e1-2.

89. Werfel SJ, Cooke SK, Sampson HA. Clinical reactivity to beef in children allergic to cow's milk. J Allergy Clin Immunol 1997;99(3):293–300.

90. Martelli A, De Chiara A, Corvo M, et al. Beef allergy in children with cow's milk allergy; cow's milk allergy in children with beef allergy. Ann Allergy Asthma Immunol 2002;89(6 Suppl 1):38–43.

91. Wal JM. Bovine milk allergenicity. Ann Allergy Asthma Immunol 2004;93(5 Suppl 3):S2–11.

92. Jarvinen KM, Chatchatee P. Mammalian milk allergy: clinical suspicion, cross-reactivities and diagnosis. Curr Opin Allergy Clin Immunol 2009;9(3):251–8.

93. Woo CK, Bahna SL. Not all shellfish "allergy" is allergy! Clin Transl Allergy 2011; 1(1):3.
94. Parekh H, Bahna SL. Infant formulas for food allergy treatment and prevention. Pediatr Ann 2016;45(4):e150–6.
95. Mourad AA, Bahna SL. Fish-allergic patients may be able to eat fish. Expert Rev Clin Immunol 2015;11(3):419–30.
96. Du Toit G. Food-dependent exercise-induced anaphylaxis in childhood. Pediatr Allergy Immunol 2007;18(5):455–63.
97. Barg W, Wolanczyk-Medrala A, Obojski A, et al. Food-dependent exercise-induced anaphylaxis: possible impact of increased basophil histamine releasability in hyperosmolar conditions. J Investig Allergol Clin Immunol 2008;18(4): 312–5.
98. Dohi M, Suko M, Sugiyama H, et al. Food-dependent, exercise-induced anaphylaxis: a study on 11 Japanese cases. J Allergy Clin Immunol 1991;87(1 Pt 1): 34–40.
99. Asaumi T, Yanagida N, Sato S, et al. Provocation tests for the diagnosis of food-dependent exercise-induced anaphylaxis. Pediatr Allergy Immunol 2016; 27(1):44–9.
100. Paparo L, Nocerino R, Di Scala C, et al. Targeting food allergy with probiotics. Adv Exp Med Biol 2019;1125:57–68.
101. Fiocchi A, Burks W, Bahna SL, et al. Clinical use of probiotics in pediatric allergy (CUPPA): a world allergy organization position paper. World Allergy Organ J 2012;5(11):148–67.
102. Tang ML, Lahtinen SJ, Boyle RJ. Probiotics and prebiotics: clinical effects in allergic disease. Curr Opin Pediatr 2010;22(5):626–34.
103. Yao TC, Chang CJ, Hsu YH, et al. Probiotics for allergic diseases: realities and myths. Pediatr Allergy Immunol 2010;21(6):900–19.
104. Pan SJ, Kuo CH, Lam KP, et al. Probiotics and allergy in children–an update review. Pediatr Allergy Immunol 2010;21(4 Pt 2):e659–66.
105. Albuhairi S, Rachid R. Biologics and novel therapies for food allergy. Immunol Allergy Clin North Am 2021;41(2):xx.
106. Sampson HA, Leung DY, Burks AW, et al. A phase II, randomized, doubleblind, parallelgroup, placebocontrolled oral food challenge trial of Xolair (omalizumab) in peanut allergy. J Allergy Clin Immunol 2011;127(5):1309–10.e1.
107. Jones SM, Sicherer SH, Burks AW, et al. Epicutaneous immunotherapy for the treatment of peanut allergy in children and young adults. J Allergy Clin Immunol 2017;139(4):1242–52.e9.
108. Wood RA, Kim JS, Lindblad R, et al. A randomized, double-blind, placebo-controlled study of omalizumab combined with oral immunotherapy for the treatment of cow's milk allergy. J Allergy Clin Immunol 2016;137(4):1103–10.e1.
109. Vickery BP, Berglund JP, Burk CM, et al. Early oral immunotherapy in peanut-allergic preschool children is safe and highly effective. J Allergy Clin Immunol 2017;139(1):173–81.e8.
110. Kim EH, Yang L, Ye P, et al. Long-term sublingual immunotherapy for peanut allergy in children: Clinical and immunologic evidence of desensitization. J Allergy Clin Immunol 2019;144(5):1320–6.e1.

Moving?

Make sure your subscription moves with you!

To notify us of your new address, find your **Clinics Account Number** (located on your mailing label above your name), and contact customer service at:

Email: journalscustomerservice-usa@elsevier.com

800-654-2452 (subscribers in the U.S. & Canada)
314-447-8871 (subscribers outside of the U.S. & Canada)

Fax number: 314-447-8029

Elsevier Health Sciences Division
Subscription Customer Service
3251 Riverport Lane
Maryland Heights, MO 63043

*To ensure uninterrupted delivery of your subscription, please notify us at least 4 weeks in advance of move.